SUCCESS IN MEDICAL SCHOOL

INSIDER ADVICE
FOR THE
PRECLINICAL YEARS

SAMIR P. DESAI MD
RAJANI KATTA MD

FROM THE AUTHORS OF THE SUCCESSFUL MATCH

PUBLISHED BY

MD2B
HOUSTON, TEXAS

www.MD2B.net

Success in Medical School: Insider Advice for the Preclinical Years is published by MD2B, PO Box 300988, Houston, TX 77230-0988.

www.MD2B.net

Printed in the United States of America

9781937978006

Dedication

To our families

It takes more than just two individuals to write a book. We would like
to thank our families for making all of this possible.

To Teja and Shaan,
who bring us such inspiration and joy

For each book sold, two books will be donated to organizations
supporting literacy

ABOUT THE AUTHORS

Samir P. Desai, M.D.

Dr. Samir Desai serves on the faculty of the Baylor College of Medicine in the Department of Medicine. He is actively involved in medical student and resident education, and is a member of the Clerkship Directors in Internal Medicine. He is the recipient of multiple teaching awards. He is an author and editor, having written twelve books that together have sold over 150,000 copies worldwide.

In 2009, he co-authored *The Successful Match: 200 Rules to Succeed in the Residency Match*, a well-regarded and highly acclaimed book that has helped thousands of residency applicants match successfully. His commitment to helping medical students reach their professional goals led him to develop the website, TheSuccessfulMatch.com. The website's mission is to provide residency applicants with a better understanding of the residency selection process.

He is also the co-author of *Success on the Wards: 250 Rules for Clerkship Success*. This book has helped thousands of medical students make the difficult transition from the preclinical to clinical years of medical school. *Success on the Wards* is a required or recommended resource at many U.S. medical schools, providing proven strategies for success in patient care, write-ups, rounds, and other vital areas.

With Dr. Rajani Katta, he writes a regular column for the Student Doctor Network called "The Successful Match." Dr. Desai keeps residency applicants abreast of key information at The Successful Match blog (www.TheSuccessfulMatch.blogspot.com). He is also the founder of www.ImgAssist.com, a website providing guidance to international medical graduates (IMGs) seeking residency positions in the United States.

His other books include the best-selling *Clinician's Guide to Laboratory Medicine: Pocket*. This resource, widely used by students, residents, and other healthcare professionals, offers a unique step-by-step approach to lab test interpretation.

After completing his residency training in Internal Medicine at Northwestern University in Chicago, Dr. Desai had the opportunity of serving as chief medical resident. He received his M.D. degree from Wayne State University School of Medicine in Detroit, Michigan, graduating first in his class.

Rajani Katta, M.D.

Dr. Rajani Katta is an Associate Professor in the Department of Dermatology at Baylor College of Medicine. She has authored over 40 scientific articles and chapters, and lectured extensively both nationally and locally on dermatology and contact dermatitis to students, residents, and physicians. She serves as the course director for dermatology in the basic science years, and has served as the clerkship director for the dermatology rotation. In these capacities, she has seen firsthand the importance of outstanding clinical evaluations in securing a position in a competitive specialty, and her insight in this area has helped students seeking these types of competitive positions.

Having advised many students over the years regarding the dermatology match process, she was determined to become expert in this area and share her knowledge, insight, and perspective. In 2009, she co-authored *The Successful Match: 200 Rules to Succeed in the Residency Match*. This book has quickly become the best-selling title in this field. She also contributes regularly to www.studentdoctor.net with a recurring column on topics specific to the residency match, including a series of interviews with decision-makers.

She is also the co-author of *Success on the Wards: 250 Rules for Clerkship Success*. This book has helped thousands of medical students make the difficult transition from the preclinical to clinical years of medical school. *Success on the Wards* is a required or recommended resource at many U.S. medical schools, providing proven strategies for success in patient care, write-ups, rounds, and other vital areas.

After graduating with honors from Baylor College of Medicine and completing her internship in Internal Medicine, she completed her dermatology residency at the Northwestern University School of Medicine.

CONTENTS

Chapter 1

Introduction

The preclinical years of medical school are extremely challenging, and that may be understating the reality. At one medical school, faculty assigned "29,239 pages of reading for the 12 basic science modules that were scheduled during 71 weeks."[1]

As you begin med school, you'll hear a lot of advice.

- "If you thought the MCAT was tough, wait until you see the USMLE."

- "The material it took you a semester to cover in college? You'll get through that in a week in med school."

- "If you want to go down the ROAD, you'd better start planning now, figure out your research, and make your connections early - and you'll have to maximize that first summer off." [ROAD = Radiology, Ophthalmology, Anesthesiology, Dermatology]

There is at least some truth in every one of those statements.

Medical school is extremely challenging, and not just in the ways that you'd assume. The sheer volume of material covered is staggering. And most importantly, unlike in some of your college courses, much of it builds upon prior material. Your study methods therefore have to ensure long-term retention. In Chapter 2 [Preclinical Courses], you'll hear advice from students, faculty, and experts, as well as the results of research, on how to learn such a large volume of material, and how to ensure retention. In one study, researchers found that "in general, study skills are stronger predictors of first-semester total grades than aptitude as measured by the MCAT and undergraduate GPA."[2] The importance of long-term retention of basic science material is emphasized by the United States Medical Licensing Exam. The USMLE Step 1 exam is taken at the end of the preclinical years, and your score on this single exam can influence the course of your career. The exam tests your ability to take the basic science material covered over two years in medical school and apply it to clinical situations. In Chapter 3, you'll learn about the exam itself, as well as the most common mistakes that students make when preparing. You'll learn about resources that can aid your preparation, and you'll learn about the importance of this single score in the residency application process. Chapter 4 provides specifics about the COMLEX Level 1 exam. This exam, taken by osteopathic students, is of similar importance.

While mastering such a large amount of basic science material is extremely challenging, unfortunately that's not enough. Your skills in the hands-on art and science of patient care will be critical. Learning about a disease and its manifestations in the classroom does not ensure that you'll know what to do when faced with a patient in the clinic. It is widely believed that physicians' examination skills have deteriorated over the years. While a number of factors may be responsible, it is believed that clinical skills training may play a role. In fact, if you don't adequately learn certain skills and techniques during your preclinical courses [Introduction to Clinical Medicine or Physical Diagnosis], you may never learn them, not even during clerkships. "Surveys have indicated that less than 16% of attending time may be spent at the patient's side."[3] This has important ramifications for patient care. When researchers observed interns and residents, they noted frequent errors in physical exam technique, including improper use of instruments. In Chapters 5 [Taking a Patient History] and 6 [Physical Examination], you'll learn how to make the most of your history and physical exam education.

The challenges of the preclinical years extend beyond the well-known. Chapters 11 and 12 provide some startling statistics on medical student well-being and issues of professionalism. Physicians are challenged on a daily basis with the stressors of clinical patient care, and the coping mechanisms and buffering strategies you develop now, as a preclinical student, will be vital throughout the course of your career.

Several chapters highlight the significant opportunities available to medical students. Medical schools, organizations, and individual medical students have all been able to impact medical practice or their communities in significant ways, and their accomplishments are inspiring. Chapters on Community Service, Extracurricular Activities, and Research serve as a guide on how to get started, and highlight the numerous opportunities for preclinical students to become involved and thus have the opportunity to make a meaningful impact. Chapters on teaching, awards, and international experiences provide details on further opportunities.

Throughout these challenges, you do have to consider your future. As the residency selection process for certain fields becomes ever more competitive, students who have at least started strategizing early in their education will be at an advantage. Chapter 16 [Choosing a Specialty] reviews the process of strategizing in detail. For the most competitive specialties, great grades and high USMLE scores are not enough. You'll need great letters of recommendation and support from faculty advocates. In Chapter 10 [Mentoring], you'll learn ways in which preclinical students can approach established faculty members and obtain their assistance and guidance. You'll also need additional distinctions. Most applicants to the competitive specialties will have performed research, and many will have publications or presentations to their name. Chapter 7 [Research] reviews the process, demonstrates how students can begin, details what to seek in a research project, and provides specifics on research, publication, and presentation opportunities available to medical students. Some residency programs also seek additional factors of distinction, such as involvement in extracurricular activities, evidence of leadership, and commitment to service. In "Choosing a Specialty," you'll learn how to start the process of exploring a specialty. The chapter also includes specifics about identifying research opportunities, locating specialty-specific mentors, seeking out community service projects within the field, and other specialty-specific opportunities.

Throughout the next 300+ pages, we'll review each of these areas in detail. From grades and exams, to the art of patient care, to strategizing for your career, you'll learn specific, detailed information relevant to the preclinical medical student. These reviews and recommendations are based on the experiences of students, residents, and faculty, as well as a thorough review of the scientific literature in the areas of medical education and patient care. This combination of insider information and evidence-based advice is utilized to help you gain the strongest foundation as you face the challenges of medical school. Your goal is to become the best doctor possible, and that process begins on day one of medical school.

Preclinical courses/grades

At one medical school, faculty assigned "29,239 pages of reading."[1]

The core of this chapter centers on one vital question related to that startling fact. How can a student read and retain such a large volume of information?

In Chapter 2, you'll learn what students, faculty, and experts advise on how to get through the mountain of material a med student is expected to master. The most common mistake that med students seem to make? They assume that studying longer and harder will be enough to succeed.

It's not.

The students who are able to excel in medical school have learned how to effectively strategize and utilize the techniques of active learning, among other study strategies. Reading and highlighting material, even multiple times, won't be enough to ensure the long-term retention that medical school requires.

Upperclassmen at the University of Alabama Birmingham School of Medicine offer the following advice to new students: "The material is rarely difficult; there is just a mountain's worth to cover. A normal medical school exam seems like a cumulative final in the most strenuous science course you took in undergraduate. You simply cannot learn the material overnight or with one quick read-through of the scripts."[4]

Prior to med school, you no doubt heard about the heavy academic workload. The volume of material to be covered is truly enormous, and while students expect this, it doesn't fully sink in until the first week when you receive lecture materials, syllabi, and books. Consider the following comments made by new medical students:

- "I was worried that I wouldn't be able to keep up."

- "What scared me most was the amount of information I was asked to master."

- "It was all so overwhelming. How could I possibly learn it all? After all, I could barely carry it."

While the preclinical curriculum will vary among medical schools, most schools will focus on the same core subjects. In 2006, the

International Association of Medical Science Educators convened a group of respected medical educators to answer some key questions about the role and value of the basic sciences in medical education.[5] The educators identified eight sciences - anatomy, physiology, biochemistry, neuroscience, microbiology, immunology, pathology, and pharmacology – as "vital foundations of medical practice." Also deemed critical to a strong foundation was education in behavioral sciences, genetics, epidemiology, molecular biology, and biostatistics.

Given the significant challenges of learning and retaining this much material, what is the best way for students to approach their preclinical courses? In this chapter, you'll learn the differences between top and average performers, and you'll learn about study strategies that have led to success. In one study, researchers found that "in general, study skills are stronger predictors of first-semester total grades than aptitude as measured by the MCAT and undergraduate GPA."[2] You'll learn about common mistakes that students make when approaching the basic sciences, and how to avoid those mistakes. You'll also hear suggestions from students who have successfully navigated these challenges.

USMLE Step 1 Exam

The USMLE Step 1 exam is a critical factor in the residency selection process. While there's a lot that can be said about preparation for this exam, it can be summarized in one sentence: typical study methods don't work for this exam.

To become an allopathic physician with the license to practice in the United States, you must pass the three-part United States Medical Licensing Exam, referred to as the USMLE. Medical students typically take the first part of the USMLE (Step 1 exam) at the end of the second year of medical school. The Step 1 score is also an important criterion used by residency programs in the selection process. In a 2006 survey of over 1,200 residency program directors across 21 medical specialties, the USMLE Step 1 score was found to be the second most important residency selection factor, following only grades in required clerkships.[6]

In competitive specialties such as dermatology, plastic surgery, ophthalmology, otolaryngology, radiology, neurosurgery, orthopedic surgery, and urology, many programs have a cut-off, or threshold, USMLE Step 1 score. Highly sought-after programs in less competitive specialties may also have threshold scores. Applicants who score above the cut-off are considered for interviews. Those below the cut-off may be removed from consideration.

"Many medical students that we have talked to underestimate the amount of clinical material on the USMLE Step 1 examination.... Furthermore, many students also leave the exam feeling somewhat intimidated regarding the clinical slant of how the basic science material is tested." - Drs. Tao Le and Chirag Amin, authors of the popular book *First Aid for the USMLE Step 1*.[7]

The National Board of Medical Examiners (NBME), which administers the exam, states that the USMLE Step 1 exam "assesses whether you can understand and apply important concepts of the sciences to the practice of medicine, with special emphasis on the principles and mechanisms underlying health, disease, and modes of therapy."[8]

While strong factual knowledge is necessary for exam success, most questions seek to determine your ability to apply basic science knowledge to clinical problems, rather than regurgitate isolated facts. In a recent posting at www.usmle.org, the National Board of Medical Examiners announced a further reduction in the number of Step 1 items presented without a clinical vignette.

This focus on clinical applications, rather than rote memorization, makes the USMLE a distinctive and challenging exam for most students. Adding to the challenge is the amount of information that students are expected to master. The content of the exam is drawn from the following disciplines: Anatomy, Physiology, Biochemistry, Pathology, Pharmacology, Microbiology, Behavioral Sciences, and Nutrition/Genetics/Aging. The Step 1 exam, therefore, covers information that requires 2 years of medical school to learn. Most students devote a 6 week block of time to review material and prepare for this exam. Cramming, obviously, won't work.

In Chapter 3, you'll learn the basics of the Step 1 exam. What material does it cover, and what material do you need to review? Does the curriculum offered by your school provide adequate preparation? Most schools adhere to a disciplines-based, organ-based, or problem-based curriculum, or a combination thereof. Researchers have utilized AAMC [Association of American Medical Colleges] data to determine what effects, if any, the curricular approach had on USMLE scores.

What are the mistakes that students make when preparing for the exam? Dr. Judy Schwenker, Kaplan's Curriculum Director, has identified the five most common mistakes students make when preparing for the Step 1 exam.[9] These include passive studying, insufficient practice with questions, memorizing without understanding the material, inappropriate test day strategies, and misreading or misinterpreting questions. In this chapter, we provide suggestions on exam preparation that avoid these common mistakes.

How should you study for an exam of this importance that's so distinct from other exams? Drs. Helen Loeser and Maxine Papadakis, Deans at the UCSF School of Medicine, advise: "Use active learning methods as you integrate your knowledge and apply basic science information to clinical vignettes."[10] Research has shown that active learning leads to better long-term retention of information and easier retrieval of information when needed. In this chapter you'll learn about techniques of active learning, and resources that can aid in your preparation.

COMLEX Level 1 Exam

For osteopathic students, the route to licensure requires passage of the three-level COMLEX. These parts include COMLEX Level 1, COMLEX Level 2 (further subdivided into Level 2 Cognitive Evaluation or CE and Level 2 Performance Evaluation or PE), and COMLEX Level 3. Osteopathic students typically take the COMLEX Level 1 exam near the end of the second year, while both components of the Level 2 exam are taken in the fourth year.

According to the National Board of Osteopathic Medical Examiners (NBOME), which administers the exam, the COMLEX Level 1 exam "emphasizes the scientific concepts and principles necessary for understanding the mechanisms of health, medical problems and disease processes."[11] Information about the content of the exam is available at their website (see Bulletin of Information), and should be reviewed carefully. In contrast to the USMLE, the COMLEX examination incorporates osteopathic principles, including the use of osteopathic manipulative treatment.

Like the USMLE, the COMLEX Level 1 exam is used by programs in the residency selection process. This process can be divided into two phases – screening and ranking. In the screening phase, programs whittle down a large applicant pool into a smaller group. The members of this group will be offered interview invitations. The COMLEX Level 1 score is frequently used in the screening process by allopathic and osteopathic residency programs. In 2010, a survey of several thousand allopathic residency program directors representing multiple specialties was performed by the National Resident Matching Program. The survey found that the Level 1 score was the factor used most commonly in the screening process.[12]

In competitive specialties such as dermatology, plastic surgery, ophthalmology, otolaryngology, radiology, neurosurgery, orthopedic surgery, and urology, many programs have a cut-off or threshold COMLEX Level 1 score. Highly sought-after programs in less competitive specialties may also have threshold scores. Applicants who score above the cut-off are considered for interviews. Those below the cut-off may be removed from consideration.

In this chapter, you'll learn about how the COMLEX Level 1 score is used by residency programs in the selection process. You'll learn about ways to identify your strengths and weaknesses, as well as indicators that you may be at risk for a low COMLEX score. You'll also hear tips to help you prepare for the exam. For example, the NBOME offers students the opportunity to take the Comprehensive Osteopathic Medical Self-Assessment Exam (COMSAE) as a means to assess readiness for the COMLEX Level 1 exam. The format and structure of the Phase 1 COMSAE resembles that of the Level 1 exam. Furthermore, scoring and reporting of the two exams are similar. In a study performed by the NBOME, the organization found that the two scores were highly related. While candidates can take a timed or untimed COMSAE, the data seems to suggest that the timed exam has higher self-assessment value.

While we review the role of the COMLEX in the residency selection process, in this chapter you'll learn that this score, by itself, may not be sufficient for all residency programs. In recent years, an increasing number of osteopathic students have applied to residency programs approved by the Accreditation Council for Graduate Medical Education (ACGME). According to Drs. Cummings and Sefcik, Deans at the Michigan State University College of Osteopathic Medicine, "in 2006, more than two of every three DOs [6,629 of 9,618] in postdoctoral training were in an ACGME program."[13] Since ACGME-accredited programs are less familiar with the COMLEX score, these programs often recommend that osteopathic applicants take the USMLE Step 1 exam. This allows programs to make easier comparisons between MD and DO student applicants.

Taking a Patient History

It's well-known that the transition between learning about medicine in the classroom and actually applying that knowledge in the care of real patients is quite challenging. Studies have confirmed that students have high levels of stress and anxiety as they move from the preclinical to clinical years of medical school.[14]

Clinical skills, including the history and physical exam, are often mentioned as a major struggle in the transition period. One student described her discomfort. "I felt uncomfortable talking to the patient and trying to come up with methodical ways of asking questions and making sure I didn't miss things, not just jumping around all over the place."[15]

Traditionally, preclinical students have had limited contact with patients. In recent years, however, schools have placed new emphasis on clinical skills training in early medical education. Some schools now even introduce students to patients as soon as the first week or month of medical school.

Medical organizations have also recognized the importance of an early emphasis on clinical skills, including communication. In 2004, the Institute of Medicine made the acquisition and development of communication skills a top priority during medical education. That same year, the National Board of Medical Examiners (NBME) began requiring students to take a clinical skills exam (USMLE Step 2 CS) as a means to assess competence in communication. The hope is that through education on effective communication, students will be better versed in how to listen, question, counsel, and motivate patients.

Your efforts to improve communication skills will also impact your clerkship performance. In a survey of clerkship directors, while over 95% felt that students require an intermediate to advanced level of communication skills, approximately 30% felt that new clerkship students aren't sufficiently prepared.[16]

Medical schools evaluate communication skills in different ways. One is through comprehensive clinical skills assessment using standardized patients. Researchers have interviewed faculty members responsible for helping those students who don't perform well in these assessments. Some of the issues have focused on patient histories.[17] "Many low-scoring students focused prematurely, failing to ask open-ended questions or adequately characterize the chief complaint. Respondents also observed students being too focused on the history of present illness, omitting or incompletely exploring the pertinent past medical, social, or family history, particularly as they related to the chief complaint." Some students failed to explore the patient's perspective on the illness. The authors wrote that "these students treated standardized patients as symptoms or diagnoses rather than as people with feelings or concerns."

In Chapter 5, you'll learn how to make the most of your clinical skills education. You'll learn about the deficiencies that have been documented in the physician-patient communication literature with respect to history taking, and how educators have developed benchmarks to guide medical students in their acquisition of important communication skills. As you develop your history taking skills, you'll learn how to use these benchmarks, solicit feedback to assess your progress, and reflect on your own performance in order to improve your skills.

Physical Examination

Although 80% of diagnoses are made based on the history and physical examination, evidence indicates that the physical exam skills of physicians today are inadequate. It is widely believed that physicians' examination skills have deteriorated over the years. While advances in technology, including laboratory testing and radiologic imaging, are partly to blame for this decline, clinical skills training during medical school and residency are also factors. According to Dr. Sal Mangione, Director of the Physical Diagnosis Curriculum at Jefferson Medical College, too little time is spent during medical school learning these skills. "Surveys have indicated that less than 16% of attending time may be spent at the patient's side."[18]

Physical exam skills have important, obvious ramifications for patient care, and the education you receive in this area during medical school is critical. If you don't learn certain skills at this stage of your education, you may never have the opportunity to do so. In one study, researchers observed interns and residents, and noted frequent errors in physical exam technique.[19] Errors included improper manual technique or use of instruments. The authors asserted that these errors resulted from a failure to learn the necessary psychomotor skills during the preclinical years.

In the real world of medicine, these deficiencies in skills have serious consequences. In a study of interns and residents on a general medicine service, at least one serious physical exam error was made for nearly two-thirds of the patients examined. The errors included failure to detect splenomegaly or focal neurological signs, findings that once discovered led to significant changes in diagnosis and treatment.[20]

While clinical courses such as "Introduction to Clinical Medicine" and "Physical Diagnosis" teach these skills, this is one area where students cannot rely on passive learning. In Chapter 6, you'll learn how to make the most of your physical exam education. These skills aren't easy to learn. While a recent study showed that third-year med students felt quite confident about their ability to measure blood pressure, students were significantly less confident in their ability to assess retinal vasculature, detect a thyroid nodule, or measure jugular venous pressure.[21]

You'll also learn the importance of soliciting preceptor feedback. If errors aren't picked up at this stage of your education, they may never be. While you might expect that your future residents or attendings would be able to correct your performance, the literature has shown that students on clerkships often aren't observed while performing physical exams. They are typically assumed to already possess the necessary skills.

The chapter also addresses other facets of physical exams, including the patient's comfort. You'll learn how to approach an often uncomfortable situation in a manner that most reassures the patient. In the article "Learning to Doctor," Conrad aptly describes the concerns of students:[22]

Students tell patients twice their age to get undressed, and then cross conventional barriers of interpersonal space to inspect the intimacies of their bodies. In addition to anxiety about doing it right, students frequently must deal with their own reactions to their patient as well as discomforting feelings of being invasive.

Research

In a presentation to medical students titled "Research in Medical School," Dr. Daniel West discussed reasons why students should consider involvement in research. Dr. West noted that participation in research allows medical students to explore a specialty in more depth, enhance critical thinking and other related skills, assess suitability for a career in academic medicine, and strengthen credentials for residency positions.[23] Medical students recognize these benefits as well. In a survey of students at three medical schools, 83% agreed that participation in research was valuable within their medical education.[24]

In Chapter 7, we'll discuss these benefits in more depth. There are significant benefits to participation in research, and while barriers exist, many medical students are able to overcome these barriers, enhance their own skills and education, and make contributions to the scientific literature.

Research training leads to better critical thinking skills. The ability to critically appraise the literature is essential to the practice of evidence-based medicine. The University of Arizona College of Medicine writes that "as future physicians, being able to critically read a scientific journal along with keeping abreast of new medical innovations is an important facet of practice that can profoundly impact patient outcomes."[25] In a recent article, Mayo researchers wrote about how research benefits medical students.[26] "Studies have shown that students who had conducted research during medical school reported gains in knowledge and skills in appraising the literature, analyzing data, and writing for publication, along with more positive attitudes toward future research." Students report significant benefits from learning the process of research, from conception of an idea to publication and presentation. It is important for all physicians to learn about literature review, hypothesis generation, study methodology, and data analysis.

Research also has known benefits in the residency selection process. Dr. Scott Pretorius, former Radiology Residency Program Director at the University of Pennsylvania, wrote that "in this competitive market for radiology residency slots, medical students with research backgrounds...allow themselves the opportunity to stand out in a field of increasingly highly qualified applicants. As an advisor of medical students, I routinely recommend that students intending to apply for radiology residency seek out a research mentor and undertake some kind of research project."[27] In a survey of University of Tennessee medical students, 63% reported that research experience was beneficial in helping them secure a residency position.[28]

As you're applying for residency positions, it's important to know your competition. Among dermatology applicants, nearly 95% had participated in at least one research project, with over 80% claiming at least one abstract, publication, or presentation.[29] In radiation oncology, among U.S. senior applicants, only 9 of the 152 applicants reported not having a single abstract, publication, or presentation. While it's not a prerequisite for students applying to competitive fields, a student may stand out due to their lack of any research experience in these fields.

While students recognize the benefits of research, many find the barriers to involvement daunting. Difficulty finding a research supervisor can be a significant barrier, with only 44% of students in one study reporting that it was easy to identify one.[24] In this chapter, you'll learn how to identify research opportunities at your institution. We highlight ways to identify the "right" research mentor, as well as what to discuss with potential mentors and how to evaluate potential research projects.

In evaluating research experience during medical school, residency programs will look closely at the level of your involvement. Did you merely collect data? Or were you involved through all phases of the project (design of the project, data collection, analysis of the data, and writing the manuscript)? Programs also assess your productivity. Did your work result in a tangible measure, such as an abstract, manuscript, or presentation at a meeting? For many students involved in research, a publication or presentation resulting from their work would be ideal. While this isn't always possible, in this chapter you'll learn how to approach the issue of publication and learn about journals that are targeted to medical students.

You'll also learn about possibilities for presentation, even if those opportunities aren't initiated by your research mentor. Students may seek out opportunities to present their work at local, regional, national, and international meetings. At Stanford University School of Medicine, 52% of medical students had presented at a national meeting.[30] Symposiums and meetings geared to medical student research presentations include the National Student Research Forum (NSRF), Eastern-Atlantic Student Research Forum (ESRF), and Western Student Medical Research Forum (WSMRF). The NSRF is held at the University of Texas Medical Branch in Galveston, and provides a forum for students to give either poster or oral presentations.[31] Over 30 awards are given at this annual event.

Time has been reported as a major barrier to pursuing research in medical school. Many students become involved in research in the summer between the first and second years of medical school. Opportunities for summer research may also be available for newly admitted students who haven't yet started medical school. At the Mt. Sinai School of Medicine, 54 to 65% of students participated in summer research between 2001 and 2004.[32]

Some students are interested in a more substantial research experience, and in this chapter you'll learn about some of the "year-out" opportunities available to students across the country. The Clinical Research Fellowship for Medical Students, sponsored by the Doris Duke Charitable Foundation, offers one-year fellowships at one of 12 selected institutions in the U.S. The HHMI – NIH (Howard Hughes Medical Institute - National Institutes of Health) Research Scholars Program and NIH Clinical Research Training Program allow participants the opportunity to work on the NIH campus. Research Training Fellowships through the HHMI are also available to students, and support one year of research at a variety of academic institutions. This chapter highlights a number of other opportunities that are available for students interested in more substantial research experience.

Extracurricular Activities

As in college, the learning environment in medical school extends beyond the classroom, and institutions offer valuable opportunities to participate in a variety of extracurricular activities. For example, at the Case Western Reserve University, there are over 40 medical student organizations.[33]

Involvement in these organizations provides a number of opportunities and benefits, and in Chapter 8 you'll learn more about the opportunities available. One of the most important is the further development of skills that are directly applicable to success as a physician. A few examples of vital skills in the daily life of a physician are teamwork, self-discipline, time management, and leadership, all of which are strengthened outside of the classroom through extracurricular involvement. Involvement in organizations is a way to develop and strengthen bonds with classmates, and since student organizations often have a faculty advisor or sponsor, students have extraordinary opportunities to work closely with faculty members. Such opportunities are usually unavailable to students during the preclinical years.

Some students are awarded recognition for their involvement. Every year, the American Medical Association honors 15 students with AMA Foundation Leadership Awards. These awards recognize students who have demonstrated "strong, nonclinical leadership skills in advocacy, community service, public health, and/or education."[34] Many other organizations recognize student involvement as well. When evaluating a student's contributions, organizations seek evidence of leadership, commitment, and the ability to make meaningful contributions to the goals of an organization. Some students, after reviewing the opportunities available at their school, commit to starting a new organization or founding a new chapter of a national organization. In this chapter, you'll learn what questions to ask, and what resources are available, as you review your opportunities.

Involvement may also help students reach their professional goals. Extracurricular activities "might provide evidence for non-cognitive attributes that predict success," writes Dr. Andrew Lee, Chairman of the Department of Ophthalmology at The Methodist Hospital.[35] "Leadership skills demonstrated by being an officer in extracurricular activities or being an Eagle Scout, or a leader or founder of a new organization or club are all looked upon favorably. The second goal is to look for evidence of non-cognitive attributes that might make a superior ophthalmologist (conflict resolution, team work, leadership ability, communication skills, performance under stress, maturity, seriousness of purpose, prior scholarly activity). Finally, programs are looking to graduate (and thus select) residents who will make the program proud."

In fact, extracurricular activities do serve as a significant nonacademic factor in the residency selection process. In a recent NRMP survey of 1,840 program directors representing the nineteen largest medical specialties, 59% of respondents cited volunteer/extracurricular experiences as a factor in selecting applicants to interview.[36]

Evidence suggests that meaningful contributions in extracurricular activities, particularly leadership, may serve as a predictor of residency performance. In one study of emergency medicine residency program directors, having a "distinctive factor" such as being a championship athlete or medical school officer, was one of three factors most predictive of residency performance.[37] In a study to determine predictors of otolaryngology resident success using data available at the time of interview, candidates having an exceptional trait such as leadership experience were found to be rated higher as residents.[38]

Community Service

In researching community service opportunities for medical students, we found ourselves amazed and inspired by the accomplishments of medical schools, medical school organizations, and individual medical students. In Chapter 9, you'll hear about the significant contributions made by students. You'll learn about opportunities for participation in community service, the impact your participation can have on the health of the community, and how your involvement can help you grow personally and professionally.

According to Dr. Aaron McGuffin, Senior Associate Dean for Medical Education at Marshall University School of Medicine, "there has been 2,700 hours of community service donated from the medical school students in the past 12 months. That is a lot of time in addition to doing their medical school work."[39] In 2008, the AAMC found that a significant percentage of medical school applicants had been involved in community service.[40] Sixty-three percent of the applicants reported nonmedical volunteer experience, while medical volunteer experience was reported by 77% of applicants. "They have a real sense of service, commitment, and discovery that I know we all want in a future doctor at our bedside," said Dr. Darrell Kirch, the AAMC President.[41]

While the provision of community service has been a major area of emphasis at U.S. medical schools for years, educators have recently stressed the importance of fostering education in community service among medical students. In 1998, Seifer defined service learning as "a structured learning experience that combines community service with preparation and reflection."[42] The Liaison Committee on Medical Education (LCME), which is responsible for the accreditation of medical schools, recommends that schools should not only provide students with sufficient opportunities "to participate in service-learning activities," but also "encourage and support student participation."[43]

Many schools provide such opportunities for service learning. In 2001, the Morehouse School of Medicine established the Center for Community Health and Service - Learning to engage students and other healthcare professionals in community service and service learning. Partnering with other organizations in the Atlanta area, the center aims to address the health disparities affecting underserved populations. At the University of New Mexico School of Medicine, community service is a key priority.[44] Educators have gone beyond just encouragement by freeing students in the afternoons during the first year for service engagement.

At other schools, student organizations have been able to make significant contributions to their communities. The AAMC's Medicine in the Community Grant Program (formerly known as Caring for Community) offers grant awards to medical students who wish to initiate, develop, and run a community service project.[45] According to the AAMC, "Medicine in the Community will help students to translate great ideas into meaningful service by contributing needed start-up and supplemental funds." Past recipients of the grant include the Medical College of Wisconsin Hmong Health Education Program. HHEP is an effort to improve health education and healthcare services for Wisconsin's Hmong population through educational workshops, outreach programs, support groups, and public service announcements. Another past recipient is the University of New Mexico School of Medicine Community Vision Project. Through the use of mobile eye clinics, basic vision care services are provided to American Indian and Hispanic populations.

For students wishing to make significant contributions to their communities, a number of organizations provide grants and assistance. In this chapter, you'll learn about grants and resources available to students who wish to initiate their own service project, as well as hear about other successful projects. For example, the Medical Student Section of the AMA (AMA-MSS) has created a list and description of projects that AMA-MSS chapters across the country have developed and implemented.[46] Since the 1970s, *Project Bank: The Encyclopedia of Public Health and Community Projects*, a tool offered by the AMA Alliance, has served as a useful compendium of community service projects conducted by state and county Alliances.[47]

Student-run health clinics have been initiated at many medical schools, and such involvement can have a significant impact on the personal and professional growth of medical students. At the University of California Davis, 85% of medical students volunteer in student clinics during their tenure in medical school.[48] "Students are often changed in unexpected, profound, and lasting ways after experiencing firsthand healthcare delivery to the poor, underserved, and marginalized," explains Dr. Ed Farrell, a physician volunteer at the Stout Street Clinic, which is run by students attending the University of Colorado School of Medicine.[49]

Not all schools have initiated such clinics. For motivated students, a number of resources are available for those wishing to establish a student-run health clinic. In an article published in JAMA, Cohen wrote "Eight Steps for Starting a Student-Run Clinic."[50] Another useful resource, "25 Steps to Starting a Student-Run Clinic," is available at the Society of Student-Run Free Clinics website.[51]

Community service provides known benefits to students as well. Research has shown that volunteering increases positive feelings, improves mental health, reduces the risk of depression, and lowers stress levels.[52-54] Participation may also improve communication skills, a vital skill in medicine. Community service is also a significant nonacademic factor in the residency selection process. Once accepted for an interview, the depth and breadth of your involvement in community service may help you stand out in a sea of academically qualified applicants.

Mentoring

The further we've progressed in our own careers, the more it becomes apparent how many individuals have helped us along the way. To achieve professional success in almost any field requires help. This may not be initially obvious to medical students, who are used to studying hard and achieving high grades on their own. Reaching medical school though, definitely required help. Professors who provided help outside of the classroom, researchers who offered the opportunity to participate in their project, advisors who provided letters of recommendation: the list goes on.

Succeeding in medical school, and succeeding in the residency match itself, requires even more assistance. At this next stage of your career, informed guidance and advice becomes even more important. For more competitive specialties or programs, you'll also require additional qualifications, which may mean approaching faculty members for research opportunities, in addition to the critically important letters of recommendation.

The definition of a mentor is one who "takes a special interest in helping another person develop into a successful professional."[55] Information, advice, and guidance from a knowledgeable faculty member is invaluable, and has the potential to impact your career in significant ways.

Sometimes the hardest part of initiating an effective relationship is just knowing how to get started. You'll be approaching respected, accomplished, busy individuals, and it can be difficult to know how to approach faculty members without appearing intrusive or presumptuous. For most students, asking for help from individuals in a position of authority can be intimidating. As a preclinical student, you also may have had limited experience in dealing with faculty on an individual level, and knowing what's acceptable can be hard to determine. Therefore, we provide advice from faculty experienced in this area. Certain approaches would be considered acceptable and non-intrusive by most faculty.

Some medical schools have formal mentoring programs. If such a program doesn't exist at your school, then you'll need confidence and possibly persistence to initiate a relationship. In one study, 28% of students met their mentors during inpatient clerkships, 19% through research activities, and 9% during outpatient clerkships.[56]

Local, regional, and state medical societies may have established mentoring programs. For example, the Santa Clara County Medical Association has a Mentor Program for Stanford medical students.[57] National organizations are committed to mentoring future doctors also. The Society of Academic Emergency Medicine (SAEM) has a medical student virtual advisor program open to students at all institutions.[58] Through this program, students can query experienced individuals about a variety of issues, including the EM residency application process. Dr. Joshua Grossman reminds students that mentors don't have to be in close proximity to you. "Your mentor does not need to be someone involved with your residency program that you see on a daily basis. By sharing your experience with someone removed from the situation you may be able to gain a different and beneficial perspective.[59]

While many of us have worked with assigned advisors during our education, a mentoring relationship is unique, and can be hard to delineate. In Chapter 10, you'll hear from mentors and organizations about the best way to develop such a relationship, and specifics on expectations and etiquette. The Association of Women Surgeons writes "A mentor is a unique individual to you: neither friend, nor colleague, but something of a combination of these and more. Because the relationship differs from those you have with others in your department, you may feel more relaxed and less constrained by professional protocol. This is acceptable to a point, but make certain that you respect the relationship."[60]

What do students talk about with a mentor? Issues may include those related to specialty choice, career satisfaction, wellness, work/life balance, residency selection process, research, interpersonal skills, professionalism, ethics, and courses. Once they have a firm idea of career choice, many students schedule meetings to discuss match strategy, seeking advice on steps they can take at their level to establish their credentials and strengthen their applications.

It can be intimidating and challenging to seek advice from qualified, well-informed faculty members. Is it worth seeking a mentor? While mentors can prove helpful throughout medical school, they can provide invaluable guidance during the process of preparing for the residency match. In researching our companion book, *The Successful Match: 200 Rules to Succeed in the Residency Match*, we asked applicants what they found most difficult about the residency application process. A number of applicants commented on the same issue. "There's so much conflicting information out there. How do you know what to believe? Who should you listen to?" Applicants with mentors have a decided advantage. Students benefit greatly when the wisdom, experience, and perspective of a knowledgeable faculty member are used to help them. Having a mentor to guide you through the complex residency application process is recognized by students as an important factor in boosting the strength of their application.

Well-being

In the past, issues of medical student well-being weren't a priority. Today, though, medical educators recognize that the intense pressures of medical school can have serious consequences for a medical student's physical health and emotional well-being. Research has demonstrated that these aren't just soft issues; they have real ramifications for patient care as well. In a recent study of pediatric residents, 20% of participants met criteria for depression, and these residents made over six times as many medication errors as their non-depressed colleagues.[61]

It's clear that medical school can be intensely stressful. In a survey of medical students, Wolf asked students to rate medical school stressors on a scale of 1 (not stressful) to 7 (extremely stressful).[62] The top four stressors, out of 16 ranked, were examinations, amount of classwork, financial responsibilities, and lack of time for recreation and entertainment. In a survey of medical students at 16 U.S. schools, 60% of first-year students reported either "moderate" or "a lot" of stress in the last two weeks.[63] This stress can lead to physician burnout, a condition which is characterized by emotional depletion from one's work, depersonalization, and the perception that one's work is inconsequential. In a survey of medical students in Minnesota, 45% had burnout.[64]

We chose to emphasize issues of medical student well-being within this chapter for several reasons. One was to highlight the impact of med school stressors on a student's health and well-being. Evidence indicates that this impact can be significant, and it is common for medical students to be affected. Even more importantly, in this chapter you'll learn how to buffer this stress. You'll learn about effective coping strategies identified by researchers. There is significant evidence that sleep, exercise, and the maintenance of strong social connections can provide strong buffers against the stressors of med school. Many students let these activities go first, though, in their efforts to focus on coursework and exams. However, studies indicate that these strategies, and others, should actually be priorities at times of intense stress. In a cross-sectional study of medical students, approximately 77% suffered some degree of anxiety.[65] Anxiety symptoms were considerably less common in students exercising at least 30 minutes three times a week. Another study revealed that "strong social ties was the factor most positively related to better health and life satisfaction" among a group of first-year medical students.[66]

It's important to develop effective coping strategies during the preclinical years, as the clinical care of patients only adds to stress. Dr. Liselotte Dyrbye, a faculty member at the Mayo Clinic, has performed extensive research in this area. She states that medical students need to have "the skills necessary to assess personal distress, determine its effects on their care of patients, recognize when they need assistance, and develop strategies to promote their own well-being. These skills are essential to maintain perspective, professionalism, and resilience through the course of a career..."[64]

In this chapter, you'll learn more about coping strategies. One effective strategy is problem-focused coping, in which efforts are made to solve or manage the problem causing the distress. Emotion-focused coping is another effective strategy, among many others. As a new med student, it's helpful to learn about how you cope with issues. In 1997, Charles Carver, a professor at the University of Miami, developed the brief COPE questionnaire, which can be used as a tool to help determine the coping strategies that you tend to use.[67] If your total scores are higher in the coping strategy categories of self-distraction, denial, substance abuse, or self-blame, you'll need to learn how to develop and use healthier and more effective coping skills. Dr. Julie Gentile, Director of Medical Student Mental Health Services at the Boonshoft School of Medicine at Wright State University, states that medical school "is a critical period in which to develop and utilize functional and effective coping strategies"[68]

Professionalism

What is professionalism, and why does it matter?

Consider the following observation made by a student:

Two doctors were down the hall from each other, and there were people around. One said to the other, "Did you hear about Mr. X?" And the other doctor said no, and he made a face like a dead face...sticking his tongue out, crossing his eyes, and tilting his head to the side. If anybody had noticed they wouldn't have been too happy with it.[69]

Students must be prepared to deal with issues of professionalism in their peers, in members of the healthcare team, and even in their teachers. Researchers found that exposure to unprofessional behavior began early in the medical education process and increased in each successive year. In Year 1 of medical school, 66% of students had "heard derogatory comments not in patient's presence" and 35% had "observed unethical conduct by residents or attending physicians."[70]

Why else does professionalism matter?

The vast majority of the students we meet have core values and a strong sense of personal integrity. Many therefore assume that issues of professionalism, while they may impact others around them, don't have any relevance to their own behavior. This is due to the common assumption that our core values regarding unethical behavior are stable over time. Studies of medical students contradict this assumption.

In one study, medical students were given a list of 11 unprofessional behaviors, and asked "Is the following behavior unprofessional for a medical student?"[71] Students were surveyed before matriculation and again six months into their first year of medical school. Researchers found that behaviors originally considered unprofessional rapidly became more acceptable. Medical students were also presented with four different scenarios, and asked "Must one do the following to be professional?" For the scenario "Report Cheating to a Professor or Administrator," 69% of students originally answered "yes." Six months into medical school, only 41% answered "yes."

There are therefore two core reasons to focus on this field. If you're a medical student, you are likely to witness lapses in professionalism in patient care, and you need to be prepared to deal with those lapses and protect your patients. You also need to define and protect your own core values and personal integrity.

What is professionalism? The foundation of the medical profession rests upon the trust that patients place in their physicians. Professionalism focuses on this foundation of trust. Although it's been defined in various ways, the core values and elements agreed upon include honesty, integrity, compassion, empathy, ability to communicate effectively with patients, and respect for others. Professionalism is a hot topic in undergraduate medical education. A number of medical education organizations, including the American Board of Internal Medicine, the Association of American Medical Colleges, and the National Board of Medical Examiners, have established professionalism as a required competency across the spectrum of medical education. Medical schools, in turn, have made it a point to educate preclinical students.

Many students, when hearing about a curriculum on professionalism, have similar reactions. "I already hold these values. Why should any of this concern me?" The studies that we describe in this chapter provide a definitive answer to that question. Most students are surprised to learn that the stresses and challenges of medical school can affect attitude, behavior, and conduct. However, this conclusion is clearly supported by a number of studies.

Even though medical students may actually harm patients when they act unethically, such actions persist. In a survey of students at a single medical school, 13 to 24% admitted to cheating during the clinical years of medical school.[72] Examples included "recording tasks not performed" and "lying about having ordered tests." In another study, students were asked whether they had heard of or witnessed unethical behaviors on the part of their student colleagues.[73] In response, 21% had personal knowledge of students "reporting a pelvic examination as 'normal' during rounds when it had been inadvertently omitted from the physical examination."

As students, you are likely to witness lapses in professional behavior, and may witness outright unethical behavior and fraud. These issues affect every level of our profession, and therefore you have to be prepared. You must guard against lapses in your own behavior, and be prepared to deal with lapses in colleagues or supervisors. As physicians, our goal is to treat and protect the patient, and this can be challenging in the real world of clinical medicine.

In a survey, third-year students at the University of Texas Medical Branch at Galveston were asked to evaluate their physicians' professionalism.[74] Although this review of nearly 3,000 evaluation forms revealed significant praise for positive faculty role modeling, negative comments were not infrequent. The majority dealt with "issues of language use, inappropriate use of humor, disrespectful treatment of patients or colleagues, and apparent disinterest in teaching."

Although we think of physicians as highly compassionate and ethical individuals, ethical lapses can extend to the highest levels of our profession. In a stunning case of scientific fraud, Dr. Scott Reuben, a highly regarded anesthesiologist whose research has significantly impacted how physicians treat surgical patients for pain, was found to have fabricated results in over 20 published studies.[75] In some cases, he is alleged to have even invented patients.

Choosing a Specialty

For many students, having just arrived at med school and facing voluminous amounts of material to be learned and retained, the focus will be on just making it through. Why, then, have we devoted a large chapter to the topic of choosing and exploring a specialty?

Those medical students who are able to plan and strategize for the residency match have a decided advantage. For the most competitive specialties, great grades and high USMLE scores are not enough. You'll need great letters of recommendation and support from faculty advocates. You'll also need additional distinctions. Most applicants to the competitive specialties will have performed research, and many will have publications or presentations to their name. Some programs look for additional factors of distinction, such as involvement in extracurricular activities, evidence of leadership, and commitment to service.

We present this information not to scare you, but to prepare you. These are the realities of the residency match today, and students who are prepared for these realities have a definite advantage. Your preparation doesn't need to be an overwhelming experience, either. It can start with the basics, such as exploring different specialties by shadowing faculty or speaking to residents. You may choose to take an aptitude test to help guide you in your exploration of specialties. Many students maximize their free summer after first year by participating in research. Those who are knowledgeable can obtain research grants from organizations to fund their research. This has tangible benefits. It results in research experience, an awarded research grant, and the opportunity to develop a relationship with a research mentor who may be able to support your application down the road.

In this chapter, you'll learn more about how to approach the process of choosing a specialty. You'll learn how to approach your target department, and how to cultivate opportunities. You'll gain from the insider knowledge presented in this section, as the chapter outlines, for each and every specialty, detailed specifics about medical student opportunities. These include mentorship programs, research grants targeted to medical students, and information about national meetings.

Why is it important to at least start thinking about your specialty choice now? While many med students wait until the clinical years to assess fit, this approach can be problematic. At most schools, students are required to rotate through the major or core specialties (internal medicine, general surgery, pediatrics, psychiatry, family medicine, obstetrics & gynecology) before pursuing clerkships in other fields. After completing these core rotations during the third year, students aren't left with much time. Most have two to three months of elective time to explore other specialties before they need to decide, since residency applications are typically submitted in September of the fourth year. For example, in a survey of med schools, it was found that anesthesiology is an elective rotation in 66% of schools.[76] For most students, this means that unless you attend a school with a flexible clerkship curriculum, you won't be able to rotate through the specialty until the beginning of your fourth year.

This can have a decided impact on a student's career. In one study of medical students, 26.2% were unsure of their specialty choice at matriculation.[77] Surprisingly, a similar proportion remained undecided at graduation. According to Gwen Garrison, Director of Student and Applicant Services at the AAMC, 30% of residents "either switch from their intended specialty after a transitional or preliminary year or switch outright during their specialty residency."[78] Dr. George Blackall, Director of Student Development at Penn State University College of Medicine, offers some reasons why residents switch. "Residents primarily switch because they a) realize their initial choice is not as interesting as another specialty, or b) desire a different lifestyle, level of flexibility, or income."[78]

In this chapter, you'll learn how to start the process of exploring a specialty. During the preclinical years, one way to assess fit for specialties is by completing personality-type inventories. The premise of this approach is that people are most satisfied professionally when there is a good match between their specialty choice and their values, skills, and interests. Commonly used assessment methods include the AAMC Careers in Medicine program and the Glaxo Wellcome Pathway Evaluation Program. The AAMC Careers in Medicine (CiM) is a structured program designed to help students gain a better understanding of their personality, values, skills, and interests. The program also allows for exploration of different specialties. The AAMC writes that "as you work through the CiM program, you'll gain the tools to make an informed decision, based on guided self-reflection and the information you'll gather about many career options available to you."[79] Another resource is the Medical Specialty Aptitude Test, an online test developed by the University of Virginia School of Medicine.[80] It is based on content and material from the book, *How to Choose a Medical Specialty*, by Anita Taylor. The website indicates that "you will be asked to rate your tendencies compared to the tendencies of physicians in each specialty. The higher your score for a given specialty, the more similar you are to the physicians in that specialty."

What is the most important factor in choosing a specialty? In a recent survey of graduating medical students, approximately 97% reported that fit with personality, skills, and interests was moderately or strongly influential in choosing which specialty to pursue as a career.[81] No other factor was given as much importance.

For many students, work/life balance also plays an important role. In the 2010 AAMC Medical School Graduation Questionnaire, over 11,000 graduating students were asked, "How influential was work/life balance in helping you choose your specialty?"[81] Over 70% of respondents reported work/life balance as being either moderately or strongly influential in their decision-making process. In 1989, Schwartz introduced the term *controllable lifestyle* to refer to "specialties that offer regular and predictable hours."[82] These specialties are often characterized by fewer hours spent at work and less frequent on-call duties, allowing for greater personal time and flexibility to pursue other activities. Specialties that are generally felt to offer a controllable lifestyle include anesthesiology, dermatology, neurology, ophthalmology, otolaryngology, pathology, psychiatry, and radiology.

Research has shown that efforts to explore specialties during the preclinical years can increase the certainty of specialty choice.[83] In this chapter, you'll learn about multiple avenues to learn more about specialties during the preclinical years. Examples include:

- Identify and work with a mentor
- Volunteer for clinical experiences (e.g., shadowing)
- Perform specialty-specific research
- Meet and speak with as many physicians as you can in your specialties of interest
- Attend local and national specialty organization meetings
- Join specialty interest groups (e.g., Internal Medicine Interest Group, Emergency Medicine Interest Group)

For each of these avenues, we've included specifics on how to proceed. Medical students value mentoring relationships, but identifying and working with a faculty member can be difficult. According to Dr. Gus Garmel, Co-Program Director of the Stanford-Kaiser Emergency Medicine Residency Program, finding a mentor is not easy.[84] "How students find faculty mentors is challenging, because their exposure to a broad selection of emergency medicine faculty may be limited early in their training." We've provided suggestions on how to proceed for each of the specialties. For example, the American College of Physicians (ACP) has created a Mentoring Database. To access the database, which includes program directors, clerkship directors, chairs of medicine, practicing internists, and residents, you must be a member. Mentors are available to answer "specific questions about scheduling your summer preceptorships, getting through the match, and preparing for clerkships and residency interviews..."[85]

We've also included further information about identifying research opportunities. For many of the most competitive specialties, such as dermatology and radiation oncology, your competition will almost all have performed research. Therefore, if you're considering dermatology as a career, you may wish to participate in research between the first and second years of medical school. Research experience has significant educational benefits. Beyond those benefits, research allows a student the chance to develop a relationship with their research supervisor.

In this chapter, you'll gain from the insider knowledge presented for each and every specialty, with detailed, specific information about medical student opportunities.

References

[1] Klatt E, Klatt C. How much is too much reading for medical students? Assigned reading and reading rates at one medical school. *Acad Med* 2011; 86(9): 1079-83.

[2] West C, Sadoski M. Do study strategies predict academic performance in medical school? *Med Educ* 2011; 45(7): 696-703.

[3] Collins G, Cassie J, Daggett C. The role of the attending physician in clinical training. *J Med Educ* 1978; 53: 429-31.

[4] University of Alabama Birmingham School of Medicine. Advice from MS-2 Students. Available at: http://main.uab.edu/uasom/2/show.asp?durki=111766. Accessed October 22, 2011.

[5] Finnerty E, Chauvin S, Bonaminio G, Andrews M, Carroll R, Pangaro L. Flexner revisited: the role and value of the basic sciences in medical education. *Acad Med* 2010; 85 (2): 349-55.

[6] Green M, Jones P, Thomas J. Selection criteria for residency: results of a national program directors survey. *Acad Med* 2009; 84(3): 362-7.

[7] Medscape. The USMLE: Ten Questions. Available at: http://www.medscape.com/viewarticle/403686. Accessed October 19, 2011.

[8] NBME. Available at: http://www.nbme.org. Accessed October 29, 2011.

[9] University of Utah School of Medicine. Preparing for Step 1. Available at: medicine.utah.edu/learningresources/usmle/step1.htm. Accessed October 19, 2011.

[10] University of California San Francisco School of Medicine. Rx for Success on STEP 1 of The Boards. Available at: http://medschool.ucsf.edu/medstudents/documents/step1success.pdf. Accessed October 19, 2011.

[11] NBOME. Available at: http://www.nbome.org. Accessed November 4, 2011.

[12] NRMP. Available at: http://www.nrmp.org. Accessed September 12, 2011.

[13] Cummings M, Sefcik D. The impact of osteopathic physicians' participation in ACGME-accredited postdoctoral programs, 1985-2006. *Acad Med* 2009; 84(6): 733-6.

[14] Moss F, McManus I. The anxieties of new clinical students. *Med Educ* 1992; 26: 17-20.

[15] O'Brien B, Cooke M, Irby D. Perceptions and attributions of third-year student struggles in clerkships: do students and clerkship directors agree? *Acad Med* 2007; 82(10): 970-978.

[16] Windish D, Paulman P, Goroll A, Bass E. Do clerkship directors think medical students are prepared for the clerkship years? *Acad Med* 2004; 79(1): 56-61.

[17] Hauer K, Teherani A, Kerr K, O'Sullivan P, Irby, D. Student performance problems in medical school clinical skills assessments. *Acad Med* 2007; 82(10): S69-S72.

[18] ACP Internist. Good diagnostic skills should begin at the bedside. Available at: http://www.acpinternist.org/archives/2001/02/diagnostics.htm. Accessed February 1, 2012.

[19] Wiener S, Nathanson M. Physical examination: frequently observed errors. *JAMA* 1976; 236(7): 852-5.

[20]Wray N, Friedland J. Detection and correction of house staff error in physical diagnosis. *JAMA* 1983; 249: 1035-7.

[21]Wu E, Fagan M, Reinert S, Diaz J. Self-confidence in and perceived utility of the physical examination: a comparison of medical students, residents, and faculty internists. *J Gen Intern Med* 2007; 22(12): 1725-30.

[22]Conrad P. Learning to doctor: reflections on recent accounts of the medical school years. *Journal of Health and Social Behavior* 1988; 29(4): 323-32.

[23]University of California Davis School of Medicine. Available at: http://mdscholars.ucdavis.edu/Research%20in%20Medical%20School.ppt. Accessed February 9, 2012.

[24]Siemens D, Punnen S, Wong J, Kanji N. A survey on the attitudes towards research in medical school. *BMC Med Educ* 2010; 22: 10: 4.

[25]University of Arizona Medical Student Research Program. Available at: http://www.msrp.medicine.arizona.edu/dist_guidrat.htm. Accessed February 9, 2012.

[26]Dyrbye L, Davidson L, Cook D. Publications and presentations resulting from required research by students at Mayo Medical School, 1976-2003. *Acad Med* 2008; 83(6): 604-10.

[27]Pretorius E. Medical student research: a residency director's perspective. *Acad Radiol* 2002; 9(7): 808-9.

[28]Solomon S, Tom S, Pichert J, Wasserman D, Powers A. Impact of medical student research in the development of physician scientists. *J Investig Med* 2002; 51(3): 149-56.

[29]National Resident Match Program Charting Outcomes in the Match. www.nrmp.org. Accessed August 1, 2010.

[30]Jacobs C, Cross P. The value of medical student research: the experience at Stanford University School of Medicine. *Med Educ* 1995; 29(5): 342-6.

[31]National Student Research Forum. Available at: http://www.utmb.edu/nsrf/. Accessed February 9, 2012.

[32]Zier K, Friedman E, Smith L. Supportive programs increase medical students' research interest and productivity. *J Investig Med* 2006; 54(4): 201-7.

[33]Case Western Reserve University School of Medicine. Available at: http://casemed.case.edu/. Accessed February 12, 2012.

[34]American Medical Association. Available at: http://www.ama-assn.org/ama/pub/about-ama/ama-foundation/our-programs/public-health/excellence-medicine-awards.page. Accessed February 12, 2012.

[35]The Successful Match: Getting into Ophthalmology. Available at: http://studentdoctor.net/2009/08/the-successful-match-interview-with-dr-andrew-lee-ophthalmology/. Accessed February 12, 2012.

[36]NRMP 2010 Program Director Survey. Available at: http://www.nrmp.org/data/index.html. Accessed February 12, 2012.

[37]Hayden S, Hayden M, Garnst A. What characteristics of applicants to emergency medicine residency programs predict future success as an emergency medicine resident. *Acad Emerg Med* 2005; 12(3): 206-10.

[38]Daly K, Levine S, Adams G. Predictors for resident success in otolaryngology. *J Am Coll Surg* 2006; 202 (4): 649-54.

[39]Joan C. Edwards School of Medicine at Marshall University. Available at: http://www.marshallparthenon.com/news/med-students-earning-cash-for-community-service-1.1936252. Accessed September 12, 2011.

[40]Association of American Medical Colleges. Available at: http://www.aamc.org/newsroom/pressrel/2008/enrollmentdata2008.pdf. Accessed July 23, 2011.

[41]American Academy of Family Physicians. Available at: http://www.aafp.org/online/en/home/publications/news/news-now/resident-student-focus/20081119med-school-enroll.html. Accessed February 12, 2012.

[42]Seifer SD. Service-learning: community-campus partnerships for health professions education. *Acad Med* 1998; 73(3): 273-7.

[43]Liaison Committee on Medical Education (LCME) Available at: http://www.lcme.org/standard.htm#servicelearning. Accessed February 12, 2012.

[44]University of New Mexico School of Medicine. Available at: http://hsc.unm.edu/som/. Accessed February 22, 2012.

[45]AAMC Medicine in the Community Grant Program. Available at: http://www.aamc.org/about/awards/cfc/start.htm. Accessed February 12, 2012.

[46]American Medical Association Medical Student Section. Available at: http://www.ama-assn.org. Accessed February 12, 2012.

[47]AMA Alliance Project Bank. Available at: http://www.amaalliance.org/site/epage/40331_625.htm. Accessed February 12, 2012.

[48]University of California Davis School of Medicine. Available at: http://www-med.ucdavis.edu/. Accessed September 12, 2011.

[49]American Medical Association Virtual Mentor. Available at: http://virtualmentor.ama-assn.org/2005/07/medu1-0507.html. Accessed February 12, 2012.

[50]Cohen J. Eight Steps for starting a student-run clinic. *JAMA* 1995; 273: 434-5.

[51]Society of Student-Run Free Clinics. Available at: http://www.studentrunfreeclinics.org/index.php?option=com_content&view=article&id=65&Itemid=144. Accessed February 12, 2012.

[52]Thoits P, Hewitt L. Volunteer work and well-being. *Journal of Health and Social Behavior* 2001; 42(2): 115-31.

[53]Van Willigen M. Differential benefits of volunteering across the life course. *The Journals of Gerontology Series B: Psychological Sciences and Social Sciences* 2000; 55B(5): S308-S318.

[54]Rietschlin J. Voluntary association membership and psychological distress. *J Health Soc Behav* 1998; 39; 348-55.

[55]Adviser, teacher, role model, friend. Available at: http://stills.nap.edu/readingroom/books/mentor. Accessed March 13, 2008. Washington, DC: National Academy Press; 1997.

[56]Aagaard E, Hauer K. A cross-sectional descriptive study of mentoring relationships formed by medical students. *J Gen Intern Med* 2003; 18: 298-302.

[57]Santa Clara County Medical Association Mentor Program for Stanford medical students. Available at: http://med.stanford.edu/mentors/. Accessed February 9, 2012.

[58]Society of Academic Emergency Medicine (SAEM). Available at: http://www.saem.org/e-advising-faqs-students. Accessed February 9, 2012.

[59]American College of Physicians. Finding the right mentor for you. Available at: http://www.acponline.org/medical_students/impact/archives/2010/11/feature/. Accessed February 9, 2012.

[60]Association of Women Surgeons. Available at: https://www.womensurgeons.org/CDR/Mentorship.asp. Accessed February 9, 2012.

[61]Fahrenkopf A, Sectish T, Barger L, Sharek P, Lewin D, Chiang V, Edwards S, Wiedermann B, Landrigan C. Rates of medication errors among depressed and burnt out residents: prospective cohort study. *BMJ* 2008; 336(7642): 488-91.

[62]Wolf T, Faucett J, Randall H, Balson P. Graduating medical students' ratings of stresses, pleasures, and coping strategies. *J Med Educ* 1988; 63(8): 636-42.

[63]Compton M, Carrera J, Frank E. Stress and depressive symptoms/dysphoria among US medical students: results from a large, nationally representative survey. *J Nerv Ment Dis* 2008; 196(12): 891-7.

[64]Dyrbye L, Thomas M, Huntington J, Lawson K, Novotny P, Sloan J, Shanafelt T. Personal life events and medical student burnout: a multicenter study. *Acad Med* 2006; 81 (4): 374-84.

[65]Hussein E, Gabr A, Mohamed A, Hameed A. Physical exercise and anxiety among medical students at Ain Shams University. Presented at the 13th Annual International Ain Shams Medical Students' Congress, Feb 14-16, 2005.

[66]Parkerson G, Broadhead W, Tse C. The health status and life satisfaction of first-year medical students. *Acad Med* 1990; 65(9): 586-8.

[67]Carver C. You want to measure coping but your protocol's too long: consider the brief COPE. *International Journal of Behavioral Medicine* 1997; 4: 92-100.

[68]Gentile J, Roman B. Medical student mental health services; psychiatrists treating medical students. *Psychiatry* 2009; 6(5): 38-45.

[69]Baernstein A, Oelschlager A, Chang T, Wenrich M. Learning professionalism: perspectives of preclinical medical students. *Acad Med* 2009; 84(5): 574-81.

[70]Satterwhite W, Satterwhite R, Enarson C. Medical students' perceptions of unethical conduct at one medical school. *Acad Med* 1998; 73(5): 529-531.

[71]Humphrey H, Smith K, Reddy S, Scott D, Madara J, Arora V. Promoting an environment of professionalism: The University of Chicago "Roadmap." *Acad Med* 2007; 82(11): 1098-1107.

[72]Dans P. Self-reported cheating by students at one medical school. *Acad Med* 1996; 71 (1, suppl): S70-72.

[73]Anderson R, Obenshain S. Cheating by students: findings, reflections, and remedies. *Acad Med* 1994; 69(5): 323-332.

[74]Szauter K, Turner H. Using students' perceptions of internal medicine teachers' professionalism. *Acad Med* 2001; 76(5): 575-6.

[75]Kowalczyk L. Doctor accused of faking studies. *The Boston Globe*; March 11, 2009.

[76]Lin S, Strom S, Canales C, Rodriguez A, Kain Z. The impact of the anesthesiology clerkship structure on medical students matched to anesthesiology. Abstract presented at the 2010 Annual Meeting of the American Society Anesthesiologists. A1106.

[77]Kassebaum D, Szenas P. Medical students' career indecision and specialty rejection: roads not taken. *Acad Med* 1995; 70(10): 937-43.

[78]Association of American Medical Colleges. Available at: http://www.aamc.org/students/cim/august10choices.pdf. Accessed November 21, 2011.

[79]Association of American Medical Colleges (AAMC). Available at: http://www.aamc.org/students/cim/about.htm. Accessed September 23, 2011.

[80]University of Virginia School of Medicine Medical Specialty Aptitude Test. Available at: http://www.med-ed.virginia.edu/specialties. Accessed January 24, 2012.

[81]2010 AAMC Medical School Graduation Questionnaire. Available at: http://www.aamc.org. Accessed August 13, 2011.

[82]Dorsay E, Jarjoura D, Rutecki G. Influence of controllable lifestyle on recent trends in specialty choice by US medical students. *JAMA* 2003; 290(9): 1173-8.

[83]Weinstein P, Gipple C. Some determinants of career choice in the second year of medical school. *J Med Educ* 1975; 50(2): 194-8.

[84]Garmel G. Mentoring medical students in academic emergency medicine. *Acad Emerg Med* 2004; 11(12): 1351-7.

[85]ACP Mentoring Database. Available at: http://www.acponline.org/residents+fellows/mentors/. Accessed January 25, 2012.

Chapter 2

Preclinical Courses / Grades

Upperclassmen at the University of Alabama Birmingham School of Medicine offer the following advice to new students: "The material is rarely difficult; there is just a mountain's worth to cover. A normal medical school exam seems like a cumulative final in the most strenuous science course you took in undergraduate. You simply cannot learn the material overnight or with one quick read-through of the scripts."[1]

Prior to med school, you no doubt heard about the heavy academic workload. The volume of material to be covered is truly enormous, and while students expect this, it doesn't fully sink in until the first week when you receive lecture materials, syllabi, and books. Consider the following comments made by new medical students:

- "I was worried that I wouldn't be able to keep up."

- "What scared me most was the amount of information I was asked to master."

- "It was all so overwhelming. How could I possibly learn it all? After all, I could barely carry it."

At one medical school, on average, students spent 6 hours per day reading assigned material faculty.[2]

While the preclinical curriculum will vary among medical schools, most schools will focus on the same core subjects. In 2006, the International Association of Medical Science Educators convened a group of respected medical educators to answer some key questions about the role and value of the basic sciences in medical education.[3] The educators identified eight sciences - anatomy, physiology, biochemistry, neuroscience, microbiology, immunology, pathology, and pharmacology – as "vital foundations of medical practice." Also deemed critical to a strong foundation was education in behavioral sciences, genetics, epidemiology, molecular biology, and biostatistics.

Given the significant challenges of learning and retaining this much material, what is the best way for students to approach their preclinical courses? In this chapter, you'll learn the differences between top and average performers, and you'll learn about study strategies that have led to success. In one study, researchers found that "in general, study skills are stronger predictors of first-semester total grades than aptitude as measured by the MCAT and undergraduate GPA."[4] You'll learn about common mistakes that students make when approaching the basic sciences, and how to avoid those mistakes. You'll also hear suggestions from students who have successfully navigated these challenges.

Preclinical Courses: 19 Tips for Success

No one can tell you that their approach to learning and studying is the most effective or "right way" to study. However, you can gain valuable information from your successful med student predecessors.

1 Did you cram regularly in college? This may not work in med school. First, cramming leads to poor long-term retention of information, and in med school this long-term retention is important: you'll be using this information in the care of your patients. Second, cramming may allow you to regurgitate information, but it's a poor method for developing a deeper level of understanding. Finally, the sheer amount of information may make it difficult for you to succeed on an exam by cramming.

2 Students often ask, "How many hours will I have to study?" The short answer is "a lot." When asked the number of hours spent studying on the weekend, students at the Indiana University School of Medicine offered the following advice to incoming freshmen. "The amount of time a student spends studying on the weekend completely depends on the student! Some students prefer to do all of their studying during the week, and then have their weekends free. Other students spend time relaxing after class, and use the weekends to catch up...The most important thing to find is a system that works best for you...Just be sure you don't fall behind in the beginning..."[5]

3 When educators have looked at why certain preclinical students are more successful than others, students who study efficiently and effectively are generally identified as the top performers. In other words, it's not just quantity of study time; quality matters as well.

4 Many students utilized a passive approach in their undergraduate coursework. However, simply reading your lecture handouts or books won't be sufficient in medical school. The sheer volume of material that med school requires mandates a more active approach. Dartmouth Medical School writes that "higher-level learning requires the intentional use of strategies. Without sustained effort and carefully considered techniques, your study is not likely to be very efficient, nor are you likely to learn as much. The good news is that almost everyone can learn to study smarter."[6] Strategies for active learning are presented on page 41.

5 Underachieving students tend to study in a passive manner, whereas high-achieving students use more active learning strategies. Dartmouth Medical School offers sound advice. "The more active you are—the more you DO with the information—the better your attention will be, and more you're going to learn. For example, reading is necessary, but just reading something over more than once probably won't do the trick. It's too passive. Mix it up. Try some of these approaches: reading a section to answer specific questions, re-explaining a concept (out-loud), diagramming a process, making a chart, creating an outline, presenting information to a study group or partner, mapping a lecture, making up questions, or having a study partner quiz you."[6] Your openness to learning and adopting new study habits and techniques may have a significant impact on your education and performance.

6 As you learn, you must develop ways to monitor your progress and assess your learning. Some students like to test themselves by periodically answering practice questions. Others gain insight into their level of preparation through discussions with classmates, such as in study groups. Some students make the mistake of using sheer number of hours spent studying as a method of self-assessment. However, the number of hours spent studying doesn't matter as a stand-alone factor: the quality of study time is typically more important.

7 Working on practice questions is an effective way to promote better retention of information. In one study, self-testing was one of only two study strategies "that appeared to be related to academic performance during the first semester" of medical school.[4] "Practice questions are powerful study aids because they help you to focus on topics that are likely to serve as the basis for questions," writes Dr. John W. Pelley.[7]

8 What is your preferred learning style? Many students learn best through reading, which indicates a visual learner. Some students prefer learning a subject through lectures, rather than through reading a book. This is a characteristic of an aural learner. Kinesthetic learners tend to learn best by doing. You may not have ever given much thought to your preferred learning style. However, this knowledge may provide some idea of what subjects might prove challenging. Visual learners often find anatomy easier to learn than a long list of anti-hypertensive medications. You can use knowledge of your learning style to find or develop ways to grasp challenging material.

9 New students often use the same study strategy that served them well in college. While this approach may have been sufficient for college, some students find that they now need to modify their strategy. The Office of Academic Enhancement at the University of Texas San Antonio Health Science Center recommends the following. "Try not to compare study habits with others. You've gotten this far so you know what works for you. However, don't be afraid to leave old study habits behind and try something new if you've found that the old way is not effective or efficient enough."[8]

10 In your undergraduate coursework, you probably received a well-defined syllabus that detailed the breadth and depth of topics for study. Unfortunately, in your med school courses things won't be so clear. Many students spend considerable energy, time, and effort (and a lot of worry) trying to determine precisely what they need to know. While your course will likely provide some guidance, you will ultimately decide the depth of your study, and this can be difficult to determine. You can't be too superficial in your approach, but delving too deeply into every topic means you won't get through the material.

11 What motivates you to study and learn? Motivating factors may vary greatly depending on the individual, or even depending on timing. Some students are interested in the subject matter, while others relate the subject to its clinical applicability. These insights into individual motivation can be helpful when the volume of material becomes a burden.

12 During the preclinical years, you'll spend a substantial amount of time in the classroom or lecture hall. How much time depends on the structure and curriculum of your particular medical school. It's not unusual for days to start at 8 or 9 AM and end at 4 or 5 PM. Lecture attendance is often voluntary. While some students attend regularly, others base attendance decisions on a variety of factors. In a study of first-year students at one northeastern U.S. medical school, only 17% stated that they routinely attend all lectures.[9] Most students made the decision to attend or skip a lecture on a case-by-case basis, taking into account previous experience with a particular teacher, the likelihood that the lecture would add to their own study and learning, time of lecture, and whether they had any competing commitments.

13 Students with non-science backgrounds or majors often worry that they will be at a disadvantage. However, studies have largely shown no difference in basic science academic performance between science and non-science majors. In one study, choice of college major had no significant effect on medical school performance. The endpoints included course grades and USMLE scores.[10]

14 Participation in a study group offers several advantages. Many students enjoy the sense of camaraderie, and active discussion can help with retention. Study groups also help keep you accountable and driven, since others are relying on you to be prepared. If you missed certain points, or didn't focus on certain areas during the lecture, study group can help. Having to explain material to others can be a great way to learn, enhancing your understanding of the material and highlighting any gaps in your knowledge. Also importantly, your group can share pearls, tips, and mnemonics.

15 Be alert for the common problems that can occur in study groups. Some groups can lose focus, drifting to unrelated topics. If some members are unprepared, the bulk of study group time may be used to help them. The group may be a poor fit for you; the pace may be too fast or slow, or the learning style may not match your own. Group dynamics may create unnecessary pressure to compete, while disorganized groups and late starts just waste your time.

16 The decision to join a study group is entirely based on your needs and preferences. Once you join, it's important to periodically assess effectiveness. Are you getting what you need out of the group? Since you have a limited amount of time, is the time spent in the group productive? Would you do better studying on your own? If you're not maximizing your learning through this group, then you should leave. This isn't letting anyone down; it's just acknowledging that your study needs are different.

17 Make a schedule and stick to it. It's been said that information covered in college over a two week period of time is expected to be mastered in one day of medical school. With so much information to cover in a relatively short period of time, it's recommended that students create a schedule and adhere to it. Students often have a hard time with this concept, since most didn't need to use schedules in college. However, when asked to offer advice to those just beginning medical school, comments often revolve around organization and time management. University of Washington medical students were asked "If you could do first year over again, what (if anything) would you do differently?" A sample of their responses: "Plan out my time better...Studying every weekend would have made my workload during the week more manageable." "Stay more on top of studying during the beginning of quarters so I wouldn't have to play catch up for the rest of the time."[11]

18 Do you memorize well? Probably. It's unlikely you would have achieved your level of academic success without the ability to memorize well relative to your peers. Your skills in memorization will definitely help during med school, where you'll be required to ingest and regurgitate vast amounts of information. From learning the origin and insertion of muscles to listing the names of beta-blocker medications, having a good memory will definitely help. However, that memorization alone is not enough. You must know how to apply knowledge. Not long from now, you'll be caring for patients, and your ability to apply what you've learned in the classroom will be essential. As an example, when you care for a patient with heart failure exacerbation, you'll rely on memory for a list of causes. However, you'll need to go much further than just generating a list. You'll need to determine which of these causes is most likely, which requires skills in problem-solving and critical thinking. Basic science exams are increasingly geared towards these types of skills. In the past, they tended to focus on straight recall. Increasingly, though, exams are testing higher-order thinking skills.

19 While every medical student worries about failing a class, most will complete the basic science years without any academic difficulty. However, performing at the same level they've been accustomed to can be a challenge. After all, 90% of the class won't be in the top 10%. It's important for med students to step back and think of the bigger picture. Success is not defined by how well you perform on an exam. Success is defined by utilizing the material to become the best physician possible. The advice given to new medical students at the University of Texas Southwestern Medical School states it well. "Be prepared to readjust what success means to you...Try to focus on mastery of the material, not on the grades you receive, or your performance relative to others."[12] Upperclassmen at the University of Alabama Birmingham School of Medicine have similar advice for new students. "Do not allow your grades to determine how successful you are or be your base of confidence. Chances are that you were in the top 95 percentile of your graduating college class, yet 95% of you will be below that in medical school. Accept that concept and your stress level will be much lower."[1]

10 Resources You Can Use to Transform Passive Studying Habits to Active Learning

1 In 2004, the University of New Mexico School of Medicine developed an excellent guide for new medical students titled "Learning Strategies for Success in Medical School." In the guide, Pamela Houghton DeVoe, the author, offers valuable advice. "Understanding the ways you learn best and how your learning styles can be accommodated in medical school can help with adjustment to the particular medical school curriculum, and help to prevent problems with course work."[13] The guide can be accessed at hsc.unm.edu/community/cnah/docs/handbook_2004.pdf.

2 April Apperson, Assistant Director of Student Services at the University of San Diego California School of Medicine, provides information on successful study strategies on the UCSD website. "If you're not happy with your performance, the most likely culprit is your study strategies. The material presented in medical school is not conceptually more difficult than many rigorous undergraduate courses, but the volume flow rate of information per hour and per day is much greater – it has frequently been described as 'drinking from a fire-hose.'"[14]

3 The University of Utah School of Medicine has identified seven study skills or learning tactics that students should apply to med school learning. Among the techniques and skills discussed are surveying, concept mapping, and reinforcement.[15]

4 Liza Thompson, Director of the Post-Baccalaureate Premedical Program at Johns Hopkins University, recommends that students consider adopting certain strategies. She offers details on how to effectively preview/pre-read lecture notes, take notes during lecture, review class notes, rewrite notes, and read corresponding textbook chapters using an informed and interactive approach.[16]

5 The Office of Academic Support and Student Counseling at the Albert Einstein College of Medicine encourages the use of active reading strategies. A detailed explanation of two recommended strategies – SQ3R (Survey, Question, and Read, Recite, Review) and PQRST (Preview, Question, Read, State, Test) – is available at the school's website.[17]

6 Your choice of study techniques and habits should also be based on your preferred sensory mode of learning. Although all sensory modes of learning may be used by an individual learner, one is typically preferred. VARK is an acronym for the major sensory modes of learning – visual, aural, reading/writing, and kinesthetic. Wayne State University researchers recommend adopting techniques based on your preferred mode. "For example, visual learners learn through seeing drawings, pictures, and other image-rich teaching tools. Auditory learners learn by listening to lectures, exploring material through discussions, and talking through ideas. Reading/writing learners learn through interaction with textual materials, whereas kinesthetic learners learn through touching and experiences that emphasize doing, physical involvement, and manipulation of objects."[18]

7 Many students have used mnemonics, songs, rhymes, flash cards, games, questions, and cases as means to memorize, retrieve, and understand information. According to the University of Kansas Center for Research and Learning, "there is abundant research to support the use of mnemonic devices to aid memory storage and retrieval."[19]

8 Princeton University offers ten active reading strategies, including making outlines, flow charts, and diagrams. Also recommended is the technique of writing a summary of a chapter in your own words.[20]

9 The Cornell method of taking notes, developed by Walter Pauk, is widely used. In contrast to simple note taking, the Cornell method incorporates review and summarization to promote more active learning.[21]

10 The University of Wisconsin School of Medicine and Public Health encourages students to teach what they have learned. "Explaining and teaching others is a great way to retain information."[22]

Time Management for Medical Students: 10 Important Tips

To maintain a healthy balance between studying and other aspects of your life, you need to plan well. Research has indicated that study skills are important factors affecting academic performance in medical school.[23-26] Among study strategies, evidence indicates that time management may be more important than other factors.[27] In one study performed at a single medical school, researchers found that "in general, study skills are stronger predictors of first-semester total grades than aptitude as measured by the MCAT and undergraduate GPA."[4] Of the study skills assessed, time management was one of only two study strategies "that appeared to be related to academic performance..." This is echoed by senior medical students in advice given to new students. According to the Unofficial Guide to University of Texas Southwestern developed by the school's AMSA group, "the two most important things you can do to aid in your success are to establish effective study patterns, and to stave off the desire to procrastinate."[12]

1 Start your semester by finding out the important dates in each of your courses, including quizzes, tests, due dates for assignments, and final exams. Mark these dates on your calendar.

2 Are there any important events or days unrelated to school, such as weddings or holidays? Mark these dates as well.

3 Before the start of every week, plan each day. Identify the times of each day when you'll be in class or lecture. The remaining time is your free time.

4 Plan your free time so that you can keep up with your coursework, yet still spend time with friends and family. The University of New Mexico School of Medicine recommends that you identify your high, medium, and low concentration periods.[13] Low concentration periods of time are ideal for rest, relaxation, and recreation. Time spent in these activities pays many dividends: multiple studies have shown that rest and relaxation is necessary to maintain energy and focus when working and studying.

5 Both study and personal time should be uninterrupted, but you should break longer periods of study into smaller blocks. Many students spend hours on end studying, only to realize that their concentration and energy can't be maintained for long uninterrupted stretches. Short blocks of time allow for greater focus and productivity.

6 Analyze your study methods. In her book, *Study Skills and Test-taking Strategies for Medical Students*, Deborah Shain writes that, in her years as a medical education counselor, students struggling academically often had "not learned how to manage time or material...undisciplined time use compromises your learning ability. Irregular spurts of study make you feel out of step, inadequate, guilty, and unduly anxious, which results in forgetting...success in medicine requires self-discipline, steady commitment, and a sense of humor."[28]

7 The number of study hours required varies from student to student. By the end of the first few weeks, though, you should have a good idea of how much time you'll need to spend reading and studying.

8 Don't upset your rhythms over the weekend. The University of Kansas School of Medicine reminds students to "not create artificial 'jet lag' in yourself by keeping a reasonable schedule during the week and then completely blowing the schedule during the weekend." Staying up late on weekend nights and then sleeping in most of Saturday and Sunday disrupts "psychological and physiological rhythms."[29]

9 At the end of each day, assess how you spent each hour. Your goal is to identify time wasters. Even study time can qualify. If you studied from 4-6 pm, and found that you didn't retain any of the material, then that block of time probably isn't your optimum study time.

10 Maintain flexibility in your schedule. You should be able to react to unanticipated events with minimal stress. Students with rigid schedules, though, are constantly worried that they're off schedule. In the February 2009 issue of ACP IMpact, Lavanya Viswanathan, a medical student at the Uniformed Services University of the Health Sciences, wrote that "sometimes the frustration of not being able to follow your schedule to the tee takes precious energy away and leaves us feeling like failures. Whatever the reason, we have to be able to forgive ourselves for falling off course every once in a while, in hopes that a break will allow us to get right back into the swing of things."[30]

Preclinical Grades: 9 Key Points about their Importance

In a study of medical students at the University of Colorado, University of Utah, and Vanderbilt University, participants were asked to rate the importance of sixteen residency selection criteria.[31] Approximately 42% of survey participants rated "grades in first two years" as extremely or moderately important. The reality does not quite match that statement. In this section, we discuss the importance of preclinical grades based on a review of the literature.

1 In a 2006 survey of over 1,200 residency program directors across 21 medical specialties, grades in preclinical courses were found to be twelfth in importance among a group of fourteen academic residency selection criteria.[32] The authors surmised that preclinical grades are not highly valued "because there is considerable variability in the naming and content of courses in medical schools in the preclinical curriculum, perhaps making grades difficult to interpret."

2 In a 1999 survey of program directors, while preclinical grades were not an important factor in the residency selection process, receiving a failure in a preclinical course was an area of concern.[33] Program directors were asked to rate the importance of a preclinical course failure on a scale of 1 (no concern) to 5 (very concerned). The mean score was 3.73.

3 While failing a course is a potential red flag, many students who've failed have ultimately matched. Since clerkship grades and other selection criteria are more highly valued, students who fail a preclinical course can overcome this obstacle by strengthening the rest of their application.

4 Preclinical grades may have an impact on class rank. While your individual grade in a preclinical course may have little impact in the residency selection process (assuming you don't fail), preclinical grades are used by some schools in the determination of class rank. In one survey of program directors, class rank was found to be seventh in importance among a group of fourteen academic residency selection criteria, with competitive specialties generally attaching more importance to this factor than noncompetitive specialties.[32] At the start of med school, learn your school's policy regarding class rank. Does your school have a class ranking system? If so, how is rank determined? Are preclinical grades used to determine class rank? How much weight do these grades carry relative to clerkship grades?

5 Exceptional preclinical performance can lead to medical school academic awards. In Dr. Green's survey, medical school awards were ranked 10th in importance in the residency selection process, below clerkship grades, USMLE step 1 and 2 scores, and letters of recommendation.[32] Although not as important as other criteria, winning an award can strengthen your overall residency application, and allow you to stand out from your peers.

6 Medical school academic scholarships awarded to second and third-year students are often based on superior academic performance in preclinical courses.

7 Preclinical grades may be used for AOA determination. In 1902, William Webster Root and five other medical students founded the Alpha Omega Alpha Honor Medical Society (AOA) at the College of Physicians & Surgeons in Chicago. Today, over 120 medical schools in the United States and Canada have AOA chapters. Individual specialties and residency programs attach varying degrees of importance to AOA membership. In the 2006 survey of over 1,200 residency program directors, AOA membership ranked eighth among a group of fourteen academic selection criteria.[32] Of note, AOA was more important to competitive specialties, including plastic surgery (ranked second), neurosurgery (ranked fourth), ophthalmology (ranked fifth), radiology (ranked sixth), and urology (ranked sixth). Students may be elected to AOA either in their junior or senior year of medical school. Election as a junior medical student is often heavily weighted towards academic criteria, including preclinical grades and USMLE Step 1 scores.

8 In a recent article offering advice for students interested in dermatology, arguably the most competitive of all specialties, the authors wrote about how preclinical grades may be viewed by programs. "Conventional wisdom is that preclinical grades are relatively unimportant in the application process. Whereas they may be less important as a stand-alone factor, the benefits of a sound preclinical performance trickle down to other key aspects of the application. The importance of grades largely depends on the grading system employed at your school. In a pass/fail system, simply passing is sufficient; no one will know the applicant's actual rank in a particular class. However, in schools with non-pass fail grading systems, high grades may be an important factor in class ranking and for nomination to the Alpha Omega Alpha honor society. Additionally, because the vast majority of dermatology applicants are outstanding, there is no need to take students with low basic science grades."[34]

9 A variety of grading systems are used by U.S. medical schools during the preclinical years. In recent years, a number of schools have moved to pass/fail grading, hoping that this change in grading will reduce stress and anxiety, decrease competition among classmates, and promote collaborative learning. Students at schools that have adopted pass/fail grading are concerned about the effects that this system may have on their competitiveness as a residency applicant. In one study, University of Virginia researchers found no significant difference in academic performance, clerkship grades, board scores, or residency placement following a change in grading from an A/B/C/D/E to a pass/fail system. They did find that the pass/fail system improved psychological well-being.[35] A recent University of Michigan study also explored the effects of changing to pass-fail grading. The authors wrote that "pass-fail grading can meet several important intended outcomes, including 'leveling the playing field' for incoming students with different academic backgrounds, reducing competition and fostering collaboration among members of a class, and more time for extracurricular interests and personal activities."[36]

10 Things You Must Do If You Experience Academic Difficulty

Now that you're in, you may wonder if you have what it takes to make it through medical school. The simple answer: you do. We highlight two studies that examined medical school attrition rates. In the first, the AAMC looked at graduation and attrition rates for the medical school classes of 1987, 1992, and 1995.[37] The key findings:

- Over 80% of each of the three cohorts in the study graduated in four years.
- The graduation rate rose to 91.3% within five years.
- The 10-year completion rate was 96%.

With a 10-year attrition rate of less than 4%, it's clear that once admitted, most students will successfully complete medical school and become physicians. Some students who require more than four years to complete med school do so voluntarily because they're in combined MD/JD, MD/MBA, MD/MPH, or MD/PhD programs.

Looking more closely at the group of students who left med school before graduating, it becomes clear that reasons for leaving are varied. While academic difficulty is a major cause for attrition, it is reassuring to note that less than 2% of the 47,315 students followed in the study (635 students) left medical school for academic reasons.

In another study, the American Association of Colleges of Osteopathic Medicine (AACOM) found that the 2003-2004 attrition rates for first and second-year osteopathic students were 2.2% and 2.1%, respectively.[38] Dismissal for academic failure was the most common cause of attrition. Below, we share important advice for the learner experiencing academic difficulty.

1 Approach your medical school at the first hint of trouble. If you're experiencing academic difficulty or have reasons to believe that you might perform poorly in a course, don't keep it to yourself. Seek the help and expertise of your school's administration. "Failing students have a generalized reluctance to approach appropriate academic personnel for advisement—despite their clear recognition of its importance...With earlier detection it might be possible to diminish unreasonable burdens on students, and rearrange environmental circumstances to promote success" writes Dr. Caven S. Mcloughlin.[39] It's far better to approach school officials before failure, at a time when more options are available. Once a course is failed, it becomes a permanent part of the transcript.

2 Diagnose your problem(s). An accurate diagnosis of the exact problem or problems that led to the academic difficulty is essential. Struggling students need to meet with an expert for an objective analysis, rather than relying solely on their own self-assessment. Successful remediation is often contingent on a diagnosis, followed by targeted interventions.

3 Poor time management is a common problem. In her book, *Study Skills and Test-taking Strategies for Medical Students*, Deborah Shain writes that, in her years as a medical education counselor, students struggling academically often had "no conscious system of study...undisciplined time use compromises your learning ability."[28] Dason Evans and Jo Brown, authors of *How to Succeed at Medical School*, also stress the importance of good time management. "Time management skills can be learned and are not necessarily something you are born with, and getting into good time management habits now will serve you for the rest of your life, both professionally and personally."[40]

4 "Anecdotal evidence from the University of Mississippi Medical Center's Learning Assistance Project, an academic skills counseling program for students, suggests that students who encounter difficulties in medical school often use ineffective study strategies."[41] Understand the differences between high-achieving and underachieving learners. Hendricson writes that high-achieving students "tend to be persistent and schedule a specific time block every day for reading and review. Underachievers rarely block out time for study and are easily distracted, often succumbing to social opportunities or diversionary activities like talking to friends on the phone or taking a break to watch television. High-achieving students are more likely to use active learning strategies such as writing detailed notes in class, reviewing class notes daily, interacting frequently with instructors, and self-quizzing. In contrast, underachieving students tend to approach their studies in a more passive manner."[42]

5 Major life crises involving family members can occur during medical school, and this can impact academic performance. In one study at a single medical school, 22% of graduates from 1980 to 1999 experienced a major life crisis. The most common causes were relationship stressors with spouses or significant others, illness or death of family members, and personal illness. The authors found that "experiencing a crisis was associated with lower annual grades, GPA at graduation, as well as lower USMLE Step 1 and Step 2 scores."[43]

6 Your own personal illness or health problem may affect your learning and performance. In a survey of over 1,000 students at nine U.S. medical schools, 90% of students reported "needing care for various health concerns, including 47% having at least one mental health or substance-related health issue…Students expressed varying levels of concern about academic jeopardy in association with personal illness…"[44]

7 Consider the possibility of an undiagnosed learning disability. Ten to fifteen percent of the U.S. population has a learning disability. It is believed that 3% of U.S. medical students have a learning disability. Although these often come to light before or during college, students with learning disabilities may "graduate from college without having their disability diagnosed" and "first encounter difficulty at graduate levels of education."[45] A 1997 survey of 105 U.S. and Canadian schools revealed that nearly all had services for learning-disabled students.[46]

8 Beware of the consequences of failure. Every medical school has its own policy on academic performance. You can find this information in the Student Handbook. Failing one or more courses will bring your situation to the attention of the Student Promotions Committee. This committee has the power to dismiss medical students or allow for remediation. At many schools, courses are offered only once every academic year. Therefore, a single failure may force you to repeat the entire year. However, schools may offer students with a single failure the opportunity to remediate the course during the same semester or in the summer after the academic year ends. Failure in multiple courses may make you ineligible for summer remediation. This generally means that you'll have to repeat the entire academic year, if you aren't dismissed.

9 Failure of a remedial course will again prompt referral of your case to the Student Promotions Committee, and you may be dismissed. Therefore, before remediating a course, a thorough and objective analysis of the factors that led to the course failure should be performed by a qualified professional. A firm understanding of what went wrong minimizes the risk of an unsatisfactory repeat performance.

10 Since course failure leaves you with a permanent mark on your transcript and damage to your psyche, struggling students may consider a leave of absence. It is often better to take a leave of absence than suffer multiple failures that would place you at risk for dismissal. Even if you aren't dismissed, once the courses are taken, the official grade will become a permanent part of your medical school transcript. You may be able to arrange a short-term leave of absence to deal with a difficult issue in your life. Your school may be able to accommodate your request, delay an exam, and offer you needed support. This may be precisely what's needed if you have a short-term stressor. When you return, you may find yourself in a better state, and more equipped to handle the course work. However, for students with long-term stressors, the best course of action may be to take a longer leave of absence. With longer leaves, returning students often have to repeat the entire year.

References

[1]University of Alabama Birmingham School of Medicine. Advice from MS-2 Students. Available at: http://main.uab.edu/uasom/2/show.asp?durki=111766. Accessed October 22, 2011.

[2]Klatt E, Klatt C. How much is too much reading for medical students? Assigned reading and reading rates at one medical school. *Acad Med* 2011; 86(9): 1079-83.

[3]Finnerty E, Chauvin S, Bonaminio G, Andrews M, Carroll R, Pangaro L. Flexner revisited: the role and value of the basic sciences in medical education. *Acad Med* 2010; 85 (2): 349-55.

[4]West C, Sadoski M. Do study strategies predict academic performance in medical school? *Med Educ* 2011; 45(7): 696-703.

[5]Indiana University School of Medicine. New Student FAQ. Available at: http://msa.iusm.iu.edu/StudentDevelopment/NewStudentFAQ/classes.htm. Accessed October 22, 2011.

[6]Dartmouth Medical School. Effective Study at DMS. Available at: http://dms.dartmouth.edu/admin/learnserv/effective_study.shtml. Accessed February 21, 2012.

[7]Texas Tech University Health Sciences Center School of Medicine. Success Types Survival Strategies. Available at: http://www.ttuhsc.edu/som/success/page_survival%20strategy/Survival.htm.

[8]University of Texas San Antonio Health Sciences Center. Office of Academic Enhancement. Available at: http://som.uthscsa.edu/AcademicEnhancement/index/asp. Accessed October 22, 2011.

[9]Billings-Gagliardi S, Mazor K. Student decisions about lecture attendance: do electronic course materials matter. *Acad Med* 2007; 82 (10 Suppl): S73-6.

[10]Smith S. Effect of undergraduate college major on performance in medical school. *Acad Med* 1998; 73(9): 1006-8.

[11]University of Washington School of Medicine. Managing the First Year of Medical School. Available at: http://uwmedicine.washington.edu/NR/rdonlyres/41AB4807-24F4-4944-A099-9A2D76ECA5E2/0/ManagingtheFirstYearofMedicalSchool.pdf. Accessed August 25, 2011.

[12]AMSA's Unofficial Guide to UT Southwestern 2008-2009. Available at: http://www.southwesternstudents.com/AMSAUnofficialGuidetoUTSW.pdf. Accessed October 22, 2011.

[13]University of New Mexico School of Medicine. Learning Strategies for Success in Medical School. Available at: hsc.unm.edu/community/cnah/docs/handbook_2004.pdf. Accessed February 20, 2012.

[14]University of California San Diego School of Medicine. Successful Study Strategies in Medical School. Available at: http://meded.ucsd.edu/ugme/oess/study_skills/how_to_study_actively/. Accessed February 20, 2012.

[15]University of Utah School of Medicine. Study Skills. Available at: http://medicine.utah.edu/learningresources/tools/study/index.htm. Accessed February 21, 2012.

[16]Johns Hopkins University. Study Techniques for Premedical Students. Available at: http://web.jhu.edu/prepro/health/study_skills.html. Accessed February 21, 2012.

[17]Albert Einstein College of Medicine. Reading Course Textbooks. Available at: http://www.einstein.yu.edu/oasc/page.aspx?id=19678. Accessed February 21, 2012.

[18]Lujan H, DiCarlo S. First-year medical students prefer multiple learning styles. *Adv Physiol Edu* 2006; 30: 13 - 16.

[19]University of Kansas Center for Research on Learning. Available at: www.kucrl.org/. Accessed February 21, 2012.

[20]The McGraw Center for Teaching and Learning. Active Reading Strategies. Available at: http://www.princeton.edu/mcgraw/library/for-students/remember-reading/. Accessed February 21, 2012.

[21]The Cornell Note-Taking System. Available at: http://lsc.sas.cornell.edu/Sidebars/Study_Skills_Resources/cornellsystem.pdf. Accessed February 21, 2012.

[22]University of Wisconsin School of Medicine and Public Health. Study Methods/Tutors. Available at: http://www.med.wisc.edu/education/md/resources/study-methodstutors/1191. Accessed February 20, 2012.

[23]Barker J, Olsen J. Medical students' learning strategies: evaluation of first year changes. *J Mississippi Acad Sci* 1997; 42(2)

[24]Durak H, Torun S, Abdullah S, Kandiloglu G. Description and evaluation of an innovative course on learning and study skills for first-year medical students. *Tohoku J Exp Med* 2006; 210: 231-7.

[25]Kleijn W, van der Ploeg H, Topman R. Cognition, study habits, test anxiety, and academic performance. *Psychol Rep* 1994; 75: 1219-26.

[26]Salamonson Y, Everett B, Koch J, Wilson I, Davidson P. Learning strategies of first year nursing and medical students: a comparative study. *Int J Nurs Stud* 2009; 46: 1541-7.

[27]Schumacker R, Sayler M. Identifying at-risk gifted students in an early college entrance programme. *Roeper Rev* 1995; 18(2): 126-30.

[28]Shain D. *Study Skills and Test-taking Strategies for Medical Students*. New York; Springer-Verlag: 1995.

[29]The University of Kansas School of Medicine. Available at: http://kumc.edu/som/medsos/tms.html. Accessed October 22, 2011.

[30]ACP IMpact February 2009. Medical student perspectives: time management during medical school. Available at: http://www.acponline.org/medical_students/impact/archives/2009/02/perspect/. Accessed October 22, 2011.

[31]Brandenburg S, Kruzick T, Lin C, Robinson A, Adams L. Residency selection criteria: what medical students perceive as important. *Med Educ Online* 2005; 10: 1-6.

[32]Green M, Jones P, Thomas J. Selection criteria for residency: results of a national program directors survey. *Acad Med* 2009; 84(3): 362-7.

[33]Wagoner N, Suriano J. Program directors' responses to a survey on variables used to select residents in a time of change. *Acad Med* 1999; 74: 51-8.

[34]Alikhan A, Sivamani R, Mutizawa M, Felsten L. Advice for fourth year medical students beginning the dermatology residency application process: Perspectives from interns who matched. *Dermatol Online J* 2009; 15(10): 3.

[35]Bloodgood R, Short J, Jackson J, Martindale J. A change to pass/fail grading in the first two years at one medical school results in improved well-being. *Acad Med* 2009; 84(5): 655-62.

[36]White C, Fantone J. Pass-fail grading: laying the foundation for self-regulated learning. *Adv Health Sci Educ Theory Pract* 2010; 15(4): 469-77.

[37]Association of American Medical Colleges. Available at: http://www.aamc.org/data/aib/aibissues/aibvol7_no2.pdf. Accessed July 16, 2011.

[38]2006 Annual Statistical Report on Osteopathic Medical Education. Available at:
http://www.aacom.org/resources/bookstore/2006statrpt/Documents/ASROME2 006.pdf. Accessed October 22, 2011.

[39]Mcloughlin C. Characteristics of students failing medical education: an essay of reflections. *Med Educ Online* 2009; 14. Available at: http://www.med-ed-online.org. Accessed October 22, 2011.

[40]Dason E, Brown J. *How to Succeed at Medical School*. Great Britain; BMJ Books: 2009.

[41]University of Mississippi Medical Center. Learning Assistance Project. Available at: http://msacad.org/journal/ejour2.html. Accessed February 21, 2012.

[42]Hendricson W, Kleffner J. Assessing and helping challenging students: Part One, why do some students have difficulty learning? *J Dent Educ* 2002; 66 (1): 43-61.

[43]Greenburg D, Durning S, Cruess D, Cohen D, Jackson J. The prevalence, causes, and consequences of experiencing a life crisis during medical school. *Teach Learn Med* 2010; 22(2): 85-92.

[44]Roberts L, Warner T, Lyketsos C, Frank E, Ganzini L, Carter D. Perceptions of academic vulnerability associated with personal illness: a study of 1,027 students at nine medical schools. *Comp Psychiatr* 2001; 42(1): 1-15.

[45]Rosebraugh C. Learning disabilities and medical schools. *Med Educ* 2000; 34(12): 994-1000.

[46]Faigel H. Changes in services for students with learning disabilities in U.S. and Canadian medical schools 1991-97 *Acad Med* 1998; 73(12): 1290-3.

Chapter 3

USMLE Step 1 Exam

To become an allopathic physician with the license to practice in the United States, you must pass the three-part United States Medical Licensing Exam, referred to as the USMLE. Medical students typically take the first part of the USMLE (Step 1 exam) at the end of the second year of medical school.

Steps 2 and 3 are most commonly taken during the fourth year of medical school and internship, respectively. The USMLE Step 2 is divided into two parts – Step 2 CK (clinical knowledge) and Step 2 CS (clinical skills). In this chapter, our focus is exclusively on the Step 1 exam.

While the route to licensure for osteopathic students requires passage of the three-level Comprehensive Osteopathic Medical Licensing Examination (COMLEX – USA), many osteopathic students also take the USMLE Step 1 exam. This score is important in the selection process for residency programs approved by the Accreditation Council for Graduate Medical Education (allopathic residency programs).

USMLE Step 1: 9 Things to Know about the Exam on Day 1 of Medical School

1 The USMLE Step 1 exam covers the basic sciences. However, there is nothing basic about the exam. It's a difficult test. In 2009, over 1,300 MD and DO examinees failed to pass the Step 1 exam on their first attempt.[1]

2 Among first-time test takers, 94% of MD examinees and 81% of DO examinees passed. Despite passing, however, many students are unhappy with their score results.[1]

3 While simply passing the exam is sufficient for licensure purposes, you should strive for the highest score possible. The Step 1 score is an important criterion used by residency programs in the selection process. In a 2006 survey of over 1,200 residency program directors across 21 medical specialties, the USMLE Step 1 score was found to be the second most important residency selection factor, following only grades in required clerkships.[2]

4 Unlike the MCAT, once you pass you cannot take the exam again. In other words, once you pass, that single score will be the score used by residency programs in their decision-making process.

5 In a study of medical students, participants were asked to rate the importance of sixteen residency selection criteria.[3] While 47% of survey participants rated the USMLE Step 1 score as extremely important, 53% felt that scores were either moderately, mildly, or not important at all. The results of this study show that students often underestimate the importance of the Step 1 score.

6 The residency selection process can be divided into two phases – screening and ranking. In the screening phase, programs whittle down a large applicant pool into a smaller group. The members of this group will be offered interview invitations. The USMLE Step 1 score is frequently used in the screening process. In 2010, a survey of several thousand residency program directors representing multiple specialties was performed by the National Resident Matching Program.[4] The survey found that the Step 1 score was the factor used most commonly in the screening process.

7 Certain specialties are more competitive than others, meaning they're difficult to get into. In competitive specialties, such as dermatology, plastic surgery, ophthalmology, otolaryngology, radiology, neurosurgery, orthopedic surgery, and urology, many programs have a cut-off, or threshold, Step 1 score. Highly sought-after programs in less competitive specialties may also have threshold scores. Applicants who score above the cut-off are considered for interviews. Those below the cut-off may be removed from consideration.

8 The Step 1 score is important in the ranking phase. During this phase, programs develop their rank-order list. This is a list of applicants interviewed in the order in which the program would extend offers.

9 Program directors are also interested in your USMLE Step 1 score because it offers them some insight into whether you are capable of passing the specialty board-certifying examination. "Low USMLE scores concern program directors that the applicant may have difficulty passing Step III (which is needed for medical licensure) and may ultimately have difficulty passing the pediatric board exam (which may reflect poorly on the residency program)" writes Dr. Su-Ting Li, Program Director of the pediatrics residency program at University of California Davis School of Medicine.[5] There is some data to suggest that performance on the Step 1 exam is predictive of performance on the specialty board-certifying exam. In a recent study, researchers explored the relationship between the Step 1 score and the American Board of Pediatrics board-certifying exam among a group of 70 residents.[6] The results showed that scores were significantly associated with board exam performance, with scores > 220 associated with 95% board passage rate.

USMLE Step 1 Exam Preparation: 8 General Strategies for Success

1 Following the end of second year, most students will have a block of time to study before taking the exam. One study found that examinees typically had an average of 5.8 weeks to prepare.[7] This block of time is best spent reviewing the material, not learning it. Therefore, you need to maximize your retention of material during each and every basic science course. This is echoed by Drs. Chirag Amin and Tao Le, authors of the popular book *First Aid for the UMSLE Step 1*. They state that "because the material tested on the USMLE Step 1 examination covers a large amount of information that is learned over the course of 2 years in medical school, strict cramming is usually not an effective method for USMLE preparation. Medical students who studied diligently during their first- and second-year coursework end up minimizing the stress and workload of a USMLE Step 1 review."[8] Students who do well on the Step 1 exam follow the same formula. It begins with learning, understanding, and organizing information well in each and every basic science course, followed by an effective review before the exam.

2 According to the National Board of Medical Examiners (NBME), which administers the exam, the USMLE Step 1 exam "assesses whether you can understand and apply important concepts of the sciences to the practice of medicine, with special emphasis on the principles and mechanisms underlying health, disease, and modes of therapy."[9] The content of the exam is drawn from the following disciplines: Anatomy, Physiology, Biochemistry, Pathology, Pharmacology, Microbiology, Behavioral Sciences, and Nutrition/Genetics/Aging. Information about exam content is available at the USMLE website (www.usmle.org). While it would seem obvious that students should review the content of the exam, in a 1998 survey of 1,217 examinees, only 70% had used the content description and sample items booklet made available by the NBME.[7]

3 As you study for your courses, use board review guides or books along with the lecture material supplied by your school. Many students have found this an effective approach. When it comes time for your final review, you can simply look over books you're already familiar with.

4 With hundreds of USMLE review books to choose from, how can you decide which ones to use? Start by surveying colleagues, especially senior students who've already taken the exam. Don't rely too heavily on the advice of a single student; it's important to solicit as many opinions as you can. You should be able to identify the books widely considered to be the best. Your next step is to visit your local medical bookstore. Browse the available choices, and determine which books suit your preferred learning style.

5 Concerned about how your school's curriculum might affect your Step 1 performance? Don't be. While there are different types of curricula, your school probably adheres to a disciplines-based, organ-based, or problem-based curriculum, or a combination thereof. Students often wonder whether one curricular approach is better than another for USMLE performance. In a recent study, researchers used AAMC data to determine what effects, if any, the curricular approach had on USMLE scores.[10] In their conclusion, the authors wrote that "formal medical school curricula, which reflects how schools conceptualize the relationship between basic and clinical sciences, do not have much effect on USMLE performance."

6 While strong factual knowledge is necessary for exam success, most questions seek to determine your ability to apply basic science knowledge to clinical problems, rather than regurgitate isolated facts. Authors Tao Le and Chirag Amin state that "many medical students that we have talked to underestimate the amount of clinical material on the USMLE Step 1 examination.... Furthermore, many students also leave the exam feeling somewhat intimidated regarding the clinical slant of how the basic science material is tested."[8] In fact, in a recent posting at www.usmle.org, the National Board of Medical Examiners announced a reduction in the number of Step 1 items presented without a clinical vignette.

7 As discussed earlier, your preparation for USMLE Step 1 begins on day 1 of med school. As you might expect, you will spend countless hours reading, learning, and understanding basic science material. However, while putting in sufficient time is of obvious importance, how you study is equally, if not more, important. The techniques of active learning are very important in long-term retention, and you should be utilizing these techniques throughout your basic science coursework. Drs. Helen Loeser and Maxine Papadakis, deans at the UCSF School of Medicine, advise: "Use active learning methods as you integrate your knowledge and apply basic science information to clinical vignettes."[11] Examples of active learning include taking notes, summarizing information, organizing information in the form of charts, and drawing pictures or diagrams. Research has shown that active learning leads to better long-term retention of information and easier retrieval of information when needed.

8 Dr. Judy Schwenker, Kaplan's Curriculum Director, has identified the five most common mistakes students make when preparing for the Step 1 exam. These include passive studying, insufficient practice with questions, memorizing without understanding the material, inappropriate test day strategies, and misreading or misinterpreting questions.[12]

Practice Questions to Boost Your USMLE Step 1 Score: 8 Tips

1 Practice questions are a must. Since the Step 1 exam is entirely multiple-choice, it stands to reason that practice questions would provide good preparation for the exam. These questions will help you identify your strengths and weaknesses. Students can turn to a variety of sources for practice questions. Review books with practice exams or questions abound, as do professionally developed question banks, such as Kaplan's online question bank, USMLE World, USMLE Consult, Princeton Review, USMLEasy, and Exam Master. Most popular is Kaplan's Q-Bank, a computer-based product offering over 2000 test questions. Free practice questions are available at www.4tests.com, www.histology-world.com, and www.testprepreview.com.

2 Which question bank should you choose? You'll receive recommendations from upperclassmen at your school, and you should consider their advice. Make sure that your question bank meets the following criteria:

- Your resource must have enough questions.
- The questions should be reasonably similar in content and style to the actual exam.
- Answer keys should include sound, well-written explanations.
- The website should be user-friendly, with easy navigation
- There should be no extra cost for accessing, reviewing, or repeating previously viewed questions.

3 No matter what resource you use, get into the habit of doing 50-100 questions every day. In a 2007 article written for Medscape, Dr. Fix, former Chief Resident of the Harvard emergency medicine residency program, emphasized the importance of practice questions.[13] "If there is 1 'rule' for the USMLE, it is to read many practice questions. Start reviewing questions from the beginning of your preparation period, and keep going back to them throughout...When you make mistakes, write down the correct answers and review them at the end of the day to solidify what you learned."

4 You can schedule an appointment to review sample test materials at a Prometric Test Center for a small fee. This allows you to simulate conditions of the exam in the same environment as your actual test. Note that you cannot take a practice test until you first register for the USMLE exam.

5 Regardless of whether you answer a question correctly, it is essential that you read the explanation for the answer. Reading and understanding the explanation ensures that you have a firm grasp on why a certain answer is correct and why the remaining answer choices are wrong. Refer to your review books to reinforce your knowledge and promote retention.

6 Dr. Linda Costanzo, Professor of Physiology at the Virginia Commonwealth University School of Medicine and the author of the BRS Physiology review book, reminds students that questions alone are not adequate preparation for the Step 1 exam. "Questions, great as they are, will leave gaps and will not be systematic. And, equally important, because 'just questions' is not standard preparation, you will not have that all-important confidence of having adequately prepared when you go into the exam."[14]

7 Allow 72 seconds per question. This is the amount of time you'll have per question on the actual exam.

8 If you are not used to taking an exam on the computer, consider choosing a computer-based bank of practice questions. This will help you become more comfortable reading and answering questions off a screen.

Your USMLE Step 1 Review Schedule: 10 Important Points

1 Make a day-to-day schedule for your entire study block using a calendar.

2 Incorporate catch-up days since you never know when you'll be thrown off schedule. To avoid falling behind, set aside some time every week for catching up.

3 Many students recommend reviewing major content areas (pathology, microbiology, pharmacology, physiology, biochemistry) twice in the study period, because important points and concepts are often solidified during the second review.

4 Although some subject areas are more heavily tested than others, don't neglect or avoid a subject area. Make some time in your schedule for every subject. Consider reviewing short-term memory subject areas, such as pharmacology and microbiology, towards the end of your study block.

5 Stick to your schedule.

6 Do practice questions or exams every day. Aim to do 50-100 questions. Limit yourself to 72 seconds for each question. After answering the questions, read the explanation carefully (use Tutorial Mode of your question bank resource). If necessary, turn to your resources to learn more about the topic.

7 Students often study ten to twelve hours a day. With this type of intense studying, you can easily lose your effectiveness. This becomes obvious when you've reread the same paragraph three times, and it still doesn't make sense. The most effective students schedule breaks that re-energize. Exercise, socialize with friends, hang out with family, or whatever else you feel will help you return to studying with improved focus.

8 Since you will probably take the actual exam between 8:30 AM and 4:30 PM, plan to study regularly during these hours. This will prepare and train your body and mind for peak performance during this part of the day.

9 At some point, you'll want to take one or more self-assessment exams (Comprehensive Basic Science Self-Assessment or CBSSA) offered by the NBME. You'll receive a performance profile with score interpretation guide, which will give you a better idea of your relative strengths and weaknesses. Through the expanded feedback option, you can view test items answered incorrectly and organize these items by content category.

10 End your review one or two days before the exam. By this point, you'll have put in the time, worked hard, and reviewed the subject areas thoroughly.

Preventing Anxiety from Lowering Your USMLE Step 1 Score: 10 Tips

Most students become anxious as the Step 1 exam nears. While most are able to manage their emotions, some students, overcome with fear, don't perform as well as they could. This is not due to a lack of ability or knowledge. Rather, their level of anxiety interfered with their preparation and subsequent performance on the day of the exam.

Reteguiz defined test anxiety "as an unpleasant emotional state or condition with perceived feelings of tension, apprehension, nervousness, and worry" in response to taking tests.[15] Test anxiety may lead to palpitations, nausea, dizziness, weakness, sweating, and dryness of the mouth.[16] Test anxiety may cause difficulties in information recall, concentration, and organization of thoughts. Educators largely agree that test anxiety can lower academic performance. Although this hasn't been extensively studied in medical education, one study of first-year medical students found that test anxiety did affect performance on a multiple-choice examination. Students with lower levels of anxiety performed better than those with higher levels.[17]

1 Research has shown that many students who experience high levels of test anxiety utilize different study methods. A review of your study and test-taking skills with a medical school counselor may help.

2 Students with test anxiety often engage in negative self-talk, such as "I'll be a failure if I do poorly on this test." Research has shown a reduction in test anxiety when self-defeating thoughts are replaced with more constructive thoughts.

3 There's a reason your mother told you to get enough sleep, exercise, and eat well. Physical factors can affect your performance, and have been shown to impact stress hormones. Consumption of food and drink containing caffeine, processed sugar, and alcohol may increase test anxiety. Sleep deprivation increases stress hormones, which can increase anxiety, while exercise decreases them.

4 The thought of taking the Step 1 exam incites fear in many students. Although your exam score is important in the residency selection process, it's not the only factor. Programs weigh many other components of the application, including clerkship grades, research experience, publications, letters of recommendation, and personal statements. Your future does not hinge solely on your Step 1 score. Don't place too much pressure on yourself by viewing this exam as the one factor that will "make or break" your future. It's important to remember this point as you prepare for the exam, since how you view the exam can impact your performance.

5 Yes, feelings of anxiety can be contagious. Classmates who are always on edge, tense, or panicked may transfer their feelings to you. Adjust your interactions accordingly.

6 Relaxation techniques can help alleviate symptoms of anxiety prior to and during the exam. Many studies support their utility in a number of situations. Several techniques are easy to learn and easy to implement. One technique involves closing your eyes, taking a long, deep breath, and then exhaling slowly. During the maneuver, focus entirely on your breathing. Another technique involves tightening and relaxing different muscle groups, beginning with one group at a time. Familiarity and comfort with these techniques through repeated practice, well before the exam, may lead to greater effectiveness of these techniques on the day of the exam.

7 Techniques of visualization have been studied in numerous areas, and are a well-regarded technique practiced by elite athletes. At first glance, the technique appears deceptively simple. However, there's a reason elite golfers practice this technique. Close your eyes, and picture yourself calmly and steadily working through the exam. Picture yourself excelling, and focus on this success.

8 You don't have to answer every question correctly to pass the exam. In fact, passing only requires correct answers to 60-70% of the test questions.

9 To ease the anxiety associated with Step 1 preparation, schools have developed programs to educate students about the exam. For example, the Wake Forest University School of Medicine created a seminar series.[18] At the beginning of each session, a senior medical student gives a didactic presentation. This is followed by an interactive forum in which upperclassmen share their experiences with first and second-year students, and spend time answering questions. When students were surveyed about the seminar series, a substantial number felt that they would have been more anxious had it not been for the seminars.

10 In 2004, Dr. Douglas Powell of the Harvard Medical School wrote about his experience with students who experience debilitating test anxiety (DTA), a condition that is thought to affect 2% of a medical school class.[19-20] Features of DTA include:

- Severe anxiety symptoms. These may occur before and/or during standardized exams, particularly multiple-choice tests.
- Cognitive impacts. A variety of cognitive impacts have been described, including difficulty retrieving stored knowledge, difficulty choosing among answer choices because of obsessional thinking, and difficulty in managing time. These problems are not debilitating in other arenas.
- Impacts on study habits. Anxiety may lead to procrastination, disorganization, reduced effort, and other faulty study habits.
- A history of performance issues. Students may have experienced difficulties on other standardized exams, such as the SAT, ACT, and MCAT.
- Lower scores than would be expected. Students may have standardized exam scores that are significantly lower than other measures of their academic performance.
- Failure on licensing exams. Students may fail to pass professional licensing exams such as the USMLE, despite investing considerable time, energy, and effort in preparation.
- Having a sense of being "bad" at multiple-choice exams
- A lack of other reasons for poor performance. These students do not have evidence of health problems, learning disabilities, attention-deficit hyperactivity disorder, drug or alcohol abuse,

other psychiatric illnesses, or stressors which might impact cognitive function.

- These students typically feel competent and confident in their abilities in the classroom and other professional settings.
- Excellent performance in other areas. For these students, anxiety does not impair their ability to perform or complete other demanding academic, extracurricular, or clinical activities.

The importance in recognizing DTA is that without identification and treatment, students may fail the USMLE, not just on the first attempt but on subsequent attempts. Dr. Powell writes that "unless individuals who have DTA are identified and treated, they may well continue to fail their licensing examinations and, as a result, be forced to leave their chosen field or work at a level well below their capabilities."[20]

USMLE Test Prep Courses: 3 Studies to Review Prior to Enrolling

Recognizing the importance of the Step 1 exam in the residency selection process, many students wonder if it's worthwhile to enroll in a commercial test preparation course. As a veteran of standardized tests (SAT, ACT, MCAT), you're probably familiar with test preparatory companies.

Each company touts its books, question banks, and courses as the best and most effective way to prepare for the exam. Given that the cost for these resources, particularly the courses, is easily in the thousands of dollars, it's no surprise that these companies are heavily vying for your business. Are the benefits of these courses worth their considerable expense?

1 In 1998, Thadani surveyed 1,217 first-time takers of Step 1 following the exam. Twenty-three percent of respondents had participated in a commercial test preparation course. The study revealed limited impact of these courses on test scores.[7]

2 In a study of Loma Linda medical students, researchers also found that participation in a commercial board preparation course had no significant effect on Step 1 performance. Students who studied on their own were found to have done just as well without incurring the high cost of the course.[21]

3 In a survey of medical students at the University of Miami Miller School of Medicine, Step 1 performance was not enhanced after participation in a board preparation course. However, the courses were well-received, with 97% of participants feeling that the course either definitely or somewhat helped them in their preparation. The authors suggested that the course may be useful for those needing an organized schedule for studying.[22]

The results of these studies do not make a strong argument in favor of commercial board review courses. However, for those students who need help organizing and adhering to a study schedule or staying motivated, it may be worthwhile, assuming you can afford it. Before signing up for a course, speak with upperclassmen who have taken it. Ask them about the strengths and weaknesses of the course and whether they would take it again.

Available commercial test preparation courses include:

- Kaplan Medical (www.kaptest.com)
- Exam Master for USMLE (www.exammaster.com)
- Falcon Physician Reviews (www.falconreviews.com)
- The Princeton Review (www.princetonreview.com)
- PASS program (www.passprogram.net)
- Northwestern Medical Review (www.northwesternmedicalreview.com)
- Doctors in Training (www.doctorsintraining.com)
- Cognitive Processing-Based Review for USMLE Step 1 (CPR-1)
- Institute for Board Prep (www.instituteforboardprep.com)

Scheduling the USMLE Step 1 Exam: 10 Key Points

1 Allopathic students are generally required to take the USMLE Step 1 exam at the end of the second year. Follow the policy established at your school. Seek permission if you must delay the exam beyond your school's deadline.

2 Register for the exam at www.nbme.org in the winter of your second year. Testing sites are limited, and seats fill up quickly. Signing up early will maximize your chances of securing your preferred date and location.

3 If you require special testing accommodations, early registration is particularly important. Guidelines for requesting test accommodations are available at www.usmle.org.

4 During the registration process, you will be able to indicate the three-month period of time in which you wish to take the test.

5 Your exam will take place at a Prometric Center, and you will contact them to schedule the exam date within your three-month block of eligibility.

6 Become familiar with the testing environment by scheduling a practice exam at the Center. Schedule the practice exam as soon as you've secured your exam date. Practice sessions are in great demand, and if you wait too long there may not be any time slots left.

7 A reasonable approach is to take the practice exam 1 – 2 weeks before the actual exam.

8 If you decide not to take a practice exam at the Prometric Center, visit your site several days before the actual exam. Become familiar with the drive, time required to reach the Center, traffic, parking, and restrooms.

9 Re-confirm your appointment with the Prometric Center one week before the exam.

10 If you wish to extend your period of eligibility for taking the exam (change your three-month block), contact the NBME. Before doing so, secure permission from your school.

Understanding your USMLE Step 1 Score: 5 Key Points

1 Following the exam, the NBME will determine the number of questions you answered correctly. This number is used to determine two equivalent scores, one reported on a three-digit scale and the other on a two-digit scale. Although both scores were traditionally reported on the USMLE transcript, along with a pass/fail designation, a recent change was announced. Starting in 2011, residency programs will no longer receive the two-digit score on transcripts. Only examinees and state licensing boards will receive transcripts with the two-digit score.

2 According to the USMLE, most Step 1 scores fall between 140 and 260. In recent years, the typical mean score for first-time examinees from U.S. medical schools has ranged from 210 to 230. The score required to pass is 188.[23]

3 The USMLE states that the two-digit score is "used in score reporting because some medical licensing authorities have requirements that include language describing a 'passing score of 75.' The two-digit score is derived in such a way that a score of 75 always corresponds to the minimum passing score."[23]

4 The reporting of USMLE scores on two separate scales has led to confusion among examinees. In 2005, investigators surveyed applicants to an internal medicine residency program, inquiring about their performance on the USMLE Step 1 and 2 exams.[24] They found that applicants frequently misinterpreted their scores, with many overestimating their performance. The overestimation of the score was largely due to applicants interpreting their score as a percentile.

5 According to the USMLE, the two-digit score is not a percentile. Proper interpretation of your Step 1 score is obviously of importance as you assess the strength of your candidacy for different specialties and residency programs.

7 Ways to Determine if You're at Risk for a Low USMLE Step 1 Score

1 Your past performance on standardized exams has some bearing and predictive value on your USMLE Step 1 performance. Studies have shown that MCAT scores are good predictors of USMLE scores. In a meta-analysis that examined the predictive validity of the MCAT, researchers found that scores accounted for "44% of the variance overall on the USMLE Step 1."[25] In another study, which followed over 4,000 students representing fourteen different medical schools, MCAT scores were found to be better predictors of USMLE scores than undergraduate grade-point averages.[26] Of the MCAT components, research suggests that the biological science score may be the strongest predictor of passing.[27]

2 For students who have performed well on previous standardized exams, these results may seem reassuring. However, stories abound of students who did not achieve a comparable score on the USMLE. As noted in the above meta-analysis, while MCAT scores clearly have predictive value, scores could only account for half of the variation in performance.[25] Clearly, other factors are important for Step 1 success. Chief among these is adequate preparation.

3 If you have a history of average to below average standardized test scores, now is the time to diagnose the reasons for your past performance. Don't wait until the USMLE is a few weeks away. Instead, use the substantial time that you have to your advantage. Did you have trouble finishing the exam on time? Did you know the material as well as you should have? How did you prepare? Did you do enough practice questions? Were you overcome by fear or disabling anxiety? Were you overconfident? These are just a few reasons why students may not perform up to their capabilities. Don't accept "I have always done poorly on multiple-choice exams" as an excuse. Since most medical school basic science exams are multiple-choice, attention to this area may also help you on your basic science exams.

4 Achieving a high score on the Step 1 exam requires you to be strong in all of the disciplines that make up the content of the exam. As you progress through the first and second years of medical school, make an honest and accurate assessment of your strengths and weaknesses. Have you performed poorly in a course? Did you score poorly on an NBME shelf examination? (see below) Has your academic performance been below average relative to your peers? A yes answer to any of these questions may indicate that you're at higher risk of failing or doing poorly on the Step 1 exam.

5 Traditionally, basic science departments developed their own final examination to be taken by students at the end of the course. In recent years, though, an increasing number of medical schools have opted to administer NBME Subject Examinations, also known as shelf exams, in lieu of or in addition to departmentally produced exams. Because questions on these exams tend to be similar in style and difficulty to that of the USMLE Step 1 exam, scoring poorly on one of these exams should prompt you to take steps to strengthen your knowledge in that particular subject area. In a study done to determine how well NBME Subject Exam scores predict Step 1 performance, the scores were found to be good predictors. The authors found that scores on second-year Subject Tests predicted "between 45% and 58% of the variance in USMLE Step 1 scores, while scores on first-year Subject Tests predicted slightly less (41% to 44%)."[28]

6 The NBME offers students the opportunity to take the Comprehensive Basic Science Self-Assessment (CBSSA). The CBSSA contains multiple-choice questions with content resembling that found in Step 1. According to the NBME, "there is a moderate relationship between performance on the CBSSA and subsequent step 1."[21] Following completion of the self-assessment, the NBME offers immediate feedback, which includes performance profiles indicating strengths and weaknesses in general topic areas. An assessment score is also given, with information on how this score relates to a corresponding Step 1 score. Many students find this self-assessment to be valuable in their preparation for the exam. In a study of over 12,000 U.S. and Canadian students who took the CBSSA prior to the USMLE Step 1 exam, researchers found that CBSSA "scores explained 67% of the variation in first Step 1 scores as the sole predictor variable…" The authors concluded that "examinees with low scores on CBSSA were at higher risk of failing their first Step 1 attempt."[29]

7 Major life crises can occur during medical school, and this can impact your test performance. In a study at a single medical school, 22% of graduates from 1980 to 1999 experienced a major life crisis. The most common causes were relationship stressors with spouses or significant others, illness or death of family members, and personal illness. The authors found that "experiencing a crisis was associated with lower annual grades, GPA at graduation, as well as lower USMLE Step 1 and Step 2 scores."[30]

Overcoming a low USMLE Step 1 Score: 10 Strategies

1 Although the USMLE Step 1 score is of major importance to residency programs, this score is only one component of your application. Strengthening other application components is essential to overcoming this obstacle. Dr. Andrew Lee, Chairman of Ophthalmology at The Methodist Hospital, offers the following advice. "Getting the program to ignore a subpar score is challenging but not impossible...Applicants with a subpar score should do everything possible to demonstrate their value in other ways...if you have a less optimal score you must demonstrate to the interviewer or the screener that you offer something else in your application that can justify looking away from the score alone."[31]

2 Perhaps the most common advice low-scoring applicants will hear is to take and do well on the USMLE Step 2 CK exam. This exam, which is generally taken in the fourth year of medical school, assesses clinical knowledge. Since residency programs do use the Step 2 CK score in the residency selection process, a high score on this exam can put to rest any concerns programs have about your low Step 1 score.

3 Dr. Vicki Marx, Program Director of the radiology residency program at the USC Keck School of Medicine, recommends that "the student work hard over a sustained period of time in the third year of medical school to excel on clinical rotations. Clinical rotation scores of Honors and High Pass carry significant weight in screening ERAS applications."[32] This advice is echoed by other program directors. In a 2006 survey of over 1,200 residency program directors across 21 medical specialties, clerkship grades were found to be the most important residency selection factor.[2]

4 Demonstration of leadership ability is another way to strengthen your application. A survey of emergency medicine residency program directors revealed that having a "distinctive factor", such as being a medical school officer, was one of three factors more predictive of residency performance.[33] In a survey of plastic surgery residency program directors, leadership qualities were the most important subjective criterion used to evaluate applicants during the interview process.[34] In a study done to determine the predictors of otolaryngology resident success using data available at the time of the interview, candidates having an exceptional trait such as leadership experience were found to be rated higher as residents.[35]

5 A mentor in your chosen field can be a powerful advocate for you. Dr. Roy Ziegelstein, former Program Director of Internal Medicine at the Johns Hopkins Bayview Hospital, writes that "In the modern era, sports agents have emerged as powerful figures...Modern sports figures need an agent if they are going to get the mega-contract...A medical student needs an agent too. The student has to do well in school, but that is often not enough. The student needs someone, or preferably more than one person, to trumpet his or her accomplishments."[36]

6 Letters of recommendation are an important component of the application, and you will request these letters from faculty. Preclinical students can develop relationships with faculty, and cultivating these relationships over time may lead to the development of a stronger letter later. Dr. Ziegelstein writes that the "best letter is from an individual who is very well known, who has evaluated hundreds or perhaps thousands of students over several decades, who knows you well and who believes you are one of the best students ever."[36]

7 Applicants who have a red flag in their application, such as a low USMLE score, may address the issue in their personal statement for residency. "I recommend that a student for whom a low Step 1 score is an aberration in performance explain their academic strengths very clearly up front in their personal statement" says Dr. Marx.[32] Dr. Lee offers similar advice. "Another tactic is to tackle the problem head on in the personal statement and to highlight other alternative evidence of performance and intelligence in their record."[31] For applicants who failed the Step 1, Dr. Li states that "if failure of Step 1 was due to unusual circumstances (e.g. applicant's parent died immediately prior to Step 1), the applicant should explain the unusual circumstances in their personal statement..."[5]

8 Exceptional service to the community may help overcome the low USMLE score obstacle. Community service is valued by programs, and your involvement provides information about your non-cognitive attributes, such as teamwork, leadership ability, maturity, seriousness of purpose, and conflict resolution skills. These are all skills vital to resident success.

9 Significant contributions to research are yet another way to strengthen the residency application. Although surveys of residency program directors have suggested that research is less important in the selection process, Dr. Marianne Green, Associate Dean for Medical Education at Northwestern University, writes that "Personally I believe that depth in any area can make a student stand out."[2]

10 As a clinical student, you will be able to arrange "audition", or away, electives at residency programs. Your performance during an audition rotation can have a profound impact on your chances. According to Dr. Lee, "The away elective offers the applicant the opportunity to shine at a prospective institution and introduces the student to the faculty at that specific institution in a real world setting that can create a relationship that leads to an interview or even a higher ranking for the match."[31]

Failing the USMLE Step 1 Exam: 10 Consequences

1 Nearly all allopathic schools require passage of the USMLE Step 1 exam for graduation. In a survey of U.S. medical schools, a passing score was required by 86%.[38]

2 Students who have failed the Step 1 exam are often placed on academic probation. Generally, the period of probation ends once the exam is passed.

3 Following a failed attempt, there is often a limit to the number of attempts the school will allow. Students who reach this limit may be considered for dismissal. Refer to your student handbook for your school's policy.

4 Schools may also impose a time limit for passing the exam following a failed attempt.

5 Many schools will not allow a student to begin junior clerkships until the Step 1 exam is passed. Some schools will remove students from clerkships if the failed score becomes known after the start of clerkships.

6 Medical students who fail the USMLE Step 1 exam bear a heavy emotional toll. "The biggest task in deciding what to do was dealing with the emotional side of it. I was humiliated and certainly not used to failing. In an environment filled with such bright people, it is easy to beat yourself up for not measuring up," said one student after failing the exam. She was afraid to tell her classmates but then found out that "others were in my position, and we used each other for motivation and support. The other med students were all extremely supportive as well, which was a pleasant surprise!"[39]

7 Failing Step 1 can make it difficult for you to match in a competitive specialty or program. Students who fail and then pass the Step 1 on a repeat attempt find it much more difficult to match into a competitive specialty. Over 40% of programs in dermatology, radiology, orthopedic surgery, otolaryngology, and plastic surgery never consider applicants who failed USMLE Step 1 on the first attempt.[4] Family medicine, internal medicine, obstetrics and gynecology, pathology, pediatrics, physical medicine and rehabilitation, and psychiatry are the specialties which will more often consider candidates who have failed the exam on the first attempt.

8 Although failing Step 1 will make your road to residency harder, the literature shows that most U.S. students do pass on a subsequent attempt, graduate from medical school, complete residency training, and become licensed in their chosen specialty. Researchers at a medical school in the eastern U.S. studied a group of 64 students who failed Step 1 on the first attempt.[40] Eighty-two percent of this group eventually passed the USMLE Step 1 and 2 exams. Most ultimately matched into residency and became board certified in their chosen specialty (73%).

9 The University of California Davis School of Medicine reminds students that "most of the available literature suggests that your USMLE score at best predicts how well you will perform in similar standardized tests in the future. It does NOT predict what kind of physician you will make."[41] In a recent review, the authors concluded that Step 1 "scores are not associated with measures of clinical skill acquisition among advanced medical students, residents, and subspecialty fellows."[42]

10 Realize that many students have failed before you, and then have proceeded to have successful careers in medicine. Meet with your dean to discuss the next step. When should you retake the exam? Do you have to withdraw from your present rotation or delay the start of your clerkships? These are just a few questions to address with the dean. Prior to the meeting, analyze your USMLE score report. Were you weak in a few areas or was it a global problem? Were there areas or subjects that you didn't review? Was there something going on in your life (e.g., personal or family illness) that affected your performance? Be honest in your self-assessment because an accurate diagnosis of the factors leading to the failure is crucial. Together with the dean, determine a strategy to overcome this obstacle. What will you do differently as you prepare for the repeat exam? What resources does the school have to offer you? Two USMLE preparation courses specifically geared for students who have failed include the Rosalind Franklin University of Medicine and Science CPR-1 course (Cognitive Processing-Based Review for USMLE Step 1) and the Institute for Board Prep. The CPR-1 course is "designed for U.S. medical students who have not yet been successful in passing the USMLE Step 1; especially those with multiple attempts on this exam, and whose scores have not improved significantly upon retaking the exam."[43]

References

[1]USMLE Step 1, 2009 Performance Data. Available at: http://www.usmle.org/performance-data/default.aspx#2009_step-1/. Accessed October 19, 2011.

[2]Green M, Jones P, Thomas J. Selection criteria for residency: results of a national program directors survey. *Acad Med* 2009; 84(3): 362-7.

[3]Brandenburg S, Kruzick T, Lin C, Robinson A, Adams L. Residency selection criteria: what medical students perceive as important. *Med Educ Online* 2005; 10: 1-6.

[4]NRMP 2010 Program Director Survey. Available at: http://www.nrmp.org. Accessed October 19, 2011.

[5]Student Doctor Network. The Successful Match: Getting into Pediatrics. Available at: http://www.studentdoctor.net/2011/05/the-successful-match-getting-into-pediatrics/. Accessed October 19, 2011.

[6]McCaskill Q, Kirk J, Barata D, Wludyka P, Zenni E, Chiu T. USMLE step 1 scores as a significant predictor of future board passage in pediatrics. *Ambul Pediatr* 2007; 7(2): 192-5.

[7]Thadani R, Swanson D, Galbraith R. A preliminary analysis of different approaches to preparing for the USMLE step 1. *Acad Med* 2000; 75(10 Suppl): S40-2.

[8]Medscape. The USMLE: Ten Questions. Available at: http://www.medscape.com/viewarticle/403686. Accessed October 19, 2011.

[9]National Board of Medical Examiners. Available at http://www.nbme.org. Accessed October 19, 2011.

[10]Hecker K, Violato C. Medical school curricula: do curricular approaches affect competence in medicine? *Fam Med* 2009; 41(6): 420-6.

[11]University of California San Francisco School of Medicine. Rx for Success on STEP 1 of The Boards. Available at: http://medschool.ucsf.edu/medstudents/documents/step1success.pdf. Accessed October 19, 2011.

[12]University of Utah School of Medicine. Preparing for Step 1. Available at: medicine.utah.edu/learningresources/usmle/step1.htm. Accessed October 19, 2011.

[13]Medscape. How do I prepare for the USMLE? Available at: http://www.medscape.com/viewarticle/554032. Accessed October 19, 2011.

[14]The Scoop on Step 1: A Free Guide from Lippincott.

[15]Reteguiz J. Relationship between anxiety and standardized patient test performance in the medicine clerkship. *J Gen Intern Med* 2006; 21(5): 415-8.

[16]Sartorius N, editor. Anxiety: Psychological and Clinical Perspectives. Washington: Hemisphere/Taylor and Francis; 1991.

[17]Frierson H, Hoban D. Effects of test anxiety on performance in the NBME Step 1 examination. *J Med Educ* 1987; 62: 431-3.

[18]Strowd R, Lambros A. Impacting student anxiety for the USMLE Step 1 through process-oriented preparation. *Med Educ Online* 2010; 24: 15.

[19]Powell D. Treating individuals with debilitating test anxiety: an introduction. *J Clin Psychol* 2004; 60(8): 801-8.

[20]Powell D. Behavioral treatment of debilitating test anxiety among medical students. *J Clin Psychol* 60(8): 853-65.

[21]Werner L, Bull B. The effect of three commercial coaching courses on Step One USMLE performance. *Med Educ* 2003; 37(6): 527-31.

[22]Zhang C, Rauchwarger A, Toth C, O'Connell M. Student USMLE step 1 preparation and performance. *Adv Health Sci Educ Theory Prac* 2004; 9(4): 291-7.

[23]USMLE. Available at: http://www.usmle.org. Accessed October 19, 2011.

[24]Jones R, Desbiens N. Residency applicants misinterpret their United States Medical Licensing Exam Scores. *Adv Health Sci Educ Theory Pract* 2009; 14(1): 5-10.

[25]Donnon T, Paolucci E, Violato C. The predictive value of the MCAT for medical school performance and medical board licensing examinations: a meta-analysis of the published research. *Acad Med* 2007; 82(1): 100-6.

[26]Julian E. Validity of the Medical College Admissions Test for predicting medical school performance. *Acad Med* 2005; 80(10): 910-7.

[27]Kleshinski J, Khuder S, Shapiro J, Gold J. Impact of preadmission varaiables on USMLE step 1 and step 2 performance. *Adv Health Sci Educ Theory Pract* 2007; Nov 7.

[28]Holtman M, Swanson D, Ripkey D, Case S. Using basic science tests to identify students at risk for failing step 1. *Acad Med* 2001; 76(10 Suppl): S48-51.

[29]Morrison C, Ross L, Fogle T, Butler A, Miller J, Dillon G. Relationship between performance on the NBME Comprehensive Sciences Self-Assessment and USMLE Step 1 for U.S. and Canadian medical school students. *Acad Med* 2010; 85 (10 Suppl): S98-101

[30]Greenburg D, Durning S, Cruess D, Cohen D, Jackson J. The prevalence, causes, and consequences of experiencing a life crisis during medical school. *Teach Learn Med* 2010; 22(2): 85-92.

[31]Student Doctor Network. The Successful Match: Getting into Ophthalmology. Available at: http://www.studentdoctor.net/2009/08/the-successful-match-interview-with-dr-andrew-lee-ophthalmology/. Accessed October 19, 2011.

[32]Student Doctor Network. The Successful Match: Getting into Radiology. Available at: http://www.studentdoctor.net/2010/10/the-successful-match-getting-into-radiology/. Accessed October 19, 2011.

[33]Hayden S, Hayden M, Gamst A. What characteristics of applicants to emergency medicine residency programs predict future success as an emergency medicine resident? *Acad Emerg Med* 2005; 12(3): 206-10.

[34]LaGrasso J, Kennedy D, Hoehn J, Ashruf S, Pryzbyla A. Selection criteria for the integrated model of plastic surgery residency. *Plast Reconstr Surg* 2008; 121(3): 121e-125e.

[35]Daly K, Levine S, Adams G. Predictors for resident success in otolaryngology. *J Am Coll Surg* 2006; 202(4): 649-54.

[36]Ziegelstein R. Rocking the match: applying and getting into residency. *J Natl Med Assoc* 2007; 99(9): 994-9.

[37]Student Doctor Network. The Successful Match: Interview with Dr. Marianne Green. Available at: http://studentdoctor.net/2009/05/the-successful-match-interview-with-dr-marianne-green/. Accessed March 28, 2012.

[38]Barzansky B, Etzel S. Educational programs in US medical schools, 2004-2005. *JAMA* 2005; 294(9): 1068-74.

[39]Medscape. What happens if I fail Step 1? Available at: http://www.medscape.com/viewarticle/735128. Accessed January 5, 2011.

[40]Biskobing D, Lawson S, Messmer J, Hoban J. Study of selected outcomes of medical students who fail USMLE Step 1. *Med Educ Online* 2006; 11:11.

[41]University of California Davis School of Medicine. USMLE information. Available at: http://www.ucdmc.ucdavis.edu/ome/osler/usmle.html#format. Accessed October 19, 2011.

[42]McGahie W, Cohen E, Wayne D. Are United States Medical Licensing Exam Step 1 and 2 scores valid measured for postgraduate medical residency selection decisions? *Acad Med* 2011; 86(1): 48-52.

[43]Rosalind Franklin University of Medicine and Science. Undergraduate Studies. Available at: http://www.rosalindfranklin.edu/DNN/home/CMS/EducationalAffairs/USMLE/Description/tabid/2423/Default.aspx. Accessed February 14, 2012

Chapter 4

COMLEX Level 1 Exam

The National Board of Osteopathic Medical Examiners (NBOME) is responsible for the administration of the Comprehensive Osteopathic Medical Licensing Examination – USA, also known as the COMLEX – USA. According to the NBOME, "the COMLEX – USA program is designed to assess the osteopathic medical knowledge considered essential for osteopathic generalist physicians to practice medicine without supervision" (www.nbome.org).

For osteopathic students, the route to licensure requires passage of the three-level COMLEX. These parts include COMLEX Level 1, COMLEX Level 2 (further subdivided into Level 2 Cognitive Evaluation or CE and Level 2 Performance Evaluation or PE), and COMLEX Level 3. Osteopathic students typically take the COMLEX Level 1 exam near the end of the second year, while both components of the Level 2 exam are taken in the fourth year.

Components of the three-part Comprehensive Osteopathic Medical Licensing Examination – USA		
Exam	**When is it taken?**	**What is tested?**
COMLEX Level 1	End of 2nd year	Computer-based multiple choice examination covering basic medical sciences, including anatomy, behavioral sciences, biochemistry, microbiology, osteopathic principles, pathology, pharmacology, and physiology
COMLEX Level 2 CE	4th year	Computer-based multiple choice examination covering clinical disciplines, including emergency medicine, family medicine, internal medicine, obstetrics/gynecology, osteopathic principles, pediatrics, psychiatry, and surgery
COMLEX Level 2 PE	4th year	Clinical skills (history taking, physical exam, differential diagnosis, problem solving, written communication and synthesis of clinical findings, osteopathic principles/treatment) are assessed through examinee interaction with actors trained to present clinical symptoms
COMLEX Level 3	Internship	Computer-based multiple choice examination covering clinical disciplines, including emergency medicine, family medicine, internal medicine, obstetrics/gynecology, osteopathic principles, pediatrics, psychiatry, and surgery

COMLEX Level 1: 9 Things You Must Know about the Exam on Day 1

1 All 50 states accept the COMLEX for licensure.

2 According to the National Board of Osteopathic Medical Examiners (NBOME), which administers the exam, the COMLEX Level 1 exam "emphasizes the scientific concepts and principles necessary for understanding the mechanisms of health, medical problems and disease processes."[1] Information about the content of the exam is available at their website (see Bulletin of Information), and should be reviewed carefully. In contrast to the USMLE, the COMLEX examination incorporates osteopathic principles, including the use of osteopathic manipulative treatment.

3 While simply passing the exam is sufficient for licensure purposes, students should strive for the highest score possible. The COMLEX Level 1 score is an important criterion used by residency programs in the selection process.

4 Unlike the MCAT, once you pass you cannot take the exam again. In other words, once you pass, that single score will be _the_ score used by residency programs in their decision-making process. While a higher score does not guarantee match success, it generally makes the path to reaching your career goals easier.

5 The residency selection process can be divided into two phases – screening and ranking. In the screening phase, programs whittle down a large applicant pool into a smaller group. The members of this group will be offered interview invitations. The COMLEX Level 1 score is frequently used in the screening process by allopathic and osteopathic residency programs. In 2010, a survey of several thousand allopathic residency program directors representing multiple specialties was performed by the National Resident Matching Program. The survey found that the Level 1 score was the factor used most commonly in the screening process.[2]

6 Certain specialties are more competitive than others, meaning they're more difficult to get into. In competitive specialties, many programs have a cut-off, or threshold, COMLEX level 1 score. Highly sought-after programs in less competitive specialties may also have threshold scores. Applicants who score above the cut-off are considered for interviews. Those below the cut-off may be removed from consideration.

7 The Level 1 score is important in the ranking phase. During this phase, programs develop their rank-order list. This is a list of interviewed applicants, ranked in the order in which the program would extend offers.

8 Recognizing the importance of the exam in the residency selection process, many students wonder if it's worthwhile to participate in a commercial test preparation course. A number of studies have examined the impact of commercial test prep courses on USMLE Step 1 performance. However, less data measuring the impact of these courses on COMLEX Level 1 performance is available. In one study of students at the Chicago College of Osteopathic Medicine at Midwestern University, no difference in the average COMLEX Level 1 score was found between course participants and non-participants.[3] While data is limited, when taken together with the results of the USMLE studies, it's difficult to make a strong argument in favor of commercial board review courses. However, for those students who need help organizing and adhering to a study schedule or staying motivated, it may be worthwhile (for those students who can afford it). Before signing up for a course, it would be useful to speak with upperclassmen who may have taken it. Ask them about the strengths and weaknesses of the course and whether they would take it again.

8 Program directors are also interested in your COMLEX Level 1 score because it offers them some insight into whether you are capable of passing the specialty board-certifying examination. In one study of the predictive value of the COMLEX exam, "the pass/fail status on the licensing examinations predicted 89% of the pass/fail status on the certification examination."[4]

9 A recent study found that resident competency ratings are statistically related to COMLEX-USA scores.[5]

Failing the COMLEX Level 1 Exam: 8 Consequences

1 Osteopathic schools require passage of the COMLEX Level 1exam for graduation.

2 Students who have failed the exam are often placed on academic probation. Generally, the period of probation ends once the exam is passed.

3 Following a failed attempt, there is often a limit to the number of attempts the school will allow. Students who reach this limit may be considered for dismissal. Refer to your student handbook for your school's policy.

4 Schools may also impose a time limit for passing the Level 1 exam following a failed attempt.

5 Some schools will not allow a student to begin junior clerkships until the Level 1 exam is passed.

6 Some schools will remove students from clerkships if the failed score becomes known after the start of clerkships.

7 Students who fail and then pass the Level 1 on a repeat attempt find it much more difficult to match into a competitive specialty. According to the West Virginia School of Osteopathic Medicine, "board failure is going to affect a student most in obtaining a desired residency. If a student fails one of the COMLEX exams even once, highly competitive residency programs such as dermatology, ophthalmology, surgery of all types, urology, radiology, and radiation oncology are going to be denied to him or her."[6]

8 In a survey of American Osteopathic Association-approved primary care graduate training programs, program directors indicated that nonacademic variables were the most highly valued among a group of 12 academic and 10 nonacademic variables used in residency selection. Nonacademic variables that ranked higher than Level 1 exam performance included interview, maturity, ability to work with others, and work habits. Of note, the Level 1 score was ranked thirteenth in importance. While this was not a study of competitive specialties, it does demonstrate that other variables are important in the residency selection process.[7] Although failing the exam will make your road to residency harder, most osteopathic students do pass on a subsequent attempt, graduate from medical school, complete residency training, and become licensed.

7 Ways to Determine if You're at Risk for a Low COMLEX Level 1 Score

1 Your past performance on standardized exams has some bearing and predictive value on your COMLEX Level 1 performance. Studies have shown that MCAT scores are good predictors of Level 1 scores. In a study of NYCOM students, researchers found that "physical sciences and biological sciences MCAT subscores were significantly correlated with COMLEX-USA Level 1 performance."[8] An OSU-COM study examining the predictive value of the MCAT also found the physical science subscore to be a significant predictor of Level 1 performance.[9] A positive relationship between MCAT scores and Level 1 performance was also found in a study of UMDNJ osteopathic students.[10]

2 For students who've performed well on previous standardized exams, these results may seem reassuring. However, stories abound of students who did not achieve a comparable score on the Level 1 exam. Clearly, other factors are important for success. Chief among these is adequate preparation.

3 If you have a history of average to below average standardized test scores, now is the time to diagnose the reasons for your past performance. Don't wait until the COMLEX is a few weeks away. Instead, use the substantial time that you have to your advantage. Did you have trouble finishing the exam on time? Did you know the material as well as you should have? How did you prepare? Did you work on enough practice questions? Were you overcome by disabling anxiety? Were you overconfident? These are just a few reasons why students may not perform up to their capabilities. Don't accept "I've always done poorly on multiple-choice exams" as an excuse. Since most basic science exams are multiple-choice, attention to this issue may also help you on your basic science exams.

4 Achieving a high score on the Level 1 exam requires a strong performance in all of the disciplines that make up the content of the exam. As you progress through the first and second years of medical school, make an honest and accurate assessment of your strengths and weaknesses. Have you performed poorly in a course? Has your academic performance been below average relative to your peers? A yes answer to any of these questions may indicate a higher risk of failing or performing poorly on the exam. A number of studies have sought to determine if basic science course performance might predict success on the COMLEX exam. The results are summarized below.

- In a study of osteopathic students at the West Virginia School of Osteopathic Medicine, researchers sought to determine if there was any relationship between COMLEX – USA Level 1 performance and academic performance during the first two years. The results showed that there was a "remarkable degree of agreement between these two sets of performance measures."[11]

- Researchers at the New York College of Osteopathic Medicine of the New York Institute of Technology found that COMLEX – USA Level 1 performance correlated well with year 1 and 2 GPA as well as most course grades.[8]

- A strong correlation was found between COMLEX – USA Level 1 scores and grades in the first two years among students at the University of New England College of Osteopathic Medicine.[12]

- In a study of osteopathic students at the Chicago College of Osteopathic Medicine, a significant correlation was noted between Level 1 scores and academic performance during the basic science years of osteopathic medical school. Performance in the pharmacology and pathology courses was shown to have the strongest correlation.[13]

- In one study, osteopathic medical students in the lowest quintile of GPA during the basic science years were found to be at higher risk for failing the Level 1 exam.[11]

5 Traditionally, basic science departments developed their own final examination to be taken by students at the end of the course. In recent years, some osteopathic medical schools have opted to administer NBME Subject Examinations in lieu of or in addition to departmentally produced exams. Because questions on these exams tend to be similar in style and difficulty to that of the USMLE Step 1 exam, scoring poorly on one of these exams should prompt you to take steps to strengthen your knowledge in that particular subject area.

6 The NBOME offers students the opportunity to take the Comprehensive Osteopathic Medical Self-Assessment Exam (COMSAE) as a means to assess readiness for the COMLEX Level 1 exam. The format and structure of the Phase 1 COMSAE resembles that of the Level 1 exam. Furthermore, scoring and reporting of the two exams are similar. In a study performed by the NBOME, the organization found that the two scores were highly related. While candidates can take a timed or untimed COMSAE, the data seems to suggest that the timed self-assessment exam has higher self-assessment value. The NBOME reminds osteopathic students that 5.7% of examinees who passed the Phase 1 COMSAE in the study failed the COMLEX exam:

"For any COMSAE examinee, especially those who narrowly passed COMSAE, it is important to understand that passing COMSAE does not guarantee passing COMLEX. Without extra effort, it is not guaranteed that the same performance level on COMSAE can be maintained for COMLEX." (www.nbome.og)

7 Major life crises can occur during medical school, and this can impact test performance. In a study at a single medical school, 22% of graduates from 1980 to 1999 experienced a major life crisis. The most common causes were relationship stressors with spouses or significant others, illness or death of family members, and personal illness. The authors found that "experiencing a crisis was associated with lower annual grades, GPA at graduation, as well as lower USMLE Step 1 and Step 2 scores."[14]

To Take or Not to Take the USMLE: 5 Points to Consider for Osteopathic Students

1 In recent years, an increasing number of osteopathic graduates have been applying to allopathic residency programs approved by the Accreditation Council for Graduate Medical Education (ACGME). According to Drs. Cummings and Sefcik, Deans at the Michigan State University College of Osteopathic Medicine, "in 2006, more than two of every three DOs [6,629 of 9,618] in postdoctoral training were in an ACGME program."[15] In a 2003-2004 survey of 1,353 fourth-year osteopathic medical students at 19 schools, 47% planned to pursue an allopathic residency.[16] While many allopathic residency programs accept the COMLEX, some may require or prefer you to take the USMLE Step 1 exam because it allows for easier comparison of board scores among allopathic and osteopathic applicants. The American Association of Colleges of Osteopathic Medicine writes that "each residency program determines which board scores to accept as well as acceptable scores." (www.aacom.org)

2 At allopathic residency program websites, you may encounter the following types of statements:

- "We strongly encourage you to take the USMLE exams." – Emergency medicine residency at George Washington University[17]
- "Osteopathic students and graduates must have taken USMLE Step 1 and be scheduled to take USMLE Step 2 in order to be granted an interview." – University of Chicago Illinois pediatric residency[18]
- "We will accept applications from students who have only taken COMLEX exams, but do find it additionally helpful if you have taken at least one of the USMLE exams." – Carolinas Medical Center internal medicine residency[19]

As your specialty choice becomes clear, research the specialty and programs of interest to determine if the COMLEX Level 1 exam is recognized as a USMLE equivalent. If not, you may have to take the USMLE Step 1 exam.

3 Dr. Dana Shaffer, Senior Associate Dean of Clinical Affairs at Des Moines University College of Osteopathic Medicine, offers the following advice: "For most residencies, D.O. medical students can avoid taking the USMLE exam. The exception: D.O. students planning to apply to highly competitive M.D. residency programs, such as ophthalmology, anesthesia, orthopedics, otolaryngology, and radiology."[20]

4 Some osteopathic students take the USMLE Step 1 exam well before making decisions about specialty choice. In a survey performed at the Kansas City University of Medicine and Biosciences College of Osteopathic Medicine (KCUMB) over a five-year period ending in 2004, the percentage of KCUMB students taking the Step 1 exam rose from 13.97% to 47.83%.[21] When students were asked why they chose to take the exam, a substantial number reported that they wanted to be a competitive applicant for allopathic residency programs and/or keep their options open.

5 Because programs often have difficulty making comparisons between allopathic applicants and osteopathic applicants who have only taken the Level 1 exam, researchers have studied whether COMLEX scores can be converted into USMLE scores. In one study, Dr. Slocum, Dean of the Kirksville College of Osteopathic Medicine, found a correlation between COMLEX Level 1 scores and USMLE Step 1 scores based on a formula.[22] While his work suggested that Level 1 scores "can reasonably and accurately predict USMLE Step 1" scores, he cautioned that research to explore this issue further is required, given that the research was performed at a single school. In 2010 Dr. John Gimpel, the President and Chief Executive Officer of the National Board of Osteopathic Medical Examiners (the organization that develops and administers the COMLEX Level 1 examination) commented on Dr. Slocum's study. "Although the statistical relationship between the USMLE and COMLEX-USA examinations may have been true for that particular school in 2006, it would not necessarily have been true for the national group of osteopathic medical students."[23] However, to help residency program directors, the NBOME has created a percentile conversion tool for the COMLEX-USA.

Understanding your COMLEX Level 1 Score: 5 Key Points

1 Following the exam, the NBOME will determine the number of questions you answered correctly. This number is used to determine two equivalent scores, one reported on a three-digit score scale and the other on a two-digit score scale. Both scores are reported on the COMLEX transcript along with a pass/fail designation.

2 According to the NBOME, the three-digit standard score has a mean of 500. A standard score of 400 is required to pass.[1]

3 The NBOME states that a two-digit "standard score of 75… is required to pass the examination."[1] The mean two-digit score is 82. The NBOME also emphasizes that this score is not a percentile rank, nor does it reflect the percentage of items answered correctly.

4 The reporting of Level 1 scores on two separate scales has led to considerable confusion among examinees. In our experience, applicants sometimes misinterpret their scores, with many overestimating their performance. This is often due to applicants interpreting their two-digit score as a percentile. The two-digit score is not a percentile. For candidates who wish to convert their score to a percentile, visit www.nbome.org.

5 Proper interpretation of your Level 1 score is obviously important as you assess the strength of your candidacy for different specialties and residency programs. Advisors at your school can inform you of how past students with similar Level 1 scores have fared in the residency match. According to the West Virginia School of Osteopathic Medicine, "scores below 600 will make a student much less competitive" for dermatology, ophthalmology, radiology, radiation oncology, and surgery of all types. For emergency medicine and obstetrics and gynecology, "scores below 500…will make a student much less competitive."[6] Although the Level 1 score is of major importance to residency programs, the score is only one component of your application. Students can take a number of steps to strengthen their application and overcome a low score. This was recently addressed by the American College of Physicians in the Ask the Program Director section of their IMpact newsletter. In response to the question, "How can an osteopathic medical student increase his or her chances of getting into an allopathic program?" the program director wrote that programs "are looking for students who have shown that they can excel in many areas. The more outstanding your achievements you can document, the stronger your application will be."[24] Chapters 7 – 10 and 13 – 17 provide more information on this subject.

References

[1]National Board of Osteopathic Medical Examiners. Available at: http://www.nbome.org. Accessed October 19, 2011.

[2]NRMP 2010 Program Director Survey. Available at: http://www.nrmp.org. Accessed October 19, 2011.

[3]Sefcik D, Obi C. The value of a commercial test-preparation course on COMLEX Level 1 performance. Available at: http://www.aacom.org/events/annualmtg/past/2005/Documents/Poster_Sefcik.p df. Accessed October 19, 2011.

[4]Cavalieri T, Shen L, Slick G. Predictive value of osteopathic medical licensing examinations for osteopathic medical knowledge measured by graduate written examinations. *JAOA* 2003; 103: 337-42.

[5]Langenau E, Pugliano G, Roberts W, Hostoffer R. Summary of ACOP (American College of Osteopathic Pediatricians) Program Directors' Annual Reports for First-year Residents and Relationships between Resident Competency Performance Ratings and COMLEX-USA Test Scores. E-Journal of the American College of Osteopathic Pediatricians 2010; 2(3).

[6]West Virginia School of Osteopathic Medicine. Available at: http://www.wvsom.edu/Academics/exam-center/faq. Accessed October 19, 2011.

[7]Bates B, Bates C, Tolstrup K. Selection criteria in postgraduate osteopathic medical education. *J Am Osteopath Assoc* 1998; 88(3): 391-5.

[8]Dixon D. Relation between variables of preadmission, medical school performance, and COMLEX-USA Levels 1 and 2 performance. *JAOA* 2004; 104 (8): 332-6.

[9]Evans P, Wen F. Does the Medical College Admission Test predict global academic performance in osteopathic medical school? *JAOA* 2007; 107 (4): 157-62.

[10]Meoli F, Wallace W, Kaiser-Smith J, Shen L. Relationship of osteopathic medical licensure examinations with undergraduate admission measures and predictive value of identifying future performance in osteopathic principles and practice/osteopathic manipulative medicine courses and rotations. *JAOA* 2002; 102: 615-20.

[11]Baker H, Cope M, Fisk R, Gorby J, Foster R. Relationship of preadmission variables and first- and second-year course performance on the National Board of Osteopathic Medical Examiners' COMLEX-USA Level 1 examination. *J Am Osteopath Assoc* 2000; 100(3): 153-61.

[12]Hartman S, Bates B, Sprafka S. Correlation of scores for the Comprehensive Osteopathic Medical Licensing Examination with osteopathic medical school grades. *J Am Osteopath Assoc* 2001; 101(6): 347-9.

[13]Sefcik D, Prozialeck W, O'Hare T. Characteristics of the courses that best predict COMLEX-USA level 1 performance. *J Am Osteopath Assoc* 2003; 103(10): 491-4.

[14]Greenburg D, Durning S, Cruess D, Cohen D, Jackson J. The prevalence, causes, and consequences of experiencing a life crisis during medical school. *Teach Learn Med* 2010; 22(2): 85-92.

[15]Cummings M, Sefcik D. The impact of osteopathic physicians' participation in ACGME-accredited postdoctoral programs, 1985-2006. *Acad Med* 2009; 84(6): 733-6.

[16]Teitelbaum H. Osteopathic medical education in the United States. Available at: http://www.do-online.org/pdf/acc_mededstudy05.pdf. Accessed October 19, 2011.

[17]George Washington University Department of Emergency Medicine. Available at: http://www.gwemed.edu/residency.htm. Accessed October 19, 2011.

[18]University of Chicago – Illinois Department of Pediatrics. Available at: http://www.pediatrics.uci.edu/residency/genpeds/application/application.html. Accessed October 19, 2011.

[19]Carolinas Medical Center Department of Internal Medicine. Available at: http://www.carolinasmedicalcenter.org/body.cfm?id=561&oTopID=448. Accessed October 19, 2011.

[20]Association of American Medical Colleges, Choices: The Careers in Medicine newsletter. Available at: http://www.aamc.org/students/download/184644/data/april2011choices.pdf. Accessed October 19, 2011.

[21]Punswick K, Henrie M, Avery S, McWhorter D. Osteopathic medical students and the allopathic licensing examination. *JIAMSE* 2006; 16(2): 93-9.

[22]Slocum P, Louder J. How to predict USMLE scores from COMLEX-USA scores: a guide for directors of ACGME-accredited residency programs. *J Am Osteopath Assoc* 2006; 106(9): 568-9.

[23]Gimpel J. New COMLEX-USA-to-USMLE conversion formula needed. *J Am Osteopath Assoc* 2010; 110(10: 577-8.

[24]ACP IMpact. Available at: http://www.acponline.org/medical_students/impact/archives/2011/07/ask/. Accessed October 19, 2011.

Chapter 5

Taking a Patient History

Physician communication skills can directly impact patient outcomes, and effective communication provides a number of concrete benefits. Studies have shown that good communication improves the physician-patient relationship, allows more accurate identification of patient problems, and results in fewer incidents of malpractice. It also leads to greater patient satisfaction with care, enhances compliance with therapy, and improves psychological health by diminishing patient distress.

Until relatively recently, little attention was paid to ensuring that students acquire and develop effective communication skills. However, due to a growing body of evidence showing that physician-patient communication is currently inadequate, educators have responded by increasing communication skills training during the preclinical years. In 2004, the Institute of Medicine made the acquisition and development of communication skills a top priority during medical education. That same year, the National Board of Medical Examiners (NBME) began requiring students to take a clinical skills exam (USMLE Step 2 CS) as a means to assess competence in communication. The hope is that through education students will be better versed in how to listen, question, counsel, and motivate patients.

What is the best way to teach communication skills? This question challenges medical educators. For students to learn good communication skills, it's clear that schools have to do more than simply offer general advice. Comments such as "Listen carefully to your patients" and "Have a good bedside manner" won't be enough. Having recognized this, schools have developed a variety of teaching strategies and methods. These include small-group discussions and seminars (91%), lectures/presentations (82%), student interviews with simulated patients (79%), student observation of faculty with real patients (74%), and student interviews with real patients (72%).[1]

Traditionally, preclinical students have had limited contact with patients. In recent years, however, schools have made patient contact an emphasis in early medical education. Some even introduce students to patients as early as the first week or month of med school. As a result, you'll have the opportunity to take the classroom principles of effective physician-patient communication and apply them to the real world. You'll begin to learn these skills during the preclinical years, but will hone these skills throughout your professional career.

Your efforts to improve communication skills will also impact your clerkship performance. In a survey of clerkship directors, while over 95% felt that students required an intermediate to advanced level of communication skills, approximately 30% felt that new clerkship students aren't sufficiently prepared.[2] In focus groups and interviews with clinical students at 10 U.S. medical schools, students reported a variety of struggles during the transition to clerkships.[3] The area of clinical skills was one of the five most common areas of difficulty. One student wrote:

I felt uncomfortable talking to the patient and trying to come up with methodical ways of asking questions and making sure I didn't miss things...not just jumping around all over the place...

Communication skills training is valuable, and you should take full advantage of your school's resources to maximize your education. Not all students do. Some students maintain that such training is "all common sense" or "too soft." However, research has shown that student attitudes to this type of training can impact the development and acquisition of these skills. In a recent study of student attitudes, researchers wrote that "since attitudes are often important predictors of behavior, medical students who have negative perceptions of communication skills training may devalue the importance of these skills, and ultimately they may decide that they are not important enough to develop or practice when interacting with patients."[4] It's fine to be confident in your ability to communicate. However, you still need to build on what you've already learned through the acquisition of skills specific to the physician-patient encounter. For example, giving bad news to a patient is an example of a higher order communication skill which requires considerable instruction, repeated practice on your part, and adjustment in your technique based on appropriate feedback.

Your First Patient Encounter: 7 Important Points

1 It's only natural to feel anxious as your first patient encounter nears. In the book *Surviving Medical School*, one student described how he felt after early encounters with patients.[5] "I have a lot of trouble knowing how to approach patients. I feel funny. I'm not a doctor, but I have to walk in there and 'play' doctor."

2 Another student described feelings related to her first patient experiences in medical school.[6] "My pulse is high, stomach is upside down, how can I manage all this? I know nothing and I am so mixed up as there are so many things to remember."

3 In a survey of third-year medical students before any contact with patients occurred, researchers learned that students had a number of concerns regarding communication with patients.[7] Students were asked to rate concerns on a scale of 1 (not at all serious) to 5 (very serious). Among the highest rated items were "the patient starts crying or becomes angry with me" (4.1), "the patient is in pain or emotional distress" (4.0), "not understanding the patient" (3.7), "not knowing the answer to the patient's questions" (3.5), "appearing nervous or incompetent" (3.3), and "drying up, not knowing what to ask next" (3.2). By the end of the term, all concerns were rated less serious as students gained experience in the clinical setting. With time, effort, and experience, students do become more confident in their interactions with patients.

4 Dr. Sharon Dobie, a faculty member at the University of Washington School of Medicine, wrote the following about her first patient encounter as a medical student:[8]

It was my first patient interview in Introduction to Clinical Medicine (ICM) as a first-year medical student. I remember how I felt: humble, privileged, actually in awe that someone was going to share their story with me just because I asked. It was a gift, because what did I have to offer this person? They were giving me their time, opening their life story to share with me so I could learn. Now, each fall, I hear the students in my ICM group express the same thoughts, rousing that palpable memory.

5 Medical students should always inform patients that they are, in fact, students. While this is important, it doesn't always happen. In 1976, Maguire and Rutter found that 80% of medical students failed to introduce themselves properly.[9] While this has improved over the years, more recent studies have indicated that student attitudes are not uniformly in line with recommendations. In one study of preclinical and clinical students at five Philadelphia area medical schools, researchers found that most preclinical students felt that it was important to introduce themselves as medical students and to request patients' permission before proceeding with the encounter.[10] However, clinical students attached less importance to informing patients of their student status.

6 Making clear your status as a student preserves the patient's right to refuse your participation in their care. However, most patients, once informed of your status, will still readily agree to your participation. Patients often enjoy taking an active role in educating tomorrow's doctors and gain considerable satisfaction through these interactions. In a survey of 199 patients in an academic general internal medicine ambulatory clinic, researchers studied patient attitudes toward medical student participation.[11] Nearly 90% of patients enjoyed or were neutral to medical student participation. Only 10% of patients disliked their encounter. Similar results regarding patient attitudes have been found in other specialties.

7 At the Medical and Public Health Law Site, the Louisiana State University Law Center writes that "the practice of introducing a medical student to patients as 'doctor,' 'young doctor,' or a 'student doctor' is fraud.[12] A reasonable person introduced to a doctor in a medical setting assumes that this term denotes a licensed physician with a doctoral degree in medicine."

Meeting and Greeting Patients: 5 Tips Based on Research

Pay attention to the first few moments of the patient encounter. The way in which you meet and greet patients has a number of ramifications. Patients report that healthcare professionals often don't introduce themselves properly or clarify their roles, according to a recent study by Northwestern University researcher Dr. Gregory Makoul.[13] In this survey of patients, published in 2007, Dr. Makoul and colleagues ascertained patient expectations for greetings. Over 400 patients were surveyed regarding preferences for shaking hands and the use of patient and physician names during the initial part of the encounter. Researchers also videotaped patient visits to learn about patterns of greeting behavior demonstrated by physicians. The results are summarized below.

1 Handshake: The majority of patients wanted the physician to shake hands with them; only 18% did not. Only 9 of 19 physicians shook hands with every patient.

2 Use of patient name: Over half of patients wanted physicians to use their first name, 17% wanted their last name, and 24% wanted both first and last names to be used. In over 50% of encounters, however, physicians didn't mention <u>any</u> patient names at all. When patient names were used, there was a tendency to only use the last name.

3 Use of physician name: Most patients prefer that physicians introduce themselves using their first and last names. Thirty-three percent expect physicians to only use their last name. Seven percent prefer that physicians use their first name only. Most physicians use both their first and last names and, when doing so, generally leave out the title "Dr." Thirty percent only used their last name, prefacing it with "Dr." Of note, 11% did not introduce themselves at all.

4 Based upon the study's findings, researchers recommended that physicians shake hands with patients. However, since nearly 20% of patients didn't want the physician to shake hands, physicians should be sensitive to the patient's body language. The authors also suggest using the patient's first and last names initially, along with their own first and last names when introducing themselves.

5 Survey participants were also allowed to comment on other aspects of the greeting. Patients' other preferences for physician behavior included:

- Smiling
- Friendly, personable, polite, and respectful
- Attentive/calm/making the patient feel like a priority
- Making eye contact

The study results led Dr. Makoul to conclude that "the first few moments of a medical encounter are critical to establishing rapport, making the patient feel comfortable, and setting the tone of the interview."

For preclinical students, it can be difficult to know exactly how to begin their interaction with a new patient. We've included a sample script on the next page.

Beginning the student-patient encounter

Step	Script
Step 1: Ask for permission to enter the patient's room. Confirm the patient's identity.	Good afternoon, are you Mr. Larry Jones? May I come in?
Step 2: Introduce yourself properly, leaving no ambiguity about who you are and what you will be doing.	My name is Katie Litton. I'm a second-year medical student here at ____ learning how to perform a history and physical exam. I believe that Dr. Ran informed you that I would be stopping by.
Step 3: Express appreciation for the patient's participation and request permission to proceed	I really want to thank you for helping me improve my skills in performing a history and physical exam. Is this a good time for us to talk?
Step 4: Inform the patient that he or she is not obligated to participate.	Mr. Jones, if there are any parts of the history or physical exam that you would rather not do, please feel free to tell me at any time. Also, if at any point you want to stop, that's perfectly fine too.
Step 5: Explain to the patient how any information gathered during the encounter will be used	I wanted you to know that your information will be kept confidential. With your permission, I would like to present your case to Dr. Ran later. Would that be okay with you?
Step 6: Inquire about patient's comfort or needs before beginning the interview	Before we start, are there any questions that I can answer for you? Is there anything you need before we begin?

Taking the Patient's History: 10 Tips

Following the introduction, you'll move on to the reason that prompted the patient's visit or hospitalization. This often begins by asking the patient "What brought you in today?" This is known as the chief complaint, and after eliciting the chief complaint, you'll delve into the history of present illness (HPI). The HPI is essentially the patient's story of the problem or problems he or she is experiencing. In a 1992 study, Peterson found that 76% of diagnoses made by clinicians are suggested or established by the history.[14] Therefore, it's critical that medical students learn how to elicit a proper history from the patient.

In 2003, the organization Clerkship Directors of Internal Medicine (CDIM) surveyed its members to ascertain what clinical skills students should possess at the end of their second year.[15] It was widely agreed (> 90% of respondents) that end-of-second year students should be able to obtain the history of present illness (HPI), characterize the patient's symptom(s), gather the past medical history (PMH), social history, and family history, and obtain a complete review of systems (ROS).

Your school will teach you how to obtain these elements of the history during your preclinical years, and you'll hone these skills as a clinical student and later as a resident. The foundation that you build now, as a preclinical student, may impact the quality of your clinical skills later.

1 Let the patient speak. In an often-cited study, Beckman and Frankel found that physicians frequently interrupted patients and prevented them from completing their opening statements.[16]

- Interruptions occurred after a mean time of just 18 seconds.
- Few patients (23%) were able to complete their statement.
- Waiting longer before interrupting led the patient to share more concerns.
- The order in which patients presented their concerns was not related to clinical importance.
- In 34 of 51 patient encounters, physicians interrupted patients after the patient shared his or her first complaint, assuming that this complaint was the patient's chief concern. This may or may not have been true.

- The number of late-arising concerns was significantly reduced when patients were allowed to complete their opening statement.

- Patients who were not interrupted usually completed their statement in less than 60 seconds. No patient took longer than 150 seconds.

2 Allow the patient to fully disclose his or her agenda. In studies done in the fields of primary care, pediatrics, and internal medicine, researchers have found that patients often have more than one concern in both new and return visits. However, physicians often don't allow patients to fully disclose their agenda. In a qualitative study of general practice, only 4 of 35 patients were able to voice all of their concerns.[17] This has obvious effects on patient satisfaction. In addition, this will directly impact hypothesis generation and testing. In other words, not letting the patient speak will hamper the physician's ability to make accurate diagnoses and appropriate treatment decisions.

3 Ask about the physical, emotional, and social impact of your patients' problems. Many physicians are uncomfortable asking these questions, due to a concern that the ensuing emotions may be difficult to handle or may increase the patient's level of distress. Many physicians aren't comfortable with patient emotions, and some even demonstrate blocking behaviors. These include switching topics, ignoring the expressed emotion to focus solely on the physical aspects of the illness, and explaining away distress as normal. If a patient expresses an emotion, it should be acknowledged and further explored. If you put yourself in your patient's shoes, you can imagine how you would feel if your doctor ignored or minimized your fear, sadness, frustration, or anger.

4 Use open-ended and closed-ended questions appropriately. Closed-ended questions are those that require patients to provide specific answers. A question that asks for a "yes or no" answer is one example. Another is "how many times have you felt this stabbing pain?" Contrast this with an open-ended question or statement which allows patients to elaborate. "Tell me about your back pain" is an example. It's recommended that physicians begin with open-ended questions, which allow the patient to tell his or her story fully. This can then be followed by closed-ended questions. Unfortunately, physicians sometimes transition too quickly to closed-ended questions in an effort to obtain information more efficiently. However, this "physician-dominated" rather than "patient-centered" approach has been shown to be far less effective. In an observational study of medical interns and residents, errors in the medical interview were common.[18] Trainees often did not allow the patient to tell the story of their illness. "A series of rapidly fired questions often led to a disjointed, discontinuous story, or to a series of yes and no answers." Trainees often incompletely characterized major symptoms, "with data on the setting, chronology, and alleviating or exacerbating circumstances being the most frequent omissions."

5 Utilize the techniques of active listening. This includes both nonverbal actions, which may include eye contact and appropriate body position, as well as verbal techniques, such as using words of encouragement. While we often focus on what is said in the physician-patient encounter, there is no denying the importance of nonverbal communication. The "right" body language can enhance communication. Research on the nonverbal behaviors of physicians has shown that a comfortable degree of eye contact, head nodding, forward lean, and more direct body orientation with uncrossed arms and legs is viewed positively by patients.[19]

6 Learn how to ask patients about sensitive information. Research has shown that physicians often don't elicit key components of the history, including the family history, smoking history, and history of alcohol or illicit drug use. In the Direct Observation of Primary Care study, 138 community physicians were observed in over 4,000 outpatient encounters. Family histories were only discussed in 51% of new patient visits.[20] While up to 50% of emergency room visits involve illegal drugs or alcohol, Dr. Gail D'Onofrio, Chief of Emergency Medicine at Yale-New Haven Hospital, states that typically "we don't ask it. It makes no sense whatsoever."[21] Many physicians fail to inquire about smoking. In one study, patients were asked if they smoked at 67% of all visits.[22] While there are many reasons for this, among the major reasons cited is lack of confidence in obtaining this information. Some have suggested that this lack of confidence is the result of inadequate or insufficient training in the preclinical years, followed by poor reinforcement during clerkships and postgraduate training.

7 Make it a priority to learn how to take a patient history in potentially sensitive areas. As a preclinical student with little medical experience, it is awkward to ask patients to reveal intimate or sensitive information. As this student describes:[23]

As the questions shifted away from medically safe subjects like pain to more intimate questions about her family, I began to feel extremely uncomfortable, almost as though I were a "Peeping Tom." Why should she be asked to unlock the secrets of her family life to me? It could not possibly be relevant to her illness, or could it?

8 Medical schools typically conduct comprehensive clinical skills assessments of their students using standardized patients. Researchers have interviewed faculty members responsible for remediation of problems identified in these assessments. Some of the issues have focused on patient histories.[24] "Many low-scoring students focused prematurely, failing to ask open-ended questions or adequately characterize the chief complaint. Respondents also observed students being too focused on the history of present illness, omitting or incompletely exploring the pertinent past medical, social, or family history, particularly as they related to the chief complaint." Some students failed to explore the patient's perspective on the illness. The authors wrote that "these students treated standardized patients as symptoms or diagnoses rather than as people with feelings or concerns."

9 To make the most of your communication skills training, you should prepare carefully for each session, practice the skills repeatedly, and solicit feedback. The latter is particularly important. Specific and timely feedback will help you attain these new skills.

10 In addition to soliciting feedback with all of your patient encounters, it's important to reflect on the encounter. This means noting what went well, what could have gone better, and how you can apply what you've learned to the next encounter. This has been increasingly emphasized as educators realize that reflection can play a major role in helping students learn from clinical experiences.[25] At the University of Washington School of Medicine, students "are asked to reflect on what they experience and what they learn about themselves after a variety of experiences in their first- and second-year ICM courses."[8]

References

[1]Association of American Medical Colleges. Contemporary issues in medicine: communication in medicine (Report III of the Medical School Objectives Project). Washington, DC: Association of American Medical Colleges; 1999.

[2]Windish D, Paulman P, Goroll A, Bass E. Do clerkship directors think medical students are prepared for the clerkship years? *Acad Med* 2004; 79(1): 56-61.

[3]O'Brien B, Cooke M, Irby D. Perceptions and attributions of third-year student struggles in clerkships: do students and clerkship directors agree? *Acad Med* 2007; 82(10): 970-8.

[4]Wright K, Bylund C, Ware J, Parker P, Query J, Baile W. Medical student attitudes toward communication skills training and knowledge of appropriate provider-patient communication skills: a comparison of first-year and fourth-year medical students. *Med Educ Online* 2006; 11: 18.

[5]Robert Holman Coombs. *Surviving Medical School*. Thousand Oaks, California; Sage Publications, 1998.

[6]Pitkala K, Mantyranta T. Feelings related to first patient experiences in medical school: a qualitative study on students' personal portfolios. *Patient Educ Couns* 2004; 54(2): 171-7.

[7]Hajek P, Najberg E, Cushing A. Medical students' concerns about communicating with patients. *Med Educ* 2000; 34: 656-8.

[8]Dobie S. Reflections on a well-traveled path: self-awareness, mindful practice, and relationship-centered care as foundations for medical education. *Acad Med* 2007; 82(4): 422-7.

[9]Rutter D, Maguire G. History-taking for medical students. *Lancet* 1976; 2 (7985): 558-60.

[10]Silver-Isenstadt A, Ubel P. Erosion in medical students' attitudes about telling patients they are students. *J Gen Intern Med* 1999; 14(8): 481-7.

[11]Simons R, Imboden E, Mattel J. Patient attitudes toward medical student participation in a general medicine clinic. *J Gen Int Med* 2005; 10(5): 252-4.

[12]LSU Law Center's Medical and Public Health Law Site. Available at: http://biotech.law.lsu.edu/books/lbb/x477.htm. Accessed January 20, 2012.

[13]Makoul G, Zick M, Green M. An evidence-based perspective on greetings in medical encounters. *Arch Intern Med* 2007; 167 (11): 1172-6.

[14]Peterson M, Holbrook J, Von Hales D, Smith N, Staker L. *West J Med* 1992; 156: 163-5.

[15]Clerkship Directors in Internal Medicine. Available at: http://www.im.org/CDIM/. Accessed January 30, 2012.

[16]Beckman H, Frankel R. The effect of physician behavior on the collection of data. *Ann Intern Med* 1984; 101(5): 692-6.

[17]Barry C, Bradley C, Britten N, Stevenson F, Barber N. Patients' unvoiced agendas in general practice consultations: qualitative study. *BMJ* 2000; 320 (7244): 1246-50.

[18]Wiener S. Nathanson M. Physical examination: frequently observed errors. *JAMA* 1976; 236(7): 852-5.

[19]Beck R, Daughtridge R, Sloane P. Physician-patient communication in the primary care office: a systematic review. *JABFP* 2002; 15(1): 25-38.

[20]Hayflick S, Eiff M, Carpenter L, et al. Primary care physicians' utilization and perceptions of genetics services. *Genet Med* 1998; 1: 13-21.

[21]Neergaard L. Helping doctors ask about drug, alcohol problems. Available at: http://www.physorg.com/news/160675177.html. Accessed January 30, 2012.

[22]Thorndike A, Rigotti N, Stafford R, Singer D. National patterns in the treatment of smokers by physicians. *JAMA* 279(8): 604-8.

[23]Conrad P. Learning to doctor: reflections on recent accounts of the medical school years. *Journal of Health and Social Behavior* 1988; 29(4): 323-32.

[24]Hauer K, Teherani A, Kerr K, O'Sullivan P, Irby, D. Student performance problems in medical school clinical skills assessments. *Acad Med* 2007; 82(10): S69-S72.

[25]Grant A, Kinnersley P, Metcalf E, Pill R, Houston H. Students' views of reflective learning techniques: an efficacy study at a UK medical school. *Med Educ* 2006; 40: 379-88.

Chapter 6

Physical Examination

Although 80% of diagnoses are made based on the history and physical examination, evidence indicates that the physical exam skills of physicians today are inadequate. It's widely believed that physicians' exam skills have deteriorated or eroded over the years. The decline in these skills is thought to be partly related to increased dependence on laboratory testing and radiologic imaging. In fact, some have even argued that it's appropriate for such tests to supplant the history and physical exam, since findings obtained from the physician-patient encounter are commonly ambiguous.

While today's technology has certainly advanced medicine, tests should be ordered and interpreted in the context of the patient's history and physical examination, rather than as a surrogate for the patient encounter. Dr. Christopher Feddock, a faculty member in the Department of Internal Medicine at the University of Kentucky, reminds us that history-taking and physical examination skills "serve as the foundation for all clinical decision-making."[1] He further writes that "indiscriminate use of new technology will not improve health care but will only contribute to spiraling health care costs."

While advances in technology are partly to blame for the decline in examination skills, clinical skills education and training during medical school and residency are also factors. According to Dr. Sal Mangione, Director of the physical diagnosis curriculum at Jefferson Medical College, too little time is spent during medical school learning these skills.[2] "Surveys have indicated that less than 16% of attending time may be spent at the patient's side."

In response to this, medical schools have renewed emphasis on the teaching of physical examination skills. In this chapter, we discuss how you can make the most of your education in this important area.

Physical Examination: 9 Tips Before Your First One

Examining a patient for the first time often invokes feelings of discomfort, awkwardness, insecurity, and even fear. In the article "Learning to Doctor," Conrad aptly describes the concerns of students:[3]

Students tell patients twice their age to get undressed, and then cross conventional barriers of interpersonal space to inspect the intimacies of their bodies. In addition to anxiety about doing it right, students frequently must deal with their own reactions to their patient as well as discomforting feelings of being invasive.

With continued patient interaction, you will become more comfortable and gain confidence in your abilities. In a study assessing self-confidence of medical students and physicians by training level, Fagan found that overall self-confidence increased with level of training.[4] We provide some recommendations as you prepare for your first physical examination.

1 Prepare well before the exam takes place. How will you approach the patient? What will you say to begin? How will you make the patient comfortable during the exam?

2 If you'll be performing a complete physical exam, think about the order in which you'll proceed. It's generally recommended that you move from head to toe, being careful throughout to not subject your patient to frequent position changes.

3 Before the examination, wash your hands. Do so in front of the patient.

4 Inform the patient beforehand that the exam will take longer than what he or she is accustomed to.

5 Reassure the patient that extra time spent listening to the heart or lungs does not indicate an abnormal finding.

6 One of the first steps you should take is to note the environment. Since you'll need a quiet setting, ask the patient or roommate if they can lower the volume on the TV or radio. Adjust the height of the bed or table according to your needs, and don't forget to lower it at the end of the exam.

7 Show concern for the patient's privacy and comfort throughout the examination. Close the door and slide the curtain. Adjust the pillow as needed.

8 As you proceed with the exam, tell the patient what you're doing, or ask permission. For example, "I'd like to listen to your lungs now."

9 As you examine each organ system or body area, keep other areas covered with a sheet. It's important to convey to the patient that you respect their privacy and recognize how intrusive a physical exam can be.

Physical Examination Skills of Medical Students, Residents, and Physicians: 10 Shocking Statistics

To help you gain proficiency in physical exam skills, your school will provide considerable instruction during the preclinical years. While students continue to develop their skills in the clinical years, and then during residency, evidence indicates that the foundation you build now may impact your proficiency later.

1 In a study of interns and residents on a general medicine service, at least one serious physical exam error was made for nearly two-thirds of the patients examined. The errors included failure to detect splenomegaly or focal neurological signs, findings that once discovered led to significant changes in diagnosis and treatment.[5]

2 In an observational study of medical interns and residents, errors in physical exam technique were frequently noted, as were errors of omission, defined as failure to perform parts of the examination.[6] The errors in physical exam technique included poor ordering and organization of the exam, improper manual technique or use of instruments, and poor bedside etiquette leading to patient discomfort, embarrassment, or hostility. The authors asserted that these errors in technique are the result of failure to learn the necessary psychomotor skills during the preclinical years.

3 Other studies have also demonstrated deficiencies in the physical exam skills of residents and physicians. In fact, studies have suggested that as students advance into residency and practice, physical exam skills do not necessarily improve. To compare the cardiac auscultatory proficiency of medical students and residents, Dr. Sal Mangione had participants listen to 12 cardiac events directly recorded from patients.[7] Study participants were asked to identify the condition on a multiple-choice questionnaire. On average, residents identified approximately 20% of the conditions, which was not significantly different than the percentage identified correctly by students.

4 Similar results were found when Stanford researchers tested the cardiac exam skills of a group of medical students, residents (internal medicine and family practice), physicians, and cardiology fellows.[8] While mean scores did improve from the preclinical to clinical years, no improvement was noted when clerkship students were compared to residents or physicians. The authors concluded that "cardiac examination skills do not improve after MS3."

5 In a study of over 300 internal medicine residents from the United States, Canada, and England, researchers tested the cardiac auscultatory skills of the participants. Residents listened to 12 prerecorded cardiac events and then completed a multiple-choice questionnaire. Auscultatory proficiency was poor among residents in all three countries, with mean identification rates ranging from 22% in American residents to 26% in Canadian residents.[9]

6 Medical students, residents, and pulmonary fellows were asked to listen to 10 pulmonary events recorded directly from patients. They then completed a multiple-choice questionnaire. Researchers found that internal medicine and family practice residents recognized less than half of all respiratory events, on average, with little improvement per year of training. No significant difference was noted when compared to medical students.[10]

7 Internal medicine residents were assessed as to their comfort with and performance of the physical exam. Assessments were performed at the start of internship, one month into internship, and then during the third year of residency.[11] Third-year residents had higher comfort and performed better than residents at the start of internship, but not more so than residents following one month of internship. The researchers "called into question how much further learning occurs with physical examination throughout residency training."

8 The proficiency of emergency medicine residents was assessed, specifically in regard to their ability to recognize key physical exam findings in critically ill patients.[12] Proficiency was also compared to that of senior medical students and internal medicine residents. Emergency medicine residents were only found to be better than senior students or internal medicine residents in one area – ophthalmology.

9 Internal medicine residents had considerable difficulty identifying three common valvular heart diseases using a cardiology patient simulator.[13] Overall correct response rates were mitral regurgitation (52%), mitral stenosis (37%), and aortic regurgitation (54%).

10 In a study of internal medicine residents and physicians, most reported the ability to perform physical exam maneuvers involving the heart, lung, and abdomen.[14] However, residents had a high degree of difficulty performing certain parts of the exam, including musculoskeletal (back, knee, shoulder) and eye examinations.

14 Ways to Maximize Your Physical Examination Instruction

Physical exam skills are usually introduced during the preclinical years. The courses are often named "Physical Diagnosis" or "Introduction to Clinical Medicine." In a 2003 survey of clerkship directors, it was noted that over two-thirds of schools begin teaching physical exam skills during the first year of medical school.[15] The remaining schools begin during the second year.

1 Recognize where you need to be at the end of your second year. When clerkship directors were asked what clinical skills students should have at the end of their second year, 90% felt that students should be able to perform vital signs. Seventy-five percent felt that students should be able to perform a complete physical exam using only their memory. Many directors feel that new clinical students aren't as prepared in this key area as they should be. In one study, directors indicated that an intermediate to high level of ability in interviewing and physical exam skills was required.[16] However, 44% of students were thought to be underprepared in this area at the start of clerkships.

2 Learn what other students typically omit from the exam. To assess the skills of beginning third year med students, faculty were asked to observe students while they performed a focused history and physical exam on a standardized patient.[17] Students commonly omitted key aspects of the examination:

- Head & neck: frontal maxillary sinuses, cranial nerve assessment
- Cardiovascular: Capillary refill
- Thorax: Tactile fremitus
- Abdomen: Palpation of abdominal aorta
- Musculoskeletal: Range of motion spine/extremities, assessment of gait
- Neurological: Stereognosis, graphesthesia, two point discrimination

3 Put in the time. You'll be taking the Introduction to Clinical Medicine course in conjunction with other preclinical courses. Make sure you devote sufficient time to this important area. This includes preparing for each and every physical exam teaching session. Reading about the neurological exam before you attend a lecture or work with a preceptor helps maximize retention.

4 A variety of teaching strategies and methods will be used to teach the fundamentals of physical diagnosis. Learn about these methods. As expected, the structure and format of physical diagnosis courses differs from school to school. Courses typically include large group lecture and discussion, examination of one another (peer physical examinations), examination of standardized patients, simulators, and examination of real patients.

5 Students often learn physical diagnosis initially through practice on one another. In 2000, faculty at the University of Minnesota published the results of a study in which they assessed medical student attitudes and comfort level with peer physical examinations. Ninety-eight percent of students agreed that these exams "are appropriate, valuable, and a comfortable experience."[18] In a similar survey published in 2005, 95% of respondents believed that peer physical exams are valuable. Approximately 6% reported discomfort.[19] These exams have long been a component of physical diagnosis education. In a recent Slate article, the author described a conversation she had with a physician friend about his early experiences learning physical diagnosis:[20]

I talked to a 50-ish physician friend about my experiences, and he said when he was in medical school and it was time for the first rectal/genital exam, the students were told to pair off and examine each other. "So, do you pick someone you like, or someone you don't like?" he recalled. "Either way, it's lose-lose."

Today, students are no longer asked to perform breast, genital, and rectal exams on one another. While peer physical exams continue to be widely used in medical education, some schools have replaced this form of instruction with standardized patient encounters.

6 A standardized patient is generally a healthy individual who has been trained to portray a real patient. Encounters with standardized patients can help boost confidence and increase comfort in students who are just beginning to develop their interview and exam skills. According to Dr. Britta Thompson, Assistant Dean for Medical Education at the University of Oklahoma, "standardized patients allow medical students to see patients as near to reality as possible. Students can ask questions, they can take a history and conduct a physical exam. They can learn all those clinical skills before they ever even go out to practice those skills on a real patient."[21] Many standardized patients are trained in basic communication and physical exam skills. This allows them to provide feedback to students. One standardized patient described her role in the education of medical students:[20]

I was to sit on the edge of a padded table in one of those awful flapping hospital gowns, in a room equipped with recording devices in the ceiling. Each doctor had 30 minutes to conduct a standard head-to-toe physical: from my vital signs, to my nerve function, to my reflexes, etc. Then I was to go to a computer and check off whether they'd done all 45 parts of the exam, and write my comments on their bedside manner.

7 Unlike standardized patients, simulators can present abnormal findings. For example, the Harvey mannequin, first developed in 1968, allows students to gain comfort and familiarity with the cardiac exam through exposure to a spectrum of cardiac disease. Simulators may also be used to teach students how to perform certain sensitive exams, such as the breast exam. Recently, engineers at the University of Florida developed a hybrid computer/mannequin which helps students learn how to appropriately perform a breast exam. The mannequin, named Amanda Jones, is programmed to "talk" to students. This was recently described in *Science Daily*:[22]

The student must tease out Jones' medical history, listen to her concerns and respond to her questions. Just as in a real exam, this interaction occurs simultaneously with the physical examination. For that, the student must use the correct palpating technique and apply the proper pressure. Sensors within the prosthetic breast — developed by Dr. Carla Pugh at Northwestern University — provide pressure information depicted by colors on the virtual breast, guiding students in the exams. The engineers can program the system to include or exclude an abnormality — and the attendant conversation.

8 Interviewing and examining peers and standardized patients eventually leads students to the real deal – taking histories and performing exams on real patients. In a recent survey, over 60% of U.S. medical schools reported that students had 5 or more real patient encounters during the Introduction to Clinical Medicine course.[23]

9 Seek feedback on what you've learned. Physical exam maneuvers will probably be introduced in a large group setting. Following this, students are typically subdivided into smaller groups. You may be asked to pair off and practice on one another or a standardized patient. To make progress towards proficiency, you must receive regular feedback. While you should rate your own performance, don't rely solely on self-assessment. Studies have questioned physicians' ability to accurately self-assess performance. In fact, there does seem to be a tendency for physicians to overestimate their true abilities.[24] In a well-regarded article on feedback, Ende wrote about the ramifications of infrequent or no feedback.[25] When feedback is withheld, students may continue to make the same mistakes. In addition, the opportunity to reinforce what a student is doing well is lost. This can have a significant impact on the acquisition of clinical skills.

10 Note that some physical exam maneuvers are considered more difficult than others. For example, a recent study showed that third-year med students feel quite confident about their ability to measure blood pressure. However, students were significantly less confident in their ability to assess retinal vasculature, detect a thyroid nodule, or measure jugular venous pressure.[4]

11 When you're first learning a maneuver, close observation by a trained preceptor is critical. This allows instructors to identify any errors in your technique. If these errors aren't picked up early in the learning process, you'll proceed to repeat the incorrect technique, unless a teacher down the line chooses to monitor your actual performance of the exam. While you might expect that your future residents or attendings would pick up on improper technique, this is often not the case. The literature has shown that students on clerkships are often not observed while performing physical exams. If your instructor is responsible for supervising a number of students, make it a priority to bring the instructor to you. Have him or her watch as you perform the maneuver.

12 Over the years, bedside teaching has become less common during clerkships, and "rounds" are typically held in a conference room. You therefore won't have the same opportunities during clerkships that you will during the preclinical years, especially as it's expected that at this stage of your learning you'll need much more assistance. However, you may need to take the initiative to bring the attending to the bedside to observe your skills. "Dr. Smith, would you be able to set aside a few minutes to watch me assess the jugular venous pressure on my patient?" This ensures that you'll have the opportunity to demonstrate the maneuver, verify that you're performing it correctly, and correct any errors in your technique. This is one of the best reinforcements for what you've learned.

13 You may be assessed in a variety of ways. While this may be used for grading purposes, these evaluations are much more valuable, since you can use this information to directly help you become a better doctor. Medical schools assess progress using a variety of assessment methods, including multiple-choice question exams, graded practical exam/objective structured clinical examination, global evaluation by the teacher, and evaluation by trained non-physician evaluators.

14 Work hard to retain the skills you've learned. You might assume that once you know how to perform a focused neurological exam, you're set. However, studies have found that even when learned well, physical exam skills can deteriorate over time. In one study, following a second-year physical diagnosis course, students achieved 90% performance level on a physical exam that was performed on a patient instructor.[26] When students' physical exam skills were assessed at the beginning of their third-year surgery clerkship, performance was significantly poorer. The authors concluded that "deterioration of learned physical examination skills occurs from the preclinical to the clinical years and that this deficiency is not corrected by clerkship experiences." In another study, second-year students had an assessment of their ophthalmic skills following instruction in this area. When the skills were reassessed in the third and fourth years, significant erosion in the acquired skills was noted.[27]

To retain your skills, we recommend that you:

- Take advantage of each and every opportunity to practice your skills.
- Keep your eyes and ears open for patients with abnormal physical exam findings.
- Ask faculty to observe your exam.
- Solicit feedback about your performance.
- Make use of your school's resources for physical diagnosis education, such as breast and prostate models, books, videotapes, CD-ROMS, heart sound simulators, and infrared stethoscopes.

References

[1]Feddock C. The lost art of clinical skills. *Am J Med* 2007; 120(4): 374-9.

[2]ACP Internist. Good diagnostic skills should begin at the bedside. Available at: http://www.acpinternist.org/archives/2001/02/diagnostics.htm. Accessed February 1, 2012.

[3]Conrad P. Learning to doctor: reflections on recent accounts of the medical school years. *Journal of Health and Social Behavior* 1988; 29(4): 323-32.

[4]Wu E, Fagan M, Reinert S, Diaz J. Self-confidence in and perceived utility of the physical examination: a comparison of medical students, residents, and faculty internists. *J Gen Intern Med* 2007; 22(12): 1725-30.

[5]Wray N, Friedland J. Detection and correction of house staff error in physical diagnosis. *JAMA* 1983; 249: 1035-7.

[6]Wiener S, Nathanson M. Physical examination: frequently observed errors. *JAMA* 1976; 236(7): 852-5.

[7]Mangione S, Nieman L. Cardiac auscultatory skills of internal medicine and family practice trainees. A comparison of diagnostic proficiency. *JAMA* 1997; 278(9): 717-22.

[8]Vukanovic-Criley J, Criley S, Warde C, Boker J, Guevara-Matheus L, Churchill W, Nelson W, Criley J. Competency in cardiac examination skills in medical students, trainees, physicians, and faculty: a multicenter study. *Arch Intern Med* 2006; 166(6): 610-6.

[9]Mangione S. Cardiac auscultatory skills of physicians-in-training: a comparison of three English-speaking countries. *Am J Med* 2001; 110(3): 210-6.

[10]Mangione S, Nieman L. Pulmonary auscultatory skills during training in internal medicine and family practice. *Am J Respir Crit Care Med* 1999; 159: 1119-24.

[11]Willett L, Estrada C, Castiglioni A, Massie F, Heudebert G, Jennings M, Centor R. Does residency training improve performance of physical examination skills? *Am J Med Sci* 2007; 333(2): 74-7.

[12]Mangione S, Burdick W, Peitzman S. Physical diagnosis skills of physicians in training: a focused assessment. *Acad Emerg Med* 2008; 2(7): 622-9.

[13]St. Clair E, Oddone E, Waugh R, Corey G, Feussner J. Assessing housestaff diagnostic skills using a cardiology patient simulator. *Ann Intern Med* 1992; 117: 751-6.

[14]Bonds D, Mychaleckyj M, D Phil, Watkins R, Palla S, Extrom P. Ambulatory care skills: do residents feel prepared? *Med Educ Online* 2002; 7.

[15]Clerkship Directors in Internal Medicine. Available at: http://www.im.org/CDIM/. Accessed January 30, 2012.

[16]Windish D, Paulman P, Goroll A, Bass E. Do clerkship directors think medical students are prepared for the clerkship years? *Acad Med* 2004; 79 (1): 56-61.

[17]Scott and White Healthcare. Available at: http://www.sw.org/web/researchAndEducation/iwcontent/public/SimulationCenter/en_us/pdf/PhysicalExamSkills3rdTearMedStudents.pdf. Accessed July 6, 2011.

[18]Chang E, Power D. Are medical students comfortable with practicing physical examinations on each other? *Acad Med* 2000; 75(4): 384-9.

[19]Power D, Center B. Examining the medical student body: peer physical exams and genital, rectal, or breast exams. *Teach Learn Med* 2005; 17(4): 337-43.

[20]Slate. Playing doctor. Available at: http://www.slate.com/id/2169480. Accessed February 1, 2012.

[21]BCM Solutions. Available at: http://www.bcm.edu/solutions/v5i1/simulatedpatient.html. Accessed February 1, 2012

[22]University of Florida School of Medicine. "Mixed reality" human helps medical students learn to do intimate exams. Available at: http://news.ufl.edu/2009/06/23/mixed-reality-human/. Accessed February 1, 2012.

[23]2005 CDIM survey. Available at: http://www.im.org/Resources/SurveysandData/SurveyDataandReports/CDIMS urveyData/Documents/2005PlenaryIII-Durning,Steve- SurveyReport.pdf. Accessed August 21, 2011.

[24]Davis D, Mazmanian P, Fordis M, Van Harrison R, Thorpe K, Perrier L. Accuracy of physician self-assessment compared with observed measures of competence: a systematic review. *JAMA* 2006; 296(9): 1094-1102.

[25]Ende J. Feedback in clinical medical education. *JAMA* 1983; 250 (6): 777-81.

[26]Dunnington G, Reisner E, Witzke D, Fulginiti J. Teaching and evaluation of physical examination skills on the surgical clerkship. *Teach Learn Med* 1992; 2: 110-4.

[27]Lippa L, Boker J, Duke A, Amin A. A novel 3-year longitudinal pilot study of medical students' acquisition and retention of screening eye examination skills. *Ophthalmology* 2006; 113(1): 133-9.

Chapter 7

Research

Medical students at the University of Wisconsin School of Medicine and Public Health are heavily involved in research, with many performing research in the summer between the first and second years of medical school. According to Dr. Patrick McBride, Associate Dean for Students, summer research offers numerous benefits. Students gain a basic understanding of research, and their projects often lead to presentations and published manuscripts.[1]

In a presentation to medical students titled "Research in medical school," Dr. Daniel West discussed reasons why students should consider performing research, and echoed some of Dr. McBride's thoughts. Dr. West noted that participation in research allows medical students to explore a specialty in more depth, enhance critical thinking and other related skills, assess suitability for a career in academic medicine, and strengthen credentials for residency positions.[2]

Medical students recognize these benefits. In a survey of over 300 students at three medical schools, 83% agreed that participation in research was valuable within their medical education.[3] Time was reported as a major barrier to pursuing research in med school. Difficulty finding a research supervisor was also a significant barrier, with only 44% reporting that it was easy to identify one.

In this chapter, you'll learn the benefits of research in medical school, including its importance in the residency selection process. You'll also learn about ways to identify the "right" research mentor, and maximize your chances of publishing or presenting your research results.

10 Benefits of Medical Student Research

1 Participating in research is a great way to explore a particular field during the preclinical years.

2 Participation in research will expose you to how research is conducted, from conception of an idea to publication and presentation. Along the way, you'll learn about literature review, hypothesis generation, design, methodology, data collection, and data analysis.

3 Research training leads to better critical thinking skills. The ability to critically appraise the literature is essential to the practice of evidence-based medicine. The University of Arizona College of Medicine writes that "as future physicians, being able to critically read a scientific journal along with keeping abreast of new medical innovations is an important facet of practice that can profoundly impact patient outcomes."[4] In a recent article, Mayo researchers wrote about how research benefits medical students.[5] "Studies have shown that students who had conducted research during medical school reported gains in knowledge and skills in appraising the literature, analyzing data, and writing for publication, along with more positive attitudes toward future research."

4 You may discover that you're a budding researcher. Some students find the experience so intellectually satisfying that it leads them into a career with a heavy emphasis on research. In his fourth year of medical school at the University of Iowa, Dan Shivapour was asked about his interest in research. Through his participation in the Summer Research Fellowship Program, Dan realized that he "wanted clinical research to be a big part of my career going forward."[6]

5 You can see how to combine a career in research and clinical care. Dr. Wade Smith is an academic neurologist, and a great example of how a physician can combine patient care and research. "In a typical day, I see between eight and 14 patients in the ICU who are there because of stroke, intracranial hemorrhage or subarachnoid hemorrhage…I also spend about 25 percent time performing clinical research, the type of research that involves patients directly and is the closest science to directly impact patient care."[7]

6 You may have opportunities to present your research. At the University of Wisconsin, medical student research is "put on display at the annual Medical Student Research Forum."[1] At a recent forum, "more than 80 presentations covered the full spectrum of research, from basic science to public health studies." Opportunities to present are available at local, regional, national, and international conferences.

7 Research can enhance your residency application. According to Dr. Julie Parsonnet, one positive effect of research is the "possibility that participating in a scholarly activity could result in publications and/or presentations that would improve a student's ability to match into a desired field and/or into a competitive residency program."[8] In a survey of University of Tennessee medical students, 63% reported that research experience was beneficial in helping them secure a residency position.[9]

8 Your research mentor may be able to write you a strong letter of recommendation, addressing qualities that are important to residency programs such as work ethic, motivation, and interpersonal skills.

9 Some schools have developed awards of distinction for students who have been significantly involved in research. Such marks of distinction may be placed in the Medical Student Performance Evaluation (Dean's letter) or medical school transcript, and may serve to strengthen your residency application.

10 You may win an award. The University of Kentucky grants the Medical Student Research Award to a medical student "with outstanding participation in and contribution to the field of research. Recipients of this award have an exemplary record of presentations and publications documenting their hard work and achievements as researchers during their medical school career."[10]

9 Residency Program Directors Speak About The Importance of Medical Student Research

Students are often under the impression that research experience in medical school is an extremely important criterion in the residency selection process. However, in a 2006 survey of over 1,200 residency program directors across 21 medical specialties, Dr. Green and colleagues found that research experience while in medical school was ranked last among a group of 14 academic selection criteria.[11] Furthermore, a separate NRMP survey found no significant difference in research experience among U.S. seniors who did or did not match.[12]

While research experience is not highly valued relative to other academic selection criteria, the most competitive specialties do place greater importance on research experience. These residency programs are particularly impressed by published medical school research. In Dr. Green's survey, while published medical school research was next to last in overall importance, the most competitive specialties, like plastic surgery and radiation oncology, did rank it highly.

We interviewed Dr. Green for our *Successful Match* column published at www.studentdoctor.net, and asked her about these findings.[13] She stated that "Only Radiation Oncology and Plastic Surgery program directors ranked research highly; however, even among some of the less competitive specialties, research may be an important part of the student's application. In my experience advising students, those that are looking at the top 5 programs in a certain specialty are competing with other highly qualified students across the country. Scores and grades are all outstanding, so something else may be needed to highlight the student as a competitive candidate. Personally I believe that depth in any area (not necessarily research) can make a student stand out. Extensive international experience or experience in patient safety & quality outcomes are two examples from our own institutions. Certain residency programs are looking to train research scientists. Clearly a background in research will be a necessary qualification for these programs."

In evaluating research experience during medical school, residency programs will look closely at the level of your involvement. Did you merely collect data? Or were you involved through all phases of the project, including design, data collection, interpretation and analysis of data, and preparation of the manuscript? Programs also assess your productivity. Did your work result in a tangible measure, such as an abstract, manuscript, or presentation at a meeting?

Below, we share the perspectives of program directors in competitive specialties about the importance of research.

1 Dermatology: Among 2011 U.S. applicants, approximately 95% had participated in at least one research project, with over 90% claiming at least one abstract, publication, or presentation.[12] The Southern Illinois Department of Dermatology states that "exposure to research and participating in research are preferable. More importantly is attempt at publication and experience in scientific writing."[14]

2 Emergency Medicine: The Society for Academic Emergency Medicine states "Research experience helps but it is not necessary. It will strengthen an applicant's position. The research involved does not necessarily have to be in emergency medicine. Mostly, it denotes a student who goes above and beyond the expected. There may be volunteer work or other ways to show this."[15]

3 Neurosurgery: Dr. Muizelaar, Program Director at the University of California Davis, writes, "Research in medical school is highly desirable, especially in basic or clinical sciences related to neurosurgery."[16]

4 Orthopedic Surgery: Dr. Phipps, Program Director at the University of California Irvine, states that doing research in the field will "definitely improve the chances of obtaining a residency."[17]

5 Plastic Surgery: Among 19 criteria used in the residency selection process, LaGrasso found that publications were second in importance.[18]

6 Radiation Oncology: Among 2011 U.S. senior applicants, only 9 of the 181 applicants reported not having a single abstract, publication, or presentation.[12] Dr. Ryu, Program Director at the University of

California Davis, feels that research experience is highly desirable, increasing the strength of a candidate's application.[16]

7 Otolaryngology: According to the Department of Otolaryngology at UC Davis, "research experience makes the applicant more competitive."[19]

8 Urology: In the article "Specialty Spotlight: Urology," the importance of research in the residency application was addressed. "The importance of research is dependent on the program. The more academic programs will be interested in research but do not necessarily require that the research be in the field of urology.[20] Dr. Roger Low, of the Department of Urology at UC Davis, writes that "research is highly desirable; most invited for interview are involved in past research."[16]

9 Radiology: Dr. Scott Pretorius, former Radiology Residency Program Director at the University of Pennsylvania, wrote that "in this competitive market for radiology residency slots, medical students with research backgrounds...allow themselves the opportunity to stand out in a field of increasingly highly qualified applicants. As an advisor of medical students, I routinely recommend that students intending to apply for radiology residency seek out a research mentor and undertake some kind of research project."[21] Not all agree that research involvement is required, however. In the 2008 NRMP Program Director Survey, only 64% of programs cited involvement in research as a factor in selecting applicants.[22] We interviewed Dr. Vicki Marx, Program Director of the Radiology residency program at USC, and asked how she evaluates applicant research experience.[23]

I see two types of research on applications for residency: 1) real research experience leading to peer reviewed presentations and/or publications, and 2) simulated research experience that takes place in proximity to the due date for submission of the ERAS application and does not lead to a peer-reviewed work product. Real research experience has a very positive influence on candidacy for residency – particularly at institutions where faculty research productivity is high and where ongoing scholarly activity is highly valued, or even required of residents. Research done to pad an application is easily identified.

It has no negative effect on the application because it is ubiquitous in the applicant pool. It has little positive effect either.

Absence of simulated research may have a negative effect on the ERAS application for students with mediocre academic records. My own opinion is that these students should put their energy into improving their core clinical skills rather than add another activity that will dilute the focus of their efforts.

Students with excellent academic performance throughout medical school, supported by documentation in ERAS, do not need to pad their applications to succeed in the match. Will some programs exclude them from an interview on this basis? Yes, but not many.

14 Tips to Secure the Right Summer Research Experience

Many students become involved in research in the summer between the first and second years of medical school. Opportunities for summer research may also be available for newly admitted students who haven't yet started med school. At the Mt. Sinai School of Medicine, 54 to 65% of students participated in summer research between 2001 and 2004.[24]

1 Start early. An early start allows enough time to explore the opportunities that are available at your school and other institutions. Applications and proposals for summer research funding and support are often due in March or April.

2 Examine your interests. Do you enjoy the basic sciences? If so, you might consider bench research. Or does your passion lie in clinical science? Medical schools have research opportunities in many different areas, such as basic science, clinical science, translational research, epidemiology, public health, and health outcomes research. You'll be better able to target your search if you define your interests.

3 Become informed of the research opportunities at your school through class meetings and conversations with upperclassmen. Some schools have research clubs that can introduce you to the scope of research going on at your institution. The Iowa Medical Student Research Club is one example. The Ohio State University College of Medicine has a Research Information Fair. Visit your school's office of research to learn about the types of research being conducted in different departments. Often, schools have a database of faculty members open to working with students. The office may also have a list of those who are looking for help with their projects. Offices of research are often headed by a director or dean. You may consider scheduling an appointment with this individual. He or she may be able to direct you to an appropriate mentor, factoring in your interests, goals, and time availability. You may also approach your department of interest directly by calling the chairman's office. The secretary can inform you if there is a particular faculty member (research director) who oversees the research projects in the department, and how you can arrange a meeting with this person.

4 Consider your specialty of interest. If you have a particular specialty in mind, learn about the research interests of faculty in that department. Research involvement may provide you with greater exposure to the field, allowing you to make a more informed decision about its potential as a career choice. If you're considering a particularly competitive specialty, such as dermatology or plastic surgery, early research experience may be advantageous in that you'll have substantial time before applying for residency to become published in the field. You also have the opportunity to work closely with a mentor, who might then be able to write you a strong letter of recommendation.

5 There's no need to focus initially on a single person. It's often advisable to meet with several potential mentors to learn about their research opportunities.

6 Once you identify potential mentors, contact each by email, and arrange a meeting. In your email, express your interest and attach a brief description of your research experience. If the professor is unable to take on a student, don't be concerned. If you don't hear from a potential mentor or you sense any disinterest on their part, consider it a blessing. You don't want to establish a working relationship with anyone who won't be invested in your career. It's best to move to the next person on your list.

7 Before meeting with a potential mentor, learn as much as you can about the faculty member and his or her area of interest. The Robert Wood Johnson Medical School encourages students to read one of their recent research papers. "This will not only provide you with detailed information on what the lab is doing, but it will also provide background for discussions with the professor. This will also demonstrate to the professor that you are interested in his/her research and motivated."[25] Drs. Michael and Allan Detsky recommend that students research their potential research advisor. Questions should include "What is her or his track record on grants and publications with other student coauthors?" and "Has he or she been responsive and supportive to previous students?"[26] Search for articles written by faculty at www.pubmed.org. If you know of students who've worked with the faculty member, contact them.

8 At meetings with potential mentors, listen closely to their research interests and current projects. Ask how you might be able to contribute or participate. What will be your precise role? Who will directly supervise you? At this point, you should simply gather information and not make any quick decisions.

9 Be prepared to talk about yourself. In particular, be ready to discuss your prior research experiences, and the skills you've acquired.

10 Look for a match between your interests and the project. However, the project itself isn't the only consideration. You should determine if there's a good fit between yourself and your potential mentor. According to Duke University School of Medicine, "pairing of compatible mentors with students is essential."[27]

11 Consider the scope of the research project, including its length. How long will it take to complete? Basic science research projects often require the largest investment of time. You have a limited amount of time, and therefore you may wish to select a smaller project. It is possible to complete a project during a summer break. This requires selection of the appropriate project. Case studies, chart reviews, and literature reviews are just a few examples.

12 To make the most of your summer experience, ask your mentor if it's advisable to begin some work before the research experience officially begins. Should you observe some experiments or familiarize yourself with techniques? Should you attend lab meetings?

13 Discuss issues related to funding. If you'll be applying for funding through your school, will you need documentation from your mentor? Are there professional organizations or societies in your mentor's area that offer medical student research grants? If you're not able to secure funding, would your mentor be able to provide you with a stipend?

14 Dr. Daniel Albert, Director of the Eye Research Institute at the University of Wisconsin, emphasized the importance of following through or fulfilling research responsibilities.[28] "The research faculty in medical schools are well aware of the rigorous schedule medical students face and understand that only a limited amount of time can be devoted to research. Moreover, they are forgiving when genuine conflicts arise and time scheduled for research is of necessity missed....But it is disheartening for scientists to take on students who express a desire to play a meaningful research role, and accept responsibility for a portion of a project, and then fail to fulfill those responsibilities."

Publishing and Presenting Your Research: 11 Points to Consider

Students participating in research hope that their work will lead to publication in the literature and presentation at national meetings.

1 Publication isn't always possible. At the Mayo Medical School, research is required during the third year of medical school, and students spend a three-month block immersed in research with no other classroom or clinical responsibilities.[5] Researchers examined the productivity of 998 Mayo students who graduated between 1976 and 2003. In their analysis of the data, the authors wrote that only "66% of graduates had at least one research report, abstract, or research presentation." At the Mt. Sinai School of Medicine, 25% of graduating medical students in 2004 had published peer-reviewed manuscripts.[24]

2 Even one year of full-time research may not lead to publication. The Clinical Research Training Program at the National Institutes of Health (NIH) and the Doris Duke Clinical Research Fellowship are prestigious programs that immerse students in one year of full-time clinical research. In a recent study, only 23% of fellows in either program had publications in print by 6 months post-fellowship.[29] This date was chosen to indicate publications that could be included in residency applications, as fellows usually participated between their third and fourth year of medical school. Students at the Duke University School of Medicine immerse themselves in long-term research, but over one-third do not publish prior to graduation.[27] While these figures are surprising, it's important to remember that most basic science and some clinical research projects require a large investment of time. It can easily take several years to perform the research and then complete the peer-review and publication process.

3 The conclusion is that not all research experience will result in a publication to add to your CV. However, research experience that doesn't lead to publication can still be an invaluable addition to your application. It demonstrates your dedication to the field, may result in stronger letters of recommendation, and provides a topic of discussion in interviews. Most importantly, the value of research experience extends far beyond what it can do for your application.

4 Even if you don't publish, most residency programs will still value your involvement. In a survey of general surgery residency program directors, nearly 90% "considered basic science or clinical research almost always or all the time when evaluating applicants." Only 30% of program directors "rarely or never credited research unless it had been published as an abstract or paper."[30]

5 Even if your research does not lead to publication, you may be able to share your findings in an oral or poster presentation. In advice offered to dermatology applicants, the article's authors wrote that "the ability to present research in the form of posters and oral presentations at conferences is also valuable and respected."[31]

6 To make it more likely that your work will be published, try to choose a project that is smaller in scope, preferably one that you'll be able to complete within a few months. It's also wise to share this expectation with your mentor before agreeing to participate in a particular project. See below for more details on how to do so appropriately. If your mentor is aware, you may be steered away from projects that require years to yield tangible results. Instead, for example, you may be encouraged to participate in a shorter chart review.

7 Dr. Daniel Egan, Associate Director of the Emergency Medicine residency program at St. Luke's Roosevelt Hospital, recommends that students take a delicate and honest approach in discussing their goal to be published with potential mentors. "Once you have identified a person or project, don't forget about your primary goals. For most students, this means publication. Ideally, a published paper on your curriculum vitae when you are applying to residency will show motivation and academic success. However, an abstract presentation at a regional or national conference would also be impressive. Be honest with your potential mentor. Walk the fine line of expressing interest in learning about the fundamentals of research and the project, while also acknowledging that part of your goal is a tangible result (i.e., an abstract or paper). Some projects take years and are not realistic for your involvement other than an academic exercise. Others may involve short chart or record reviews that may work much better for the summer or your research elective."[32]

8 Seek out opportunities to present your work at local, regional, national, and international meetings. At Stanford University School of Medicine, 52% of medical students had presented at a national meeting.[33] Symposiums and meetings geared to medical student research presentations include the National Student Research Forum (NSRF), Eastern-Atlantic Student Research Forum (ESRF), and Western Student Medical Research Forum (WSMRF). The NSRF is held at the University of Texas Medical Branch in Galveston, and provides a forum for students to give either poster or oral presentations.[34] Over 30 awards are given at this annual event. Most schools have a medical student research day. You may be able to present an abstract, prepare a poster, or give an oral presentation on your research. This experience will also help you prepare if you'll be presenting at a larger meeting later.

9 The McGill Journal of Medicine is an international publication produced entirely by students at McGill University.[35] It "offers all students an opportunity to publish the results of their scientific research or to contribute commentaries about pressing issues of the day. The nature of the administration of the MJM makes it particularly sympathetic to contributions from students who are just beginning their careers in the medical and scientific fields." The University of Toronto Medical Journal is a student-run enterprise which publishes articles from medical professionals around the world.[36] Students at the George Washington University School of Medicine can publish their research in *Fusion*, a research journal run by students.[37]

10 Travel to national conferences to present your research can be expensive. Medical schools may have funds in the form of travel fellowships available to help you offset the cost. National organizations may also provide travel fellowships or grants.

11 Some students continue their research following the summer period, devoting several hours a week. This is recommended if you wish to see it through to publication or presentation. Remaining involved in the project will increase your chances of becoming a co-author on a publication. It's important, though, that you not let your research compromise your academic performance. "Occasionally students have been so engaged by work in their concentration that their performance in the core curriculum has suffered," writes Dr. Laskowitz of Stanford University.[27]

10 "Year Out" Research Opportunities for Medical Students

Year-out programs are available to students who wish to spend one year fully engaged in research while free of other medical school responsibilities.

1 The Clinical Research Fellowship for Medical Students, sponsored by the Doris Duke Charitable Foundation, offers one-year fellowships at one of 12 selected institutions in the U.S.

2 The HHMI – NIH (Howard Hughes Medical Institute-National Institutes of Health) Research Scholars Program and NIH Clinical Research Training Program allow participants the opportunity to work on the NIH campus.

3 Research Training Fellowships through the HHMI are also available to students, and support one year of research at a variety of academic institutions.

4 Students interested in cardiovascular research can apply to the Sarnoff Fellowship Program.

5 The Centers for Disease Control Foundation offers the CDC Experience Applied Epidemiology Fellowship.

6 For students interested in conducting research at NIH-funded research centers abroad, contact the Fogarty International Clinical Research Scholars Support Center at Vanderbilt University for information about their Overseas Fellowships in Global Health and Clinical Research.

7 The American Diabetes Clinical Scholars Award provides one year of research support to students interested in diabetes research.

8 Through the American Heart Association Pre-Doctoral Fellowship, students receive one to two years of stipend support for cardiovascular research.

9 Students interested in pharmacology research can receive up to 24 months of stipend support through the Paul Calabresi Medical Student Research Fellowship sponsored by the Pharmaceutical Research and Manufacturers of America Foundation.

10 Your own medical school may offer opportunities. Many medical schools have 1-year research tracks, some of which are degree-granting.

References

[1] University of Wisconsin School of Medicine and Public Health. Available at: http://www.med.wisc.edu/news-events/news/students-make-an-impact-on-patients-through-research/26401. Accessed February 9, 2012.
[2] University of California Davis School of Medicine. Available at: http://mdscholars.ucdavis.edu/Research%20in%20Medical%20School.ppt. Accessed February 9, 2012.
[3] Siemens D, Punnen S, Wong J, Kanji N. A survey on the attitudes towards research in medical school. *BMC Med Educ* 2010; 22: 10: 4.
[4] University of Arizona Medical Student Research Program. Available at: http://www.msrp.medicine.arizona.edu/dist_guidrat.htm. Accessed February 9, 2012.
[5] Dyrbye L, Davidson L, Cook D. Publications and presentations resulting from required research by students at Mayo Medical School, 1976-2003. *Acad Med* 2008; 83(6): 604-10.
[6] University of Iowa Carver College of Medicine. Available at: http://www.medicine.uiowa.edu/. Accessed July 12, 2011.
[7] American Academy of Neurology. Available at: http://www.aan.com/go/education/students/careers. Accessed February 9, 2012.

[8]Parsonnet J, Gruppuso P, Kanter S, Boninger M. Required vs. elective research and in-depth scholarship programs in the medical student curriculum. *Acad Med* 2010; 85(3): 405-8.

[9]Solomon S, Tom S, Pichert J, Wasserman D, Powers A. Impact of medical student research in the development of physician scientists. *J Investig Med* 2002; 51(3): 149-56.

[10]University of Kentucky College of Medicine. Available at: http://www.mc.uky.edu/meded/student_affairs/Research.asp. Accessed February 9, 2012.

[11] Green M, Jones P, Thomas J. Selection criteria for residency: results of a national program directors survey. *Acad Med* 2009; 84(3): 362-7.

[12]National Resident Match Program Charting Outcomes in the Match, 2011. www.nrmp.org. Accessed March 29, 2012.

[13]Student Doctor Network. Interview with Dr. Marianne Green. Available at: http://studentdoctor.net/2009/05/the-successful-match-interview-with-dr-marianne-green/. Accessed February 9, 2012.

[14]Southern Illinois Department of Dermatology. Available at: http://www.siumed.edu/medicine/dermatology/. Accessed February 9, 2012.

[15]Society for Academic Emergency Medicine. Available at: http://www.saem.org/. Accessed February 9, 2012.

[16]University of California Davis School of Medicine. A guide to the perplexed: residency guide. Available at: www.ucdmc.ucdavis.edu. Accessed February 9, 2012.

[17]University of California Irvine Department of Orthopedic Surgery. Available at: http://www.orthopaedicsurgery.uci.edu/. Accessed March 12, 2011.

[18]LaGrasso J, Kennedy D, Hoehn J, Ashruf S, Pryzbyla A. Selection criteria for the integrated model of plastic surgery residency. *Plast Reconstr Surg* 2008; 121 (3): 121e-125e.

[19]University of California Davis Department of Otolaryngology. http://www.ucdmc.ucdavis.edu/otolaryngology/. Accessed February 9, 2012.

[20]Ballask J. Specialty spotlight: urology. *Journal of Andrology* 2005; 26(6).

[21]Pretorius E. Medical student research: residency director's perspective. *Acad Radiol* 2002; 9(7): 808-9.

[22]Results of the 2008 NRMP Program Directors Survey. Available at: http://www.nrmp.org. Accessed March 29, 2012.

[23]Student Doctor Network. The Successful Match: Getting into Radiology. Available at: http://studentdoctor.net/2010/10/the-successful-match-getting-into-radiology/. Accessed February 9, 2012.

[24]Zier K, Friedman E, Smith L. Supportive programs increase medical students' research interest and productivity. *J Investig Med* 2006; 54(4): 201-7.

[25]Robert Wood Johnson Medical School. Available at: http://rwjms.umdnj.edu/research/mst/mentor.html. Accessed February 9, 2012.

[26]Detsky M, Detsky A. Encouraging medical students to do research and write papers. *CMAJ* 2007; 176(12) 1719-21.

[27]Laskowitz D, Drucker R, Parsonnet J, Cross P, Gesundheit N. Engaging students in dedicated research and scholarship during medical school: the long-term experiences at Duke and Stanford. *Acad Med* 2010; 85(3): 419-28

[28]Science Careers Blog. Available at:
http://blogs.sciencemag.org/sciencecareers/2010/01/what-do-researc.html.
Accessed February 9, 2012.
[29]Cohen B, Friedman E, Zier K. Publications by students doing a year of full-time research: what are realistic expectations? *Am J Med* 2008; 121 (6): 545-8.
[30]Melendez M, Xu X, Sexton T, Shapiro M, Mohan E. The importance of basic science and clinical research as a selection criterion for general surgery residency programs. *J Surg Educ* 2008; 65(2): 151-4.
[31]Alikhan A, Sivamani R, Mutizwa M, Aldabagh B. Advice for medical students interested in dermatology: perspectives from fourth year students who matched. *Dermatology Online Journal* 2009; 15 (7): 4.
[32]Medscape. How can I get involved in research? Available at:
http://www.medscape.com/viewarticle/581864. Accessed February 9, 2012.
[33]Jacobs C, Cross P. The value of medical student research: the experience at Stanford University School of Medicine. *Med Educ* 1995; 29(5): 342-6.
[34]National Student Research Forum. Available at: http://www.utmb.edu/nsrf/.
Accessed February 9, 2012.
[35]McGill Journal of Medicine. Available at: http://www.mjm.mcgill.ca/.
Accessed February 9, 2012.
[36]University of Toronto Medical Journal. Available at:
http://utmj.org/ojs/index.php/UTMJ/. Accessed February 9. 2012.
[37]Fusion Research Journal. Available at:
http://www.gwu.edu/employment/careersatgw/opportunities/research.
Accessed February 9, 2012.

Chapter 8

Extracurricular Activities

As a preclinical student, you'll be spending many, many hours in the lecture hall in order to acquire the knowledge and skills needed to become a physician. This will be your overriding focus during medical school. However, you'll also be provided with numerous educational opportunities outside of the classroom. Extracurricular activities cover a wide range of opportunities, and are offered by every medical school.

For example, at the Virginia Commonwealth University, there are at least 12 specialty interest groups, such as the ophthalmology interest group. At the Philadelphia College of Osteopathic Medicine, athletic activities include basketball, deck hockey, flag football, men's rugby, soccer, volleyball, and runner's club. Opportunities for the musically inclined include such groups as the Harvard Medical School Chamber Music Society, Chordae Tendinae at the Alpert Medical School at Brown University, and Karaoke Interest Club at the University of Wisconsin School of Medicine.

With long days, many lectures, and vast amounts of information to absorb, new students often wonder if it's even feasible to participate in extracurricular activities. Despite demanding schedules, many preclinical students are able to do just that, provided they make participation a priority. In a survey of AOA members at the University of Texas Southwestern Medical School, respondents spent an average of 3.61 hours/week during their first year engaged in extracurricular or leadership activities.[1]

Involvement in extracurricular activities may also help students reach their professional goals. Extracurricular activities "might provide evidence for non-cognitive attributes that predict success," writes Dr. Andrew Lee, Chairman of the Department of Ophthalmology at The Methodist Hospital.[2] "The first priority of a residency selection committee is insuring that the applicant does not wash out or cause trouble during their time in the program. This is sometimes referred to generically as 'fit'. Everyone wants a team player who is unselfish and working towards a common goal. Leadership skills demonstrated by being an officer in extracurricular activities or being an Eagle Scout, or a leader or founder of a new organization or club are all looked upon favorably. The second goal is to look for evidence of non-cognitive attributes that might make a superior ophthalmologist (conflict resolution, team work, leadership ability, communication skills, performance under stress, maturity, seriousness of purpose, prior scholarly activity). Finally, programs are looking to graduate (and thus select) residents who will make the program proud."

7 Benefits of Extracurricular Activities

Like college, the learning environment in medical school extends beyond the classroom. Institutions offer valuable opportunities to participate in a variety of extracurricular activities. For example, at Case Western Reserve University, there are over 40 medical student organizations.[3] Although opportunities abound for medical student involvement, always keep in mind the importance of striking the right balance between academics and other pursuits. The University of Wisconsin School of Medicine encourages students to participate in service and leadership activities, but not at the expense of academics.[4] "Participation in service and leadership activities will not compensate for low grades and/or Board scores as you move on to residency."

Involvement in extracurricular activities also offers the chance to take on leadership roles. "There are only a few leadership positions. It's not possible for everyone to be a leader" is a commonly stated belief. Our experience has shown that medical students often underestimate the number of leadership positions available in student organizations. In our recent analysis of student organizations at the University of Texas Medical School in Houston, 109 leadership positions were found in organizations ranging from Student Senate to the Wilderness Medical Society.[5] The Association of Internal Medicine Students group had five class officers, including President, Vice-president, Treasurer, Information Technology Coordinator, and Service Coordinator. At the Southern Illinois University School of Medicine, 63 different students (out of a total student body of 292) held leadership positions, either as a class officer or a committee member (medical school admissions, curriculum, and educational policy committees, among others).[6] This number does not encompass other student organizations, each of which has its own leaders.

1 Through such experiences, you can further develop skills that are directly applicable to success as a physician. A few examples of vital skills in the daily life of a doctor are teamwork, self-discipline, time management, and leadership.

2 Involvement in organizations is a way to develop and strengthen bonds with classmates.

3 Since student organizations often have a faculty advisor or sponsor, students have extraordinary opportunities to work closely with faculty members. Such opportunities are usually unavailable to students during the preclinical years.

4 Extracurricular activities are a significant nonacademic factor in the residency selection process. In a recent NRMP survey of 1,840 program directors representing the nineteen largest medical specialties, 59% of respondents cited volunteer/extracurricular experiences as a factor in selecting applicants to interview.[7] In advice given to students seeking positions in a competitive specialty, the School of Medicine at East Tennessee State University writes that "extracurricular activities, hobbies, and interests outside medicine often make the difference. Most subspecialty residencies are very small (one to three residents per year) and want to work with someone who is interesting and enjoyable, not just an encyclopedia."[8]

Evidence suggests that meaningful contributions in extracurricular activities, particularly leadership, may serve as a predictor of residency performance. In one study of emergency medicine residency program directors, having a "distinctive factor" such as being a championship athlete or medical school officer was one of three factors most predictive of residency performance.[9] In a study to determine predictors of otolaryngology resident success using data available at the time of interview, candidates having an exceptional trait such as leadership experience were found to be rated higher as residents.[10] While success as a resident requires sufficient academic ability, equally important, if not more so, is an individual's ability to work well with others. Election to a leadership position suggests that an applicant has been recognized for his or her ability to collaborate with classmates. The assumption is that a student would utilize this same ability to collaborate during residency. One general surgery residency director looks for evidence that an applicant is a team player. "This can be seen through commitment to some sort of extracurricular activity."[11]

5 Once accepted for an interview, the depth and breadth of your involvement in extracurricular activities may help you stand out in a sea of academically qualified applicants. One dermatology applicant was involved in a local environmental conservation group as well as his medical school's admissions committee. He recalls being asked "extensively about participation in these activities during his interviews." He believes that "interesting extracurricular pursuits can make a difference as residency programs attempt to sort through hundreds of extremely well-qualified applicants each year."[12]

6 Like selective colleges and medical schools, highly sought after medical specialties and residency programs look closely at extracurricular activities to gain some insight into an applicant's potential to be a leader in the field following graduation. In a survey of residency program directors in plastic surgery, respondents were asked to rank 20 items used in the evaluation of applicants during the interview process.[13] Ranked # 1 was leadership qualities.

7 What does involvement in medical student organizations say about a student? Some residency programs believe that activities chosen as a student may predict involvement during residency. An applicant who was heavily involved in community service might continue such participation as a resident. Likewise, a student who served on several medical school committees may have an interest in serving on residency committees, such as the interview host committee.

10 Leadership Awards for Medical Students

Students who have been heavily involved in student organizations as leaders may be recognized for their contributions with awards. National organizations and medical schools have established awards recognizing exceptional leadership.

1 Every year, the American Medical Association honors 15 students with AMA Foundation Leadership Awards. These awards recognize students who have demonstrated "strong, nonclinical leadership skills in advocacy, community service, public health, and/or education.[14]

2 The American Medical Women's Association bestows the Anne C. Carter Student Leadership Award to a medical student for outstanding leadership.[15]

3 The Association of American Medical Colleges awards five scholarships every year to entering third year medical students who have demonstrated leadership in "efforts to eliminate inequities in medical education and health care" and "addressing educational, societal, and health care needs of minorities in the United States."[16] To be considered for the Herbert W. Nickens Medical Student Scholarship Award, students must submit a nomination letter from the medical school dean, several letters of recommendation, personal statement, curriculum vitae, and medical school transcript.

4 AMSA members who have shown exemplary achievement in leadership and management may receive the James Slayton National Award for Leadership Excellence.[17]

5 Alpha Omega Alpha offers the Medical Student Service Leadership Project Award "to support leadership development for medical students through mentoring, observation, and service learning."[18]

6 Local and state medical societies may also grant leadership awards to students. The Wisconsin Medical Society Presidential Scholar Award is given to a medical student who exemplifies "the attributes, skills, and desire to become a medical leader in Wisconsin."[19]

7 The American Osteopathic Foundation Presidential Memorial Leadership Award is given to an osteopathic medical student "who is committed to the principles of osteopathic medicine and who has made great strides toward becoming one of the top leaders within the osteopathic profession."[20]

8 The Student Osteopathic Medical Association (SOMA) offers the Marvin H. and Kathleen G. Teget Leadership Scholarship to "benefit students pursuing a career in specialty medicine. The selection is based on the students demonstrating leadership in a specialty field."[21]

9 The AMA Foundation Minority Scholars Award Program provides scholarships to approximately 12 students every year. The award recognizes outstanding academic achievements, leadership activities, and community involvement.[22]

10 The American Academy of Family Physicians grants the Tomorrow's Leader Award to medical students who demonstrate leadership ability.[23]

5 Important Points about Extracurricular Activities

1 Don't wait until your third or fourth year to join clubs and organizations. Although the preclinical years are busy, time is even more limited during the clinical years of medical school. Participation now is possible, if you choose to make it a priority and properly budget your time.

2 Remember that your first priority in medical school is to do as well as you can in your course work. Many students are accustomed to performing at a high level academically while juggling a variety of extracurricular activities. Soon after starting med school, you'll find many opportunities to participate in different organizations and groups. While we don't want to discourage such participation, we have found that some new students overstretch. This can have consequences, especially when you're new to med school and haven't yet determined exactly what it takes to succeed in this environment. Your initial focus should always be academics. Once you're comfortable with the workload, your responsibilities, and the environment, you can take a much more active role in student organizations. A key question to ask before adding any activity: "Can I balance my involvement with my course work?" Dr. Patrick Duff, Associate Dean of Student Affairs at the University of Florida, offers important advice for medical students.[24] "Important, but definitely secondary priorities, include participating in extracurricular activities…However, if you are having difficulty in any of the 3 areas (health, family, schoolwork), you need to get back in balance. All of the altruistic activities in the world (admirable though they may be) will not compensate for a 'failure' in school, loss of your good health, or deterioration in personal relationships."

3 While certain activities may be perceived as having better "CV-building" properties, stick with activities you enjoy. As a med student, you'll have a lot less free time compared to your undergraduate years. With so many activities and limited time, which activities should you choose? A number of factors play into this decision. First and foremost, choose an activity you'll enjoy. Other important considerations: What contributions can you make to the organization? In some organizations, students may have little or no potential to make an impact. In others, students can impact outcomes or affect change. What do you gain from your participation? Gains can include development of new skills, strengthening of important skills such as communication and leadership, the ability to form relationships with other student leaders and faculty members, or just some much-needed relaxation.

4 In evaluating extracurricular activities, residency programs will look at the depth of a student's involvement. While some students believe there's strength in numbers, residency programs value the quality of involvement. Programs are interested in learning whether a student excelled in one or two activities. Were you a leader? Did you demonstrate serious commitment to an organization? Were you able to make meaningful contributions? When comparing residency applicants of equal academic ability, factors such as depth and breadth of extracurricular activities may help one student stand out.

5 As a member of an organization, you have the power to make meaningful contributions through active involvement. This can take different forms. A student can serve in a leadership capacity, such as president or vice-president. Since many groups host events, students can volunteer to spearhead or coordinate an event. Students can also head committees within the group. A residency program can easily differentiate the student who made valuable contributions to an organization from a passive participant. Sometimes this is apparent when review of the application reveals a relative lack of detail or description of the student's involvement. In other cases it becomes known at the time of the interview. In either situation, students should think about how they would describe their involvement and be able to provide examples of their impact.

Founding and Establishing a New Organization: 9 Tips

After reviewing the opportunities available at your medical school, you may find a need to start a new organization. For example, you may have an interest in anesthesiology, but your school lacks an anesthesiology interest group. If you sense a need for a new organization, you can establish one yourself. Before starting the process, access your school's student organization database to review the list of active student organizations. Look also at dormant groups to make sure the group doesn't already exist at your school.

1 Many students don't realize that, even at their level, they have the ability to create an organization. However, medical schools often have a policy in place to guide students interested in creating or registering a new organization. If you're seeking to start a local chapter of a national organization, you'll often find resources available on the organization's website. For example, the Asian Pacific American Medical Student Association has a detailed step-by-step guide for starting a new APAMSA chapter.[25]

2 Starting a new organization has the potential to impact not only students, but also the school and greater community. As an example, consider the story of Infusion. Infusion was started as a student organization at the University of Alabama Birmingham School of Medicine.[26] In 2005, a group of eight students sang at the Anatomical Donor Ceremony. This ceremony, which followed completion of the gross anatomy course, served as a way for students to express their appreciation to the families of the donors. Following the ceremony, the students decided to make it a permanent a capella group, thus leading to the birth of Infusion. The group has performed in the hospital wards at UAB and other venues, with a major goal being to raise funds for local charities.

3 For student leaders, starting a new club is an opportunity to nurture an idea from conception to fruition. Along the way, students have many opportunities to develop and strengthen skills in organization and leadership.

4 A new organization or chapter provides opportunities for other students. An organization can provide educational opportunities, skill development, and a sense of satisfaction.

5 Since many student organizations impact the community through their service projects, this provides another opportunity for the medical school members to reach out to the surrounding community.

6 Founding an organization, or starting a chapter, is not an easy endeavor. It can provide great satisfaction, but certainly can provide a number of obstacles and hassles. With your limited time, make sure you have the passion necessary to follow through on your idea.

7 Establishing a new student organization is viewed favorably by residency programs. It demonstrates initiative on your part and allows you to stand out from other applicants.

8 To help deal with the challenges of starting a new organization, seek the expertise of a faculty member. Choose a faculty member who shares your interest, and will be available to advise and help with development. A faculty sponsor can be a valuable mentor, overseeing your efforts, answering questions, and providing guidance when needed.

9 New student groups generally require the approval of the medical school. The approval process is often initiated through an application submitted to a particular dean or student organization committee. In your application, you'll provide information about the organization's goals, the benefits of the organization to students, reason for its need at the school, leadership structure, and budget required to fulfill its role.

References

[1]University of Texas Southwestern School of Medicine Survey of AOA Members. Available at: http://www.quidprolibro.com/utswaoa/Documents/BrownBag2.pdf. Accessed May 12, 2011.

[2]The Successful Match: Getting into Ophthalmology. Available at: http://studentdoctor.net/2009/08/the-successful-match-interview-with-dr-andrew-lee-ophthalmology/. Accessed February 12, 2012.

[3]Case Western Reserve University School of Medicine. Available at: http://casemed.case.edu/. Accessed February 12, 2012.

[4]University of Wisconsin School of Medicine & Public Health. Available at: http://www.med.wisc.edu/education/md/community-service/opportunitiesforstudents/157. Accessed February 12, 2012.

[5]University of Texas Medical School at Houston. Available at: http://med.uth.tmc.edu/. Accessed February 12, 2012.

[6]Southern Illinois University School of Medicine. Available at: http://www.siumed.edu/. Accessed February 12, 2012.

[7]NRMP 2010 Program Director Survey. Available at: http://www.nrmp.org/data/index.html. Accessed February 12, 2012.

[8]East Tennessee State University Quillen College of Medicine. Available at: http://com.etsu.edu/. Accessed May 12, 2011.

[9]Hayden S, Hayden M, Garnst A. What characteristics of applicants to emergency medicine residency programs predict future success as an emergency medicine resident? *Acad Emerg Med* 2005; 12(3): 206-10.

[10]Daly K, Levine S, Adams G. Predictors for resident success in otolaryngology. *J Am Coll Surg* 2006; 202 (4): 649-54.

[11]AMSA Essentials of Matching in General Surgery. Available at: http://www.amsa.org/AMSA/Libraries/Committee_Docs/Essentials_of_a_Getti ng_into_a_Surgical_Residency.sflb.ashx. Accessed February 12, 2012.

[12]Alikhan A, Sivamani R, Mutizwa M, Aldabagh B. Advice for medical students interested in dermatology: perspectives from fourth year students who matched. *Dermatology Online Journal* 15(7): 4.

[13]LaGrasso J, Kennedy D, Hoehn J, Ashruf S, Pryzbyla A. Selection criteria for the integrated model of plastic surgery residency. *Plast Reconstr Surg* 2008; 121 (3): 121e-125e.

[14]American Medical Association. Available at: http://www.ama-assn.org/ama/pub/about-ama/ama-foundation/our-programs/public-health/excellence-medicine-awards.page. Accessed February 12, 2012.

[15]American Medical Women's Association. Available at: http://www.amwa-doc.org/page3-91/AnneCCarter. Accessed February 12, 2012.

[16]Association of American Medical Colleges. Available at: https://www.aamc.org/initiatives/awards/101280/nickens_scholarship_overvie w.html. Accessed February 12, 2012.

[17]American Medical Student Association. Available at: http://www.amsa.org/AMSA/Homepage/Events/Convention/Awards.aspx. Accessed February 12, 2012.

[18]Alpha Omega Alpha. Available at:
http://www.alphaomegaalpha.org/student_service_leadership.html. Accessed
February 12, 2012.
[19]Wisconsin Medical Society. Available at:
http://www.wisconsinmedicalsociety.org/_WMS/foundation/_files/pdf/pressch
olar-app.pdf. Accessed February 12, 2012.
[20]American Osteopathic Foundation. Available at: http://www.aof-
foundation.org/index.cfm?fa=grants.detail&gid=25. Accessed February 12,
2012.
[21]Student Osteopathic Medical Association Foundation. Available at:
http://www.somafoundation.org/scholarships_and_grants.htm. Accessed
February 12, 2012.
[22]American Medical Association. Available at: http://www.ama-
assn.org/ama/pub/about-ama/ama-foundation/our-programs/medical-
education/minority-scholars-award.page. Accessed February 12, 2012.
[23]American Academy of Family Physicians. Available at:
http://www.aafp.org/online/en/home/aboutus/theaafp/scholarships/natconfschol
ar/tomorrowleader.html. Accessed February 12, 2012.
[24]University of Florida College of Medicine. Available at:
http://osa.med.ufl.edu/faq/student-advice/. Accessed February 12, 2012.
[25]Asian Pacific American Medical Student Association. Available at:
http//www.apamsa.org/membership/start-a-new-chapter. Accessed May 10,
2011.
[26]Infusion at UAB. Available at: http://www.uabinfusion.com/. Accessed
February 12, 2012.

Chapter 9

Community Service

In 2005, after watching the devastation wrought by Hurricane Katrina on the city of New Orleans, Temple medical student Zoe Maher led a group of ten students to the ravaged area during their winter break.[1] "We wanted to do something useful for the community," said Maher of her trip. "We worked with a small clinic in New Orleans' Algiers neighborhood, with first- and second-year students providing triage, and third- and fourth-year students using their clinical skills to treat patients." At medical schools across the U.S., students like Zoe are actively involved in a variety of community service projects in an effort to better their community.

While the provision of community service has been a major area of emphasis at U.S. medical schools for years, educators have recently stressed the importance of fostering education in community service. In 1998, Seifer defined service learning "as a structured learning experience that combines community service with preparation and reflection."[2] The Liaison Committee on Medical Education (LCME), which is responsible for the accreditation of medical schools, recommends that schools should not only provide students with sufficient opportunities "to participate in service-learning activities" but also "encourage and support student participation."[3]

Many schools, such as the College of Osteopathic Medicine of the Pacific, have responded by incorporating service learning as an integral part of the curriculum. In 2001, the Morehouse School of Medicine established the Center for Community Health and Service-Learning to engage students and other healthcare professionals in community service and service learning. Partnering with other organizations in the Atlanta area, the center aims to address the health disparities affecting underserved populations.

At the Duke University School of Medicine, service learning is also a key component of medical student education.[4] "Our point is to emphasize to the students the importance of becoming involved in the community and to inform them of the needs in that community," explains Dr. Caroline Haynes, Director of Student Affairs. "They're going to be learning how to practice medicine with the people in the surrounding community, so this will give them a greater appreciation of that community. We also wanted to demonstrate that people's health depends in part on their environment and educational opportunities, and is not just a product of what happens when they encounter the health system." In 2008, the AAMC found that a significant percentage of medical school applicants had been involved in community service.[5] Sixty-three percent of the applicants reported nonmedical volunteer experience. Medical volunteer experience was reported by 77% of applicants. When compared to 2002 data, the percentage of applicants participating in community service had risen. "They have a real sense of service, commitment, and discovery that I know we all want in a future doctor at our bedside," said Dr. Darrell Kirch, the AAMC President.[6] These numbers aren't surprising, considering that students often point to medicine's service orientation as a major motivating factor in their decision to pursue a career in medicine.

As a medical student, you'll have ample opportunities to participate in community service. As stated by the Dartmouth Medical School Community Service Committee, a student-run committee that sponsors about 15 community service programs: "Whether you are interested in volunteering at a clinic for underserved populations, becoming buddies with a child with special needs, or singing at hospitals and nursing homes, you will find an opportunity to contribute to your community your way."[7]

Students spend long days listening to lectures and absorbing voluminous amounts of information, and many wonder if it's actually possible to continue participation in community service. Despite demanding schedules, many preclinical students are able to do just that, provided they make participation a priority. Eighty-one percent of Dartmouth Medical School first and second year students had participated in at least one community service activity.[7] To do so and still succeed in medical school, you'll have to strike the right balance between academics and other pursuits. The University of Wisconsin School of Medicine encourages students to participate in service and leadership activities, but not at the expense of academics.[8] "Participation in service and leadership activities will not compensate for low grades and/or Board scores as you move on to residency."

In this chapter, we discuss ways in which students can participate in community service, and the impact that this participation has on the health of the community as well as on personal and professional development.

10 Benefits of Community Service for Medical Students

Although community service clearly benefits others, medical students themselves gain tremendous benefits from their involvement and participation.

1 Community service is good for your psyche. Research has shown that volunteering increases positive feelings, improves mental health, reduces the risk of depression, and lowers stress levels.[9-11]

2 Participation may improve communication skills. At the University of Minnesota Medical School – Duluth Campus, second-year medical students travel to elementary schools throughout Minnesota and northwest Wisconsin and speak to children about how the brain works.[12] "In their comments about the experience, students have described how making presentations to elementary school students helped them understand the importance of being able to explain basic disease concepts and body processes to patients at an appropriate level."

3 When Kari Geronilla, a student at the West Virginia School of Medicine, was asked if her school's community service requirement was beneficial, she was emphatic in her response.[13] "Definitely! I have had some of my best experiences during community service events…It allowed me to bond with my classmates and talk to upperclassmen." Community service involvement can help you forge bonds with classmates, enhance your interpersonal skills, and make you feel more socially connected.

4 In research done to determine if there is a relationship between students' volunteer community service hours and medical school academic and residency performance, students in the highest service group were found to have significantly better grade point averages, USMLE Step 2 scores, and residency director assessments as compared to students having no community service hours.[14] The authors cautioned readers not to assume that this was cause and effect, since academically strong students may be able to devote more time to community service while still maintaining a high degree of academic success. Struggling students, on the other hand, may spend less time providing community service because more time is needed to handle the academic rigors of medical school.

5 According to the AAMC, over 25% of U.S. medical school graduates have participated in global health experiences, many of which have involved service to the community.[15] In the article "Preparing Medical Students for the World," Dr. Kayhan Parsi at the Loyola University Chicago Stritch School of Medicine wrote about the many benefits of international health experiences.[16] "Students improve their communication and listening skills, rely less on technology and more on their clinical physical diagnosis skills, improve their knowledge of diseases prevalent in the developing world, and become more sophisticated with regard to public health issues in resource-poor settings."

6 Involvement in student-run health clinics is one of the most popular community service activities. While volunteer physicians typically see all patients, medical students are also heavily involved in patient care. Skills that preclinical students have learned include taking a medical history, performing a physical exam, using a stethoscope, administering injections, measuring blood sugar, learning how to use an oto-ophthalmoscope, and presenting patients to other healthcare professionals. Clearly, students learn valuable clinical skills, and this is a major drive for student participation. Preclinical students also report that clinic participation reminds them of why they chose to pursue a career in medicine, something that can easily be forgotten when students are immersed in basic science coursework.

7 Students may have the opportunity to take on leadership positions. In surveys of and interviews with administrative leaders, faculty physicians, and medical student leaders, Dr. Prathibha Varkey identified the necessary qualities and skills of leaders. These included emotional intelligence, confidence, humility, creativity, teamwork, communication, and time management.[17]

8 Most students who are involved in community service have a strong sense of social responsibility and are not engaged in these activities to strengthen their curriculum vitae. However, students may be recognized for their contributions in this area. National organizations have established awards recognizing exceptional service to the community. These are listed on page 173.

9 Schools may honor students who have shown dedication to community service. The Marshall University School of Medicine awards the Community Leadership Scholarship to a student who has completed an exceptional amount of community service.[18] The University of New Mexico School of Medicine Khatali Alumni Community Service Award is given to a student who has an outstanding record of service.[19] The Ohio State University gives the Student Award for Excellence in Community Service for exceptional record of community service.[20] Students at Weill Medical College of Cornell University who demonstrate exceptional dedication to community service may receive the designation of M.D. with Honors in Service on their diploma and transcript.[21]

10 Community service involvement can serve as a draw for residency programs. Community service is a significant nonacademic factor in the residency selection process. In a recent NRMP survey of 1,840 program directors representing the nineteen largest medical specialties, 56% cited community service as a factor in selecting applicants to interview.[22] Like selective colleges and medical schools, highly sought after medical specialties and residency programs look closely at the depth and breadth of community service involvement to gain some insight into an applicant's potential to be a leader in the field following graduation. Your involvement may help you stand out in a sea of academically qualified applicants.

10 Benefits of Joining Your Medical School's Student-Run Health Clinic

Student-run health clinics have been established at many medical schools, and are among the most popular community service activities for students. At the University of California Davis, 85% of medical students volunteer in student clinics during their tenure in medical school.[23] It's clear that these clinics have a significant effect on the personal and professional growth of medical students. "Students are often changed in unexpected, profound, and lasting ways after experiencing firsthand healthcare delivery to the poor, underserved, and marginalized," explains Dr. Ed Farrell, a physician volunteer at the Stout Street Clinic, which is run by students attending the University of Colorado School of Medicine.[24]

1 You will serve a vital need in the community. These clinics generally serve underserved populations, including the uninsured, homeless, and the poor. For these patients, student-run clinics may be their only access to health care. In a recent survey of allopathic schools, researchers learned that the total number of patient-physician visits to these clinics exceeded 36,000 per year.[25]

2 You will develop a better understanding of the socioeconomic and health disparities in medicine today. Georgetown University School of Medicine has the H.O.Y.A clinic, a student-run clinic which provides comprehensive care to underserved populations in the DC area.[26] The clinic has helped Georgetown medical students better understand the socioeconomic and health disparities in medicine today.

3 Stanford University medical students are involved in the Pacific Free Clinic.[27] This clinic provides basic healthcare services to the underserved population in the East San Jose area. It primarily serves the needs of immigrants with limited English proficiency. Students learn to deliver health care in a linguistically and culturally appropriate manner.

4 At the Stout Street Clinic, University of Colorado medical students provide comprehensive healthcare to the homeless and economically disadvantaged populations in Denver.[28] Through this experience, students gain an understanding of the health issues and needs of the homeless population.

5 For students, clinic involvement provides opportunities to acquire valuable skills, knowledge, and attitudes. As the words *student-run* would suggest, medical students have primary responsibility for the management of these clinics. Medical students at all levels, as well as non-student professionals, commonly volunteer at these clinics. Non-student professionals include, among others, physicians, nurses, social workers, and pharmacists.

6 While volunteer physicians typically see all patients, medical students are heavily involved in patient care. Through their involvement, preclinical students have learned such skills as administering injections, measuring blood sugar, and learning how to use an oto-ophthalmoscope. Students learn valuable clinical skills, and this is a major drive for student participation.

7 Having the opportunity to apply knowledge gained in the classroom to a real world patient care setting is a strong draw for many students. As one student remarked, "Working in the clinic makes my textbook come alive." Since patients who frequent these clinics generally have a very different background than their own, students are also exposed to the issues that affect the lives and consequently the health of these patients.

8 Other common reasons for volunteering include a desire to help the poor, a wish to spend time with patients, and simply for enjoyment. Less commonly cited reasons are interest in strengthening curriculum vitae or earning class or community service credit.[25]

9 Some student volunteers may have the opportunity to take on leadership positions in the clinic, such as serving as the clinic administrator. In this capacity, students can learn about financial planning, staff scheduling, staff recruitment, and other skills needed to operate and manage an outpatient clinic.

10 In a survey of student-run health clinics, clinic leaders indicated that 39% of their school's first year students, on average, had given their time to the clinic on at least one occasion within the past year.[25]

9 Resources to Help You Start Your Own Community Service Project

Christian Dean, a student in the Texas College of Osteopathic Medicine class of 2012, galvanized his classmates to provide monthly health screenings for Fort Worth's homeless population.[29] During each health screening session, TCOM students see dozens of patients, providing each patient with a free screening. After exploring existing community service activities or projects at your school, you may find an unmet need in the community, such as Christian did. If you choose to address that need, a number of resources are available to assist in the process.

1 The Medical Student Section of the AMA (AMA-MSS) has created a list and description of projects that AMA-MSS chapters across the country have developed and implemented.[30]

2 Since the 1970s, *Project Bank: The Encyclopedia of Public Health and Community Projects*, a tool offered by the AMA Alliance, has served as a useful compendium of community service projects conducted by state and county Alliances.[31]

3 The AAMC's Medicine in the Community Grant Program (formerly known as Caring for Community) offers grant awards to medical students who wish to initiate, develop, and run a community service project.[32] According to the AAMC, "Medicine in the Community will help students to translate great ideas into meaningful service by contributing needed start-up and supplemental funds." Some past recipients of the grant include:

- Medical College of Wisconsin Hmong Health Education Program. HHEP is an effort to improve communication of health education and healthcare services for Wisconsin's Hmong population through educational workshops, outreach programs, support groups, and public service announcements.

- University of New Mexico School of Medicine Community Vision Project. Through the use of mobile eye clinics, basic vision care services are provided to American Indian and Hispanic populations.

- UMDNJ School of Osteopathic Medicine Revitalizing Education & Advancing Camden's Health (REACH). The REACH program aims to teach preventive community health to middle school children and train youth to create community service projects.

- Vanderbilt University School of Medicine Shade Tree Community Diabetes Program. The project's goals include raising community awareness and establishing educational programs about proper diabetes care for the uninsured and underinsured population in East Nashville.

4 The Student National Medical Association Community Service Grant program is another source of financial assistance for community service projects. Funding is available to SNMA local chapters.[33] For more information, visit www.snma.org.

5 State medical societies may also offer support. Through the Medical Student Community Leadership Grant Program, the California Medical Association Foundation provides grants to California medical student organizations for service projects which will promote community health and well being.[34] Community service grants are available to medical student members of the Massachusetts Medical Society.[35] Projects must "meet objectives in community and social service, public health activism and education, or volunteer mentorship activities."

6 The AMA offers Chapter Involvement Grants (CIG) for medical student chapters interested in initiating a project.[36] "Chapters are strongly encouraged to use the grants as 'seed money' to support a project that has start-up costs, but can then be maintained for little or no money."

7 Through the Helping Hands Grant Program, the American Psychiatric Foundation provides support to medical students interested in creating and managing mental health service projects.[37]

8 Alpha Omega Alpha offers funds through the AOA Medical Student Service Project Award to students interested in establishing or expanding a service project.[38]

9 If your school does not have a student-run health clinic, consider starting one yourself. Although far from simple, there are resources available to assist interested students. In 1995, Cohen wrote "Eight Steps for Starting a Student-Run Clinic," an article published in *JAMA*.[39] In the article were the following words of inspiration: "The most important ingredient for starting a student-run clinic is motivated students willing to work hard, adapt to a variety of situations, and energize others to participate with a heart-felt vigor and teamwork." Another useful resource, "25 Steps to Starting a Student-Run Clinic," is available at the Society of Student-Run Free Clinics website.[40] Helpful information can also be found at the National Association of Free Clinics and Volunteers in Medicine websites.[41-42]

10 Awards Given to Medical Students for Community Service

Most students are involved in community service because of their strong sense of social responsibility, not because they wish to strengthen their curriculum vitae. However, students may be recognized for their contributions in this area.

1 National organizations have established awards recognizing exceptional service to the community. The Translating Osteopathic Understanding through Community Health, better known as TOUCH, is a nationally recognized award given to osteopathic medical students who have shown commitment and dedication to serving others.[43] As a national initiative of the Council of Osteopathic Student Government Presidents, awards are given to students who volunteer at least 50 hours within one year. Silver Touch and Gold Touch pin awards are given to students who participate in at least 50 and 100 hours, respectively. At a recent awards ceremony at the Ohio University College of Osteopathic Medicine, three first-year and seven second-year students received TOUCH awards.[44]

2 The Student National Medical Association's Member of the Year Award is given to a student who is nominated for contributions to the SNMA on a local, regional, or national level.[45] Nominators must indicate how the nominee enhanced the chapter's community service involvement or served as a role model to others through mentoring and outreach.

3 The American College of Emergency Physicians (ACEP) awards the Medical Student Professionalism and Service Award to a student who plans to pursue a career in emergency medicine.[46] To be eligible for the award, a student has to show "evidence of active service to medical organizations and the community that demonstrates a substantial commitment of time and effort with evidence of leadership." Of note, grades and board scores are not a factor.

4 Community service awards and prizes are bestowed to exceptional minority students through National Medical Fellowships.[47]

5 Medical student members of the American Medical Women's Association are eligible to receive the Wilhelm/Frankowski Scholarship.[48] This scholarship is given for "community service, activity in women's health issues, and participation in AMWA and other women in medicine groups."

6 Local community service awards and grants may be available in your area. Chicago medical students can apply for the Monash/Mitchell Medical Student Scholarship Program.[49] The Florida Medical Association Sanford A. Mullen, M.D. Award for Outstanding Community Service by a Medical Student is given to a student who goes "beyond the classroom or hospital and truly exhibits outstanding community service."[50]

7 The Council of Osteopathic Student Government Presidents annually presents the Student DO of the Year Award to a student for commitment to their school, community, and the osteopathic profession. Each school nominates a single student for the award. From this group, one student is selected as the National Student DO of the year.

8 Health associations and organizations may also offer community service awards. Laura Hoffman, a medical student at Des Moines University, received the 2011 Volunteer Award from the American Lung Association in Iowa.[51] Laura was recognized for her efforts and commitment to a tobacco-free world.

9 Medical school chapters of national organizations may be recognized for exceptional contributions to the community. Recently, the American Academy of Family Physicians recognized the University of Missouri Family Medicine Interest Group with an award for outstanding community service.[52]

10 The American Association of Physicians from India bestows the Most Distinguished Medical Student Award for "outstanding performance in patient care, research, and community service."[53]

14 Questions to Ask Before Starting your Community Service Project

Before moving forward with your efforts to create a new project, you should ask some key questions. Your answers to these questions will help you articulate your vision to medical school administrators, develop a plan of execution, complete paperwork at your school, and apply for internal or external funding. It is far easier, and often more enjoyable, to plan a community service project as part of a group. Tasks and assignments can be spread over group members rather than falling on the shoulders of one individual. However, responsibilities and deadlines must be clearly addressed.

1 What need is addressed by your project idea?

2 Is this service being provided by the school through any other means, such as by another student organization? If so, how is your project different?

3 Who is the intended audience? Which community will this project benefit?

4 What are the goals of the project?

5 What will students involved in the service project learn?

6 When will the project begin and end? Or is it an ongoing project? If so, why?

7 If you've planned an ongoing project, what needs to be done to make the project sustainable over the long-term?

8 Who else will be involved in the project? What will be their roles and responsibilities?

9 How will you recruit students and faculty (or other healthcare professionals)?

10 What equipment or supplies are needed?

11 How much funding will be necessary to begin and sustain the project?

12 Where will you find this funding?

13 What is the medical school's policy regarding new community service projects?

14 What challenges do you foresee with initiating and implementing the project? How will you overcome these challenges?

20 Examples of How Medical Students Have Impacted their Community through Service Activities

We have been very inspired when hearing about the ways in which medical students and schools all across the country have impacted their communities through service. These individuals and organizations demonstrate that students can take action, in concrete fashion, to benefit their communities. In doing so, they provide inspiration for us all.

1 The Family Practice Club at Albany Medical College was recently awarded the Program of Excellence Award by the American Academy of Family Physicians for its commitment to community outreach.[54] Nearly 50% of the college's medical students are involved in the club, which has been engaged in a variety of community service activities. The activities include Tar Wars, a program to foster education among elementary school children about the dangers of tobacco, and Apple Wars, an effort to prevent childhood obesity. Another major initiative of the club is Project Medscope, which provides health care to underserved populations in the Albany area.

2 In 2002, two medical students at the Texas A & M College of Medicine established the Health Circus organization to benefit the Brazos Valley community.[55] The goal of the organization is to "improve the quality of life for children and adults by focusing on preventative medicine, insurance coverage, and a positive outlook on healthcare." Events held by the Health Circus have provided free health and dental screenings, immunizations, and blood pressure and glucose checks.

3 The "Chicago Students for Sight" program was established at Loyola University Chicago Stritch School of Medicine.[56] Through this program, eye screenings are held at local health fairs in Chicago to benefit the financially disadvantaged and uninsured populations. The program is now a collaborative effort of all medical schools in Chicago.

4 More than 95% of University of Louisville medical students participate in some type of community service before graduating.[57] "Doctors want to contribute in a positive way to all of society, which they certainly can do in their everyday practices," says Dr. Toni Ganzel, Dean of Students. "But as leaders in our communities, we also need to give back through volunteerism and service projects that help meet the needs of medically underserved populations. It's simply the right thing to do."

5 After receiving an eleven million dollar grant from the state for the development of the Healthy South Carolina Initiative, the Medical University of South Carolina (MUSC) developed 28 programs to benefit the community.[58] Students were heavily involved, tutoring middle school students, repairing homes, and sponsoring blood drives. In the first three years, over 1,000 MUSC students reached more than 26,000 public school students. To recognize the exceptional service given to the community, the Association of American Medical Colleges recently awarded the Medical University of South Carolina with the Outstanding Community Service Award.

6 Tulane University medical students "annually complete over 9,500 hours of service in the community."[59] Students have provided health care and support services to homeless youth, raised funds to fight cardiovascular disease through the AHA Heart Walk, educated teens and adults on a variety of health and social issues, and trained restaurant staff on how to perform the Heimlich maneuver.

7 According to Dr. Aaron McGuffin, Senior Associate Dean for Medical Education at Marshall University School of Medicine, "there has been 2,700 hours of community service donated from the medical school students in the past 12 months. That is a lot of time in addition to doing their medical school work."[60]

8 With funding from the AMA, medical students at the University of Illinois-Rockford organized an "Organ and Tissue Donor Awareness

Day" to raise awareness in the community and recruit donors.[61] Students arranged for a transplant surgeon to speak about donation and transplant procedures. The day also included a bone marrow registration and blood drive.

9 The Philadelphia College of Osteopathic Medicine AMA chapter made monthly visits to a local middle school to educate children about the adoption of healthy lifestyles to reduce obesity.[62] Handouts were created with healthy recipes and healthy ingredient substitutions for children to take home.

10 Through Wayne State University's "Kick Butt's Postcard Campaign," students produced postcards as part of an anti-tobacco campaign.[63] The postcards, which were created by local youth, had artwork, statistics, and links to anti-tobacco resources. Wayne State's AMA-MSS section distributed these postcards throughout the community.

11 In 2009, over 50 students at the New York College of Osteopathic Medicine at the New York Institute of Technology built a house in the 9th Ward of New Orleans, an area hit particularly hard by Hurricane Katrina.[64] In addition, through fundraising efforts, students were able to give approximately $ 3000 to the New Orleans Habitat for Humanity chapter.

12 The Penn State College of Medicine places high value on service to community. Over the past year, Penn State medical students have "helped sick children smile and laugh, provided companionship for the elderly, supported battered women and their children, served as big brothers and sisters, provided support to terminally ill patients, and administered free medical care to homeless men and women."[65]

13 In 2008, the SUNY Upstate Medical University was named to the President's Higher Education Community Service Honor Roll in recognition of the contributions its students made to the community.[66] The services provided by students included collection of warm clothing and canned goods for local refugee assistance centers, assistance to faculty physicians delivering healthcare to underserved areas, mentoring of elementary school children, recruitment of bone marrow donors, and fundraising for charities through university-sponsored walks.

14 At the University of New Mexico School of Medicine, community service is a key priority.[67] Educators have gone beyond just encouragement by freeing students in the afternoons during the first year for service engagement. For its community service contributions to the state of New Mexico, the school received the 2008 Spencer Foreman Award for Outstanding Community Service, an award bestowed by the AAMC.

15 At the Lake Erie College of Osteopathic Medicine, students are reminded that "The Community is Our Campus."[68] The college has approximately 40 student clubs and academic societies through which students have volunteered thousands of hours. For its exemplary service to disadvantaged youth, the Lake Erie College of Osteopathic Medicine was named to the President's Higher Education Community Service Honor roll, the highest federal recognition a school can receive.

16 Boston University medical students participate in the Outreach Van Project.[69] Founded in 1997 by several students, the project provides services to the medically underserved population of Boston. The project provides basic necessities (food, clothing, toiletries, dental supplies, and medical care) and connects individuals to primary care and other community services, such as detoxification programs and shelters. Project Med Health, also started by students, educates public school children about key health issues and promotes healthy behaviors.

17 Several years ago, University of South Florida medical students donated considerable time to a charter middle school in an economically depressed area of Tampa.[70] Through the project USF STARS (Students Tutoring and Role Modeling Students), students tutored, organized a book drive, raised funds for school beautification, conducted an empowerment course for girls who have survived sexual abuse, and sponsored a health fair.

18 Service activities may begin as early as the first week of medical school. At the Georgetown University School of Medicine, a recent week-long orientation for new medical students ended with a Community Service Day on which students had the opportunity to participate in several different volunteer activities.[71]

19 At Duke University School of Medicine, the class received community service training on the second day of orientation.[72] This was followed by a trip to a local charter school where students spent the rest of the day painting the walls of the school in an effort to create a better learning environment for the children.

20 Orientation for the class of 2010 at the University of Rochester School of Medicine also included a community service project.[73] Students were divided into teams, and each team planned a recreational, social, or educational activity for children between the ages of 8 and 14.

References

[1]Temple University Communications. Available at: http://www.temple.edu/newsroom/2007_2008/08/stories/studentcommservice.htm. Accessed February 12, 2012.

[2]Seifer SD. Service-learning: community-campus partnerships for health professions education. *Acad Med* 1998; 73(3): 273-7.

[3]Liaison Committee on Medical Education (LCME) Available at: http://www.lcme.org/standard.htm#servicelearning. Accessed February 12, 2012.

[4]Duke University School of Medicine. Available at: https://community.duke.edu/news_events/stories/2005_stories/colormyworld_aug22_005.php. Accessed July 16, 2011.

[5]Association of American Medical Colleges. Available at: http://www.aamc.org/newsroom/pressrel/2008/enrollmentdata2008.pdf. Accessed July 23, 2011.

[6]American Academy of Family Physicians. Available at: http://www.aafp.org/online/en/home/publications/news/news-now/resident-student-focus/20081119med-school-enroll.html. Accessed February 12, 2012.

[7]Dartmouth Medical School. Available at: http://dms.dartmouth.edu/admissions/community_service/. Accessed February 12, 2012.

[8]University of Wisconsin School of Medicine and Public Health Community Service Programs. Available at: http://www.med.wisc.edu/education/md/community-service/opportunitiesforstudents/157. Accessed February 12, 2012.

[9]Thoits P, Hewitt L. Volunteer work and well-being. *Journal of Health and Social Behavior* 2001; 42(2): 115-31.

[10]Van Willigen M. Differential benefits of volunteering across the life course. *The Journals of Gerontology Series B: Psychological Sciences and Social Sciences* 2000; 55B(5): S308-S318.

[11]Rietschlin J. Voluntary association membership and psychological distress. *J Health Soc Behav* 1998; 39, 348-55.

[12]Minnesota Medicine. Available at: http://www.minnesotamedicine.com/PastIssues/PastIssues2008/December2008/ClinicalServiceDecember2008.aspx. Accessed February 12, 2002.

[13]West Virginia School of Medicine School of Medicine. Available at: http://medicine.hsc.wvu.edu/Students/Student-Profiles/MD-Degree/Kari-Geronilla-2014. Accessed February 12, 2012.

[14]Blue A, Geesey M, Sheridan M, Basco W. Performance outcomes associated with medical school community service. *Acad Med* 2006; 81 (10): S79-S82.

[15]Association of American Medical Colleges. 2007 Medical School Graduation Questionnaire: All Schools Report. Washington, DC: Assoc of American Medical Colleges Press; 2007.

[16]Parsi K, List J. Preparing medical students for the world: service learning and global health justice. *Medscape J Med* 2008; 10(11): 268.

[17]Varkey P, Peloquin J, Reed D, Lindor K, Harris I. Leadership curriculum in undergraduate medical education: a study of student and faculty perspectives. *Med Teach* 2009; 31(3): 244-50.

[18]Marshall University Community Leadership Scholarship. Available at: http://musom.marshall.edu/scholarships/communityleadership/. Accessed February 12, 2012.

[19]University of New Mexico Khatali Alumni Community Service Award. Available at: http://hsc.unm.edu/som/oss/Awards.shtml. Accessed February 12, 2012.

[20]Ohio State University School of Medicine Service-Learning Initiative. Available at: http://service-learning.osu.edu/excellence-in-community-service-and-scholarship.html. Accessed February 12, 2012.

[21]Weill Cornell Medical College. Available at: http://www.med.cornell.edu/education/admissions/cur_md_ser.html. Accessed February 12, 2012.

[22]NRMP 2010 Program Director Survey. Available at: http://www.nrmp.org/data/index.html. Accessed February 12, 2012.

[23]University of California Davis School of Medicine. Available at: http://www-med.ucdavis.edu/. Accessed September 12, 2011.

[24]American Medical Association Virtual Mentor. Available at: http://virtualmentor.ama-assn.org/2005/07/medu1-0507.html. Accessed February 12, 2012.

[25]Simpson S, Long J. Medical student-run health clinics: important contributors to patient care and medical education. *J Gen Intern Med* 2007; 22: 352-6.

[26]H.O.Y.A Clinic. Available at: http://hoyaclinic.som.georgetown.edu/The_HOYA_Clinic/The_HOYA_Clinic/index.html. Accessed February 12, 2012.

[27]Stanford School of Medicine Pacific Free Clinic. Available at: http://pacific.stanford.edu/. Accessed February 12, 2012.

[28]Colorado Coalition for the Homeless Stout Street Clinic. Available at: http://www.coloradocoalition.org/what_we_do/healthcare.aspx. Accessed February 12, 2012.

[29]North Texas Health & Science. Available at: http://www.hsc.unt.edu/news/documents/Quarterly_Fall2009_sm.pdf. Accessed February 12, 2012.

[30]American Medical Association Medical Student Section. Available at: http://www.ama-assn.org. Accessed February 12, 2012.

[31]AMA Alliance Project Bank. Available at: http://www.amaalliance.org/site/epage/40331_625.htm. Accessed February 12, 2012.

[32]AAMC Medicine in the Community Grant Program. Available at: http://www.aamc.org/about/awards/cfc/start.htm. Accessed February 12, 2012.

[33]Student National Medical Association. Available at: http://www.snma.org/index.php?pID=166. Accessed February 12, 2012.

[34]California Medical Association Foundation Medical Student Community Leadership Grant Program. Available at: http://www.thecmafoundation.org/projects/minigrant.asp. Accessed February 12, 2012.

[35]Massachusetts Medical Society. Available at:
http://www.massmed.org//AM/Template.cfm?Section=Home6. Accessed
February 12, 2012.
[36]American Medical Association Chapter Involvement Grant. Available at:
http://www.ama-assn.org/ama/pub/about-ama/our-people/member-groups-
sections/medical-student-section/community-service/frequently-asked-
questions-about-chapter-involvement.page. Accessed February 12, 2012.
[37]American Psychiatric Foundation Helping Hands Grant Program. Available
at: http://gm5-
apf.syscomservices.com/GrantAndAwards/Grants/HelpingHands.aspx.
Accessed February 12, 2012.
[38]Alpha Omega Alpha. Available at: http://www.alphaomegaalpha.org.
Accessed May 12, 2011.
[39]Cohen J. Eight Steps for starting a student-run clinic. *JAMA* 1995; 273: 434–
5.
[40]Society of Student-Run Free Clinics. Available at:
http://www.studentrunfreeclinics.org/index.php?option=com_content&view=ar
ticle&id=65&Itemid=144. Accessed February 12, 2012.
[41]The National Association of Free and Charitable Clinics. Available at:
http://www.freeclinics.us/. Accessed February 12, 2012.
[42]Volunteers in Medicine. Available at: http://www.volunteersinmedicine.org/.
Accessed February 12, 2012.
[43]Council of Osteopathic Student Government Presidents. Available at:
http://cosgp.aacom.org/. Accessed February 12, 2012.
[44]Ohio University College of Osteopathic Medicine. Available at:
www.oucom.ohiou.edu/. Accessed July 5, 2011.
[45]Student National Medical Association Member of the Year Award. Available
at: http://www.snma.org. Accessed May 16, 2011.
[46]American College of Emergency Physicians Medical Student Professionalism
and Service Award. Available at: http://www.acep.org/aboutus.aspx?id=22572.
Accessed February 12, 201.
[47]National Medical Fellowships. Available at: http://www.nmfonline.org/.
Accessed February 12, 2012.
[48]American Women's Medical Association Wilhelm/Frankowski Scholarship.
Available at: http://www.amwa-doc.org/page3-94/AwardsAndScholarship.
Accessed February 12, 2012.
[49]Monash/Mitchell Medical Student Scholarship. Available at:
http://www.nmfonline.org/programs-monash.php. Accessed February 12, 2012.
[50]Florida Medical Association Sanford A. Mullen, M.D. Award for Outstanding
Community Service. Available at:
http://www.flmedical.org/Mullen_Award.aspx. Accessed February 12, 2012.
[51]American Lung Association Volunteer Award. Available at:
http://www.lung.org/. Accessed February 12, 2012.
[52]American Academy of Family Physicians. Available at:
http://www.aafp.org/online/en/home/media/releases/2011newsreleases-
statements/fmig-poe.html. Accessed February 12, 2012.

[53]American Association of Physicians from India Distinguished Medical Student Award. Available at: http://aapiusa.org/members/awards-criteria.aspx. Accessed February 12, 2012.

[54]Albany Medical College. Available at: http://www.amc.edu/PR/PressRelease/08_27_07FP.html. Accessed February, 22, 2012.

[55]Texas A & M College of Medicine. Available at: http://medicine.tamhsc.edu/student-affairs/organizations/circus.html. Accessed February 22, 2012.

[56]Loyola University Chicago Stritch School of Medicine. Available at: http://www.stritch.luc.edu/depts/ophtha/education/ophthalmology_club.htm. Accessed February 22, 2012.

[57]University of Louisville School of Medicine. Available at: http://php.louisville.edu/news/news.php?news=602. Accessed February 22, 2012.

[58]Medical University of South Carolina. Available at: http://www.musc.edu/catalyst/archive/2001/co11-9national.htm. Accessed February 22, 2012.

[59]Tulane University School of Medicine. Available at: http://tulane.edu/government_affairs/upload/14_med.pdf10. Accessed February 22, 2012.

[60]Joan C. Edwards School of Medicine at Marshall University. Available at: http://www.marshallparthenon.com/news/med-students-earning-cash-for-community-service-1.1936252. Accessed February 22, 2012.

[61]University of Illinois College of Medicine at Rockford. Available at: http://rockford.medicine.uic.edu/. Accessed February 22, 2012.

[62]Philadelphia College of Osteopathic Medicine. Available at: http://www.pcom.edu/index.html. Accessed February 22, 2012.

[63]Wayne State University School of Medicine. Available at: http://home.med.wayne.edu/. Accessed February 22, 2012.

[64]New York College of Osteopathic Medicine. Available at: http://www.nyit.edu/nycom/. Accessed February 22, 2012.

[65]Penn State College of Medicine. Available at: http://med.psu.edu/web/md/studentaffairs/studentlife/communityservice. Accessed February 22, 2012.

[66]SUNY Upstate Medical University. Available at: http://www.upstate.edu/publicaffairs/public_media/?id=1306.htm. Accessed February 22, 2012.

[67]University of New Mexico School of Medicine. Available at: http://hsc.unm.edu/som/. Accessed February 22, 2012.

[68]Lake Erie College of Osteopathic Medicine. Available at: http://lecom.edu/. Accessed February 22, 2012.

[69]Boston University School of Medicine. Available at: http://www.bumc.bu.edu/. Accessed February 22, 2012.

[70]University of South Florida College of Medicine. Available at: http://hscweb3.hsc.usf.edu/health/now/?p=141. Accessed February 22, 2012.

[71]Georgetown University School of Medicine. Available at: http://som.georgetown.edu/. Accessed February 22, 2012.

[72]Duke University School of Medicine. Available at:
http://medschool.duke.edu/. Accessed February 22, 2012.
[73]University of Rochester School of Medicine. Available at:
http://www.urmc.rochester.edu/smd/. Accessed February 22, 2012.

Chapter 10

Mentoring

12 Ways to Find a Mentor in Medical School

The further we've progressed in our own careers, the more it becomes apparent how many individuals have helped us along the way. To achieve professional success in almost any field requires help. This may not be initially obvious to medical students, who are used to studying hard and achieving high grades on their own. However, just getting accepted to med school required assistance. Professors who provided help outside of the classroom, researchers who offered the opportunity to participate in their project, advisors who provided letters of recommendation: the list goes on.

Succeeding in medical school, and succeeding in the residency match itself, requires even more assistance. At this next stage of your career, informed guidance and advice becomes even more important. For more competitive specialties or programs, you'll also require additional qualifications, which may mean approaching faculty members for research opportunities, in addition to the critically important letters of recommendation.

The definition of a mentor is one who "takes a special interest in helping another person develop into a successful professional."[1]

Mentor relationships can prove vital in medical school and match success. However, identifying a potential mentor, and then developing an effective relationship, can be very difficult. It's difficult to know how to proceed. Students often hesitate to impose on faculty members who are already clearly very busy. While this is understandable, it's also true that there are faculty at every medical school who find mentoring and advising students both enjoyable and rewarding, and who take these responsibilities seriously. While these individuals are sometimes recognized publicly for their work, it's more typical that they get their work done diligently but quietly. As a student, it should be your goal to identify these motivated, dedicated individuals. Information, advice, and guidance from a knowledgeable faculty member is invaluable, and has the potential to impact your career in significant ways. Since it can be so difficult and intimidating to know how to even start developing such a relationship, we've provided some suggestions.

1 Some medical schools have formal mentoring programs. If such a program doesn't exist at your school, then you'll need confidence and possibly persistence to initiate a relationship. In one study, 28% of students met their mentors during inpatient clerkships, 19% through research activities, and 9% during outpatient clerkships.[2]

2 Consider your basic science lecturers. If you're particularly impressed with a lecturer, you can contact him or her. You can also stop by at the end of the lecture. "I really enjoyed your lecture and find the work that you're doing interesting. Would it be possible for me to meet with you to discuss ways in which I might become involved?"

3 Your clinical preceptor may be an excellent choice. During the preclinical years, you may be assigned to a clinical preceptor in family medicine, internal medicine, or pediatrics. You may also encounter clinicians through Physical Diagnosis and Introduction to Clinical Medicine courses. Dr. Ryan VanWoerkom, an internal medicine resident at Oregon Health Sciences University, recalled how he met his mentor in medical school.[3] In the second-year class "Doctor-Patient Relationship," Ryan was randomly assigned to his preceptor, Dr. Adler. "Dr. Adler was a gastroenterologist who had recently moved to Utah who I was eager to meet. Unfortunately, I had a sports-related traumatic brain injury and was in the hospital during my first scheduled appointment for this preceptorship! Dr. Adler was very understanding and accommodating and took me under his wing. He reminisced about his medical school days and internship experiences with fondness. He remained very interested in my education. I expressed interest in research and he mentioned that he would have a few opportunities available down the road. Two years later we were coauthors on three papers, two posters, and an up-and-coming book chapter."

4 Joining a special interest group is another way to locate a mentor. The University of Texas Medical School at San Antonio has established its Longitudinal Surgical Mentorship Program to link new students with surgical mentors from Day 1 of medical school.[4]

5 Local, regional, and state medical societies may have established mentoring programs. These organizations often have social events where members can network with one another. The Santa Clara County Medical Association has a Mentor Program for Stanford medical students.[5]

6 National organizations are committed to mentoring future doctors. The American Academy of Dermatology (AAD) has a Diversity Medical Student Mentorship program.[6] The program allows students from "ethnically and socioeconomically diverse backgrounds to gain exposure to the specialty of dermatology by providing a firsthand, one-on-one mentorship experience with the dermatologist of the student's choice." Emergency Medicine is another field where national organizations provide mentoring opportunities. There are over 2,000 osteopathic emergency medicine physicians, and the American College of Osteopathic Emergency Physicians (ACOEP) has established a mentor program for students.[7]

7 Your dean can be a great resource. Dr. Chris Pelic, Associate Dean for Students at the Medical University of South Carolina, writes that his "job is to help get students from orientation to graduation. More specifically, I serve as a mentor, supervisor, and teacher for the students."[8] Deans can also recommend specific faculty members based on your interests and goals.

8 Senior medical students and residents are very insightful. Ask about good mentors, and why they think highly of these particular faculty members.

9 Your medical school's website may have faculty bios. You can read through these to see if there's a match between the faculty member's interests and yours.

10 Your Student Affairs or Curriculum Office may have a list of course and clerkship directors. Schedule an appointment with a director in your area of interest. The director may prove to be a potential mentor, or may refer you to others in the department.

11 Your school's Alumni Association may be able to put you in contact with mentors. The Alumni Association at the University of Utah has a Mentor Program for students.[9] By partnering with alumni physicians in the Salt Lake City area, the program allows medical students the opportunity to meet mentors who can share their perspective of the practice of medicine and their specialty.

12 Some schools lack residency programs in certain specialties. That poses obvious difficulties for students applying to that specialty. One option would be to seek advisors elsewhere, and local or national organizations may provide assistance. The Society of Academic Emergency Medicine (SAEM) has a medical student virtual advisor program open to students at all institutions.[10] Through this program, students can query experienced individuals about a variety of issues, including the EM residency application process. Recognizing the importance of mentorship, the Student Doctor Network (SDN) has launched an innovative mentorship program as well.[11] Dr. Joshua Grossman reminds students that mentors don't have to be in close proximity to you. "Your mentor does not need to be someone involved with your residency program that you see on a daily basis. By sharing your experience with someone removed from the situation you may be able to gain a different and beneficial perspective.[12]

10 Qualities of a Good Mentee

1 Dr. Gail Rose, a faculty member in the Department of Psychiatry at the University of Vermont, has written extensively about mentoring in medical school. She reminds students to "be punctual." If you're unable to meet at the designated time, let your mentor know as soon as possible.[13]

2 Respect your mentor's time. Be flexible with meeting times, and come prepared so that both of you can make the most of the available time. The Association of Women Surgeons writes "A mentor is a unique individual to you: neither friend, nor colleague, but something of a combination of these and more. Because the relationship differs from those you have with others in your department, you may feel more relaxed and less constrained by professional protocol. This is acceptable to a point, but make certain that you respect the relationship."[14]

3 Determine how your mentor prefers to be contacted. The University of Washington Department of Family Medicine writes that "the relationship will do best if both agree on how to communicate and how often to communicate. It is important that both work to ensure that contact happens and they have goals or questions to discuss."[15]

4 If you're working on a project with your mentor, complete all assignments. Meet all deadlines, and if at all possible, strive to beat all deadlines.

5 Be open to constructive criticism. Use this feedback to improve your skills. Dr. Zerzan, a faculty member in the Department of Internal Medicine at the University of Colorado Denver School of Medicine, offers this advice. "Although a mentee should put forth his or her own ideas, it is critical that he or she not get defensive or argumentative when the mentor disagrees or provides constructive feedback. The relationship's ultimate goal is to help the mentee succeed, and the mentor has the mentee's best interests in mind."[16]

6 As your relationship grows, your mentor may share confidential information with you. Consider this privileged information, and don't share it with others.

7 Send periodic updates to your mentor about your progress. A quick email is often sufficient. This is an area often neglected by students who are busy with coursework, but "sharing experiences and important milestones are vital in maintaining a relationship – if a mentor is only sought 'when needed' there is the potential for them to feel 'unwanted.'"[17]

8 Meet regularly to maintain and strengthen the relationship. In her presentation, "Getting the most out of the mentor-mentee relationship," Dr. Eva Aagaard encourages mentees to discuss and determine the frequency, duration, and content of meetings.[18]

9 Before the meeting, let your mentor know the items or issues you would like to discuss. Among the issues you can discuss are those related to specialty choice, career satisfaction, wellness, work/life balance, residency selection process, research, ethics, and courses. Once they have a firm idea of career choice, many students schedule meetings to discuss match strategy, seeking advice on steps they can take at their level to establish their credentials and strengthen their applications. Show your mentor that you value his or her time by setting a clear agenda and goals for the meeting. Don't be the ill-prepared student who simply asks, "What should I do now?"

10 Thank your mentor after every meeting by sending a quick thank-you note or email. If you feel that your mentor has been exceptional, consider nominating him or her for an institutional or national mentoring award.

15 Questions to Ask Yourself When Searching for a Good Mentor

1 Is he generally interested in student education?

2 Is she approachable and easily accessible?

3 Is he dependable and reliable?

4 Is she experienced in mentoring?

5 Is he resourceful?

6 Is she willing to share her own experiences and knowledge with you?

7 Is he a good listener?

8 Is she enthusiastic?

9 Has he taken an active interest in mentoring other students?

10 Will she be honest with you?

11 Will he maintain your confidence?

12 Does she treat people with respect?

13 Is he highly professional in all interactions?

14 Will she be sensitive to your needs?

15 Will he have your best interests in mind?

Initiating a Relationship with a Mentor

Sometimes the hardest part of initiating an effective relationship is just knowing how to get started. You'll be approaching respected, accomplished, busy individuals, and it can be difficult to know how to approach faculty members without appearing intrusive or presumptuous. For most students, asking for help from individuals in a position of authority can be intimidating. As a preclinical student, you also may have had limited experience in dealing with faculty on an individual level, and knowing what's acceptable can be hard to determine. Therefore, we provide our own advice and advice from faculty experienced in this area. These approaches would be considered acceptable and non-intrusive by most faculty.

1 Consider faculty you come into contact with as lecturers, small-group facilitators, and clinical preceptors, and approach them directly. If you're particularly impressed with a faculty member, you can stop by at the end of the session and say, "I really enjoyed your [lecture] and the work that you're doing. Can I arrange a meeting with you to learn more about your work and how I might become involved?"

2 It is acceptable to send a brief email to initiate the contact. Dr. Megan Fix encourages students to send an email stating, "I am very interested in your [research or specialty or lecture topic]. I wonder if we could set up a time to meet and talk about opportunities for me to get involved."[19] While some students are hesitant, remember that many students have received invaluable opportunities and guidance through this simple approach. At the worst, you'll receive no response.

3 Before the scheduled meeting, reconfirm the time and location of the meeting with the potential mentor or her administrative assistant.

4 Learn as much as you can about your potential mentor. Read his bio, perform a PubMed search to learn about his research, and speak with others to understand how he interacts with students during rounds. Make note of his teaching awards, recognition for mentoring, and areas of clinical expertise. Give considerable thought as to why you would like this particular faculty member to be your mentor. Reflect on your interests, needs, and goals, and consider how these may be met or furthered by establishing a mentor-mentee relationship.

5 Arrive on time, and dressed for success. First impressions absolutely matter.

6 Convey your appreciation for the meeting.

7 Review your background and share your goals.

8 Listen attentively, and ask insightful questions.

9 You don't need to use the word "mentor", and in fact you may not wish to. Many believe that mentor relationships should develop organically as you continue to work together. If your potential mentor is impressed with your qualifications, or with the quality of your work [if working together on a research project, for example], and if their schedule permits, they'll often offer more assistance. While this will develop over time, at this initial meeting you should begin by asking if he or she would be willing to advise you.

10 Immediately following the meeting, send a thank-you note or email. If the faculty member is overcommitted, unreceptive, or not a good fit or match for you, you can also ask if he or she is able to recommend other potential advisors.

Mentoring: 10 Important Points

1 Finding the right mentor can be difficult. Even when a formal system for assigning mentors exists, this doesn't necessarily mean that the mentor will be the right fit for the student. Should this happen, you should seek guidance from other faculty members. Expect to invest considerable time, effort, and energy in selecting a mentor.

2 In your initial contact with a potential mentor, seek to answer several questions. Is this someone with whom I'm comfortable? Does he or she have the time to meet with a mentee? Do they have the required expertise?

3 If you begin a mentoring relationship but find that it fails to meet your needs, seek out others who are a better fit. It often takes considerable time and effort to identify the right individuals.

4 Few mentors have the answers to every question, and it's often to your advantage to have several opinions on certain issues. Having more than one perspective can be valuable in helping you make an informed decision. In addition, your interests are likely to evolve as you progress through the curriculum, and you may need the expertise of other mentors.

5 You don't have to choose the most prestigious academic faculty member or one who's a triple threat (accomplished researcher, clinician, and educator). Your mentor can be a full-time researcher, a community physician, a retired physician, or an administrator. If you sense that your potential mentor will be knowledgeable, responsive to your needs, invested in the mentoring relationship, and accessible to you, he or she should be seriously considered. Dr. Megan Fix writes that "your mentor does not have to be the most respected person in their field, but they must be someone you can talk to and be honest with about your goals."[19]

6 The Association of Women Surgeons emphasizes the importance of "personal fit." "A personal fit is important in a mentor since differences in values can seriously undermine a mentoring relationship. You will need to be able to identify with the attributes of your mentor."[20]

7 Gender is an important issue for some medical students, and in some cases may be factored into the decision-making process. Research has shown, however, that role models of either gender can be effective mentors for both male and female students.[21] What is typically far more important is how you communicate or relate to one another. However, some female medical students seek out the wisdom of female mentors who have personally dealt with issues unique or specific to women. One female medical student found it challenging to obtain advice on work-life balance as a woman physician. "My male mentors have emphasized how much they sacrificed and how many hours they worked presumably while their spouse took care of their household. Can I find someone who can give me reasonable advice on how to keep my professional aspirations while also managing my other responsibilities?"[22] We should caution you, though, not to jump to any conclusions based on gender. Many women physicians have valuable advice to give on the issue of work-life balance. Others, particularly if they're in a residency match decision-making role, may view students who emphasize work-life balance over professional contributions in a negative light.

8 Medical students may also be effective mentors. Some schools have formal peer mentoring programs, like the University of Connecticut's big brother/big sister program.[23] In this program, a second-year student is paired with a first-year student to help ease the transition to medical school. When I was a third-year medical student interested in dermatology, I received invaluable advice from two fourth-year medical students who had chosen on their own to help other students. Their advice was spot-on, and definitely made a difference.

9 In researching our companion book, *The Successful Match: 200 Rules to Succeed in the Residency Match*, we asked applicants what they found most difficult about the residency application process. A number of applicants commented on the same issue. "There's so much conflicting information out there. How do you know what to believe? Who should you listen to?" Applicants with mentors have a decided advantage. Students benefit greatly when the wisdom, experience, and perspective of a knowledgeable faculty member are used to help them achieve a successful match. Having a mentor to guide you through the complex residency application process is recognized by students as an important factor in boosting the strength of their application.

10 As you consider possible mentors, you should be aware of problems that can occur in the mentor-mentee relationship. Chief among these is the potential conflict of interest that can occur with a mentor who advises a student and also serves on the residency selection committee at a program affiliated with the student's medical school. In a survey of 740 graduating medical students from 10 U.S. medical schools, Miller found that nearly half met with their advisors during or following the interview season.[24] In these meetings, 31.8% were encouraged to rank the advisor's program highly, 10.3% were asked which programs they planned to rank highly, and 4% were asked how they planned to rank the advisor's program. Not surprisingly, students reported varying degrees of discomfort due to these questions. One respondent stated that "it felt very uncomfortable to talk to him about my own strengths and weaknesses and about which programs I preferred knowing that he would later be evaluating me in comparison with other applicants and deciding whether or not to advocate for me to be accepted."

Mentoring Programs for Under-represented Minority Medical Students

Although racial and ethnic minorities comprise over 25% of the U.S. population, only 6% of physicians in practice are of African-American, Native American, or Hispanic descent.[25] Under-represented minority physicians (URM) comprise a very small percentage of U.S. medical school faculty (< 5%), and one-fifth of URM faculty are concentrated at six schools.[26] Minority medical students may find it difficult to identify mentors of their own race or background. Although majority mentors can serve minority students well, Bickel wrote that "even well-intentioned majority mentors may be unaware of the disadvantages URMs continue to experience such as heightened pressures to serve their community [i.e., the 'black tax'], feeling socially unwelcome, being identified by appearance rather than abilities, and being assumed to represent an entire race."[22] In this section, we offer recommendations on how minority medical students can establish mentoring relationships with both majority and minority physicians.

1 Medical schools often have well-established mentoring programs for minority medical students.

2 The Student National Medical Association (SNMA) is an organization that provides support and resources for under-represented minority medical students.[27] Mentoring programs may be available through the national organization or your school chapter.

3 The Latino Medical Student Association offers support through its national organization and school chapters.[28]

4 The Association of Native American Medical Students provides a resource network for all Native Americans enrolled in health professions schools.[29]

5 Attending the SNMA Annual Conference may expose you to mentors. At a recent conference, the American Academy of Orthopedic Surgeons had a very active exhibit. Physician members of the AAOS "greeted students, engaged them in conversation, handed out diversity-related articles and mentoring program brochures, and encouraged medical students to apply to mentoring programs sponsored by the AAOS, the Ruth Jackson Orthopedic Society, and the J. Robert Gladden Orthopedic Society."[30]

6 The American Academy of Dermatology has a Diversity Mentorship program for first- through fourth-year medical students considered to be under-represented in medicine.[31]

7 The American Psychiatric Association has a Minority Medical Student Summer Mentoring Program for minority students interested in exploring psychiatry.[32]

8 Some national organizations offer research awards to minority medical students, and mentors may be identified through such experiences. In 2011, the American Society of Hematology selected 11 participants for its Minority Medical Student Award Program. "Each of the first- or second-year medical students selected for this award will receive personalized support from a research mentor and a career-development mentor, travel stipends to attend the ASH annual meeting, and a subscription to *Blood*, the official scientific journal of ASH."[33]

9 The *Journal for Minority Medical Students* is an excellent resource to help you identify physician mentors.[34]

10 Dr. Karen Hamilton, Assistant Dean of Multicultural Affairs at the University of Pennsylvania, encourages students to visit their school's Office of Minority/Multicultural Affairs.[35] The "staff might also provide you with the names of faculty or practicing physicians in the community who could be your potential mentors and could give you advice about choosing a specialty and residency program. Another way to meet people who could potentially provide support is to join one of your school's minority student organizations like the SNMA, Boricua Latino Health Organization, or the American Indian Medical Student Organization."

References

[1]Adviser, teacher, role model, friend. Available at: http://stills.nap.edu/readingroom/books/mentor. Accessed March 13, 2008. Washington, DC: National Academy Press; 1997.

[2]Aagaard E, Hauer K. A cross-sectional descriptive study of mentoring relationships formed by medical students. *J Gen Intern Med* 2003; 18: 298-302.

[3]American College of Physicians. Medical student perspectives: find a mentor that is right for you. Available at: http://www.acponline.org/medical_students/impact/archives/2010/07/perspect/. Accessed February 9, 2012.

[4]University of Texas Medical School at San Longitudinal Surgical Mentorship Program. Available at: http://surgery.uthscsa.edu/education/students/index.asp. Accessed February 9, 2012.

[5]Santa Clara County Medical Association Mentor Program for Stanford medical students. Available at: http://med.stanford.edu/mentors/ Accessed February 9, 2012.

[6]American Academy of Dermatology (AAD) Diversity Medical Student Mentorship program. Available at: http://www.aad.org/member-tools-and-benefits/residents-and-fellows/diversity-mentorship-program-information-for-medical-students. Accessed February 9, 2012.

[7]American College of Osteopathic Emergency Physicians (ACOEP) mentor program for students. Available at: http://www.acoep.org/. Accessed February 9, 2012.

[8]Medical University of South Carolina. Available at: http://academicdepartments.musc.edu/com/contact/GASA.htm. Accessed February 9, 2012.

[9]University of Utah The Mentor Program. Available at: http://medicine.utah.edu/alumni/volunteer/mentor.htm. Accessed February 9, 2012.

[10]Society of Academic Emergency Medicine (SAEM). Available at: http://www.saem.org/e-advising-faqs-students. Accessed February 9, 2012.

[11] Student Doctor Network. Available at: http://studentdoctor.net/. Accessed February 9, 2012.

[12]American College of Physicians. Finding the right mentor for you. Available at: http://www.acponline.org/medical_students/impact/archives/2010/11/feature/. Accessed February 9, 2012.

[13]Rose G, Rukstalis M, and Schuckit M. Informal mentoring between faculty and medical students. *Acad Med* 2005; 80: 344-8.

[14]Association of Women Surgeons. Available at: https://www.womensurgeons.org/CDR/Mentorship.asp. Accessed February 9, 2012.

[15]University of Washington Department of Family Medicine. Available at: http://depts.washington.edu/fammed/predoc/programs/upath/FAQs/mentorFAQ Accessed February 9, 2012

[16]Zerzan J, Hess R, Schur E, Phillips R, Rigotti N. Making the most of mentors: a guide for mentees. *Acad Med* 2009; 84(1): 140-4.

[17]Australian Medical Student Association. Available at: http://www.amsa.org.au/content/finding-mentor. Accessed February 9, 2012.

[18]Getting the most out of the mentor-mentee relationship. Available at: http://www.ucdenver.edu/academics/colleges/medicalschool/departments/medi cine/GIM/education/ContinuingEducation/Documents/TMC%202010-2011/8-10-2010_AagaardE.pdf. Accessed February 9, 2012.

[19]Medscape. How can I find a mentor? Available at: http://www.medscape.com/viewarticle/549189. Accessed February 9, 2012.

[20]Association of Women Surgeons. Available at: http://www.womensurgeons.org/home/index.asp. Accessed February 9, 2012.

[21]Ferris L, Mackinnon S, Mizgala C, et al. Do Canadian female surgeons feel discriminated against as women? *Can Med Assoc J* 1996; 154(1): 21-7.

[22]Bickel J, Rosenthal S. Difficult issues in mentoring: recommendations on making the "undiscussable" discussable. *Acad Med* 2011; 86(10): 1229-34.

[23]University of Connecticut School of Medicine Mentoring Programs. Available at: http://medicine.uchc.edu/current/mentoring/index.html. Accessed February 9, 2012.

[24]Miller J, Schaad D, Crittenden R, Oriol N. The departmental advisor's effect on medical students' confidence when the advisor evaluates or recruits for their own program during the match. *Teach Learn Med* 2004; 16(3): 290-5.

[25]AAMC Minorities in Medical Education: Facts and Figures 2005. Available at: https://www.aamc.org/. Accessed February 9, 2012.

[26]American Medical Student Association. Available at: http://www.amsa.org/AMSA/Homepage/about/priorities/diversity.aspx. Accessed February 9, 2012.

[27]Student National Medical Association. Available at: http://www.snma.org/. Accessed February 9, 2012.

[28]Latino Medical Student Association. Available at: http://lmsa.net/. Accessed February 9, 2012.

[29]Association of Native American Medical Students. Available at: http://www.anamstudents.org/. Accessed February 9, 2012.

[30]American Academy of Orthopaedic Surgeons. Available at: http://www.aaos.org/news/bulletin/aug07/youraaos8.asp. Accessed March 29, 2011.

[31]American Academy of Dermatology. Available at: http://www.aad.org/. Accessed February 9, 2012.

[32]American Psychiatric Association. Available at: http://www.psych.org/. Accessed February 9, 2012.

[33]American Society of Hematology. Available at: http://www.hematology.org/. Accessed February 9, 2012.

[34]Journal for Minority Medical Students. Available at: http://www.spectrumpublishers.com/magazine.php?id=2. Accessed February 9, 2012.

[35]American Medical Association. Getting ready: medical school years 1-3. Available at: http://www.ama-assn.org/ama/pub/about-ama/our-people/member-groups-sections/minority-affairs-section/transitioning-residency/getting-ready-medical-school-years-1.page. Accessed February 9, 2012.

Chapter 11

Well-Being

Physicians, unfortunately, will commonly encounter stress throughout their medical career. In many cases, stress is associated with psychological morbidity, including depression, anxiety, and substance abuse. In addition to causing significant emotional distress, there is a real concern that mental illness in physicians can affect patient care. "The great worry is that if a physician has a mental illness that in any way impairs judgment or the ability to be objective, the potential exists for patients to be injured," says Dr. Morton Silverman, psychiatrist and former Director of the Suicide Prevention Resource Center, in an interview with Medscape.[1]

A recent study of pediatric residents highlighted this concern. Twenty percent of participants met criteria for depression, and these residents made over six times as many medication errors as their non-depressed colleagues.[2]

Physicians' stress clearly begins during medical training. While the clinical years of medical school are considered to be more stressful, studies have shown that students experience a significant amount of stress during the preclinical years as well. This increased stress in medical school may lead to stress-associated depression, anxiety, and substance abuse.

Since stress is prevalent among students, it's important that students be aware of the stressors associated with medical school and the consequences on personal health. Most importantly, students must learn effective ways to manage stress. Dr. Liselotte Dyrbye, a faculty member at the Mayo Clinic, has performed extensive research in this area. She states that medical students need to have "the skills necessary to assess personal distress, determine its effects on their care of patients, recognize when they need assistance, and develop strategies to promote their own well-being. These skills are essential to maintain perspective, professionalism, and resilience through the course of a career..."[3]

Medical Student Emotional Well-Being: 10 Surprising Statistics

1 Stress is common among medical students. Studies have shown that students experience considerable stress right from the start of medical school. In a survey of medical students at 16 U.S. schools, 60% of first-year students reported either "moderate" or "a lot" of stress in the last two weeks.[4] Nearly 70% reported experiencing either "moderate" or "a lot" of stress in the last twelve months.

2 Recently, researchers reported the results of a study assessing depressive symptoms in students at six medical schools. Probable depression was identified in nearly 25% of students.[5] In a survey of first and second-year medical students at the University of Pennsylvania, 24% were found to be depressed using the Beck Depression Inventory.[6]

3 Over a two-year period, Dr. Laurie Raymond, Director of the Office of Advising Resources at Harvard Medical School, met with 208 medical students (approximately 25% of the student body). "Fifteen percent presented with self-described depression."[7]

4 In one study, new medical students at the University of Massachusetts were surveyed prior to matriculation and then again in the second and fourth years.[8] At the time of matriculation, students' emotional status was no different than that of the general population. However, depression scores rose over time, with women having more significant increases than men.

5 In a study done at the LSU School of Medicine in New Orleans, students were worse off psychologically at the end of the first year than when they entered.[9] In particular, positive mood decreased while negative mood, defined as depression and hostility, increased. In a study of Rush Medical College students using the Beck Depression Inventory, median scores increased threefold from the time of matriculation to the end of second year, with 25% of the class showing considerable depressive or dysphoric symptoms.[10]

6Attrition rates in medical school have ranged from 3 to 6%, with nearly half of students dropping out for nonacademic reasons.[11-14] In a large, multi-institutional study, 11% of students had given serious consideration to dropping out within the last year.[15]

7 Medical students are not immune to the personal life stressors that others experience. In a study of preclinical students at Jefferson Medical College, 42% reported financial problems, 36% had dealt with a change of health in a relative, 25% had suffered a personal injury or illness, and 15% had experienced a death in the family over the preceding year.[16] A more recent survey of students at three medical schools found that 37% had experienced at least one major negative personal life event in the previous 12 months.[3] These events included divorce, major personal illness, major illness of a loved one, and death in the family.

8 Burnout is characterized by emotional depletion from one's work, depersonalization, and the perception that one's work is inconsequential. In a survey of medical students in Minnesota, 45% had burnout.[3]

9 In longitudinal studies of medical student anxiety, baseline anxiety scores showed no major differences between men and women. Through the course of the first year, though, anxiety levels rose higher among women than men.[17-19]

10 The suicide rate among male and female physicians is higher than that of the general population. When compared to women in the general population, the suicide rate is 130% higher among female physicians.[20] In a survey of over 2000 medical students, suicidal ideation over the past year was reported by 11.2%.[21] This is considerably higher than the 6.9% rate reported for the 25-34 year old age group in the general population.[22] In a survey of 101 US medical schools, researchers learned that 15 suicides occurred between the academic years 1989 – 1994.[23]

10 Perceived Barriers That Prevent Medical Students from Accessing Mental Health Counseling, Along with the Truth About These Perceptions

Although stress and depression are common in medical school, relatively few students seek help from support services provided by their school. In a survey done at the University of Pennsylvania School of Medicine, only 22% of students with self-reported depression accessed mental health services.[6] Barriers to treatment include:

1 Lack of time. Students are often under the assumption that counseling or treatment is time-intensive. However, many treatment plans involve short-term psychotherapy with or without antidepressant medication.

2 Lack of confidentiality. To maintain confidentiality and privacy, some schools have created websites that allow students to anonymously screen themselves for depression and communicate with counselors. The ensuing dialogue has made it easier for some students to take the next step (i.e., meet face-to-face with counselors or arrange for confidential counseling services). Through these anonymous communications, students also learn that HIPAA guidelines prevent confidential health information from being disclosed to others without the patient's permission. Recognizing that confidentiality is a major barrier, some schools have placed student mental health support services off campus. The Medical College of Wisconsin allows students to "see psychologists or psychiatrists that are not directly involved in medical educating, thereby limiting problems with confidentiality."[24]

3 Concern that "No one will be able to understand my problems." Stress, depression, and anxiety are, unfortunately, common among medical students. Over a two-year period, Dr. Laurie Raymond, Director of the Office of Advising Resources at Harvard Medical School, met with 208 medical students (approximately 25% of the student body). "Fifteen percent presented with self-described depression."[7]

4 Stigma associated with using mental health services. Medical schools are increasingly addressing stress and depression, and their consequences, during orientation. Medical school leaders and deans are encouraging students to maintain their personal well-being during medical school and to seek help if needed.

5 Feeling that "My problems are not important." Stress is common among physicians throughout their medical career, and is associated with psychological morbidity, including depression, anxiety, and substance abuse. In addition to causing significant emotional distress, there is a real concern that mental illness in physicians can affect patient care. A recent study of pediatric residents highlighted this concern. Twenty percent of participants met criteria for depression, and these residents made over six times as many medication errors as their non-depressed colleagues.[2] Since stress is prevalent, it's important for students to be aware of the stressors of medical school and the consequences of stress on personal health. Most importantly, students must learn effective ways to manage stress.

6 Cost. At some schools, counseling and mental health services are provided free of charge. Up to 12 sessions of free psychiatric counseling are offered to students at the Baylor College of Medicine.[24]

7 Fear that "Using services will mean that I am weak." In an article published in the AAMC Reporter, one student described the difficulty she experienced seeking help for her depressive symptoms.[25] Initially, she was scared to seek help. "If the medical school knew that I had this depression, I thought they'd think I was a sub-par student and that I wasn't qualified to become a doctor." After eventually undergoing effective treatment, she even started a peer group where students could discuss these issues with one another. "This gives me the confidence to know I am not the only one out there with these issues – it's not that everyone else is excelling and I alone am underachieving."

9 Fear of documentation on academic record. Dr. Holly Crisp-Han has extensive experience in the evaluation and treatment of medical students and residents in the Baylor Student and Housestaff Counseling Center. She also conducts workshops for physicians on burnout, professionalism, and balancing work and family. She states that "students are often fearful that if they seek treatment their problems will be documented in their academic record, or that their residency matching and medical licensing will be impacted. Unfortunately, the impact of not seeking necessary treatment has much greater long-term consequences on medical careers and personal lives. In general, disclosure of one's feelings and experiences in the context of a specific treatment relationship with a psychiatrist, psychologist, or social worker is a confidential and protected relationship. One's medical records and confidential treatment cannot be disclosed to the Dean without specific release from the student to do so, unless there is a life-threatening emergency situation."[26]

10 Difficulty with access to care / lack of availability of services. In a recent survey of U.S. medical schools, 100% of respondents indicated the availability of mental health services for medical students.[27]

16 Stressors of Medical School Ranked from Most to Least Stressful

In a survey of 71 medical students, Wolf asked students to rate medical school stressors on a scale of 1 (not stressful) to 7 (extremely stressful).[28] The results are shown below, ranked from most to least stressful.

1 Examinations

2 Amount of class work

3 Financial responsibilities

4 Lack of time for recreation and entertainment

5 Patient care

6 Relationships with clinical supervisors

7 Peer competition

8 Fear of failure in medical school

9 Personal psychological health

10 Sleep

11 Exercise

12 Personal physical health

13 Nutrition

14 Sex

15 Relationships with classroom instructors

16 Relationships with roommate

Coping Strategies in Medical School: 7 Important Points

1 Students respond to stressors in different ways. Dr. Laura Dunn, a psychiatrist at the University of California San Francisco, writes that "at matriculation, some individuals have more coping reserve than others; some students are inherently more resilient, with greater buffering ability; others are more susceptible to anxiety or depression. The latter group of students may experience even small stressors as major threats or crises."[29]

2 Without the "right" coping strategies in place, these stressors can have negative effects on students, adversely affecting academic performance and health and making them more prone to the development of depression and anxiety. While stress cannot be avoided, your coping mechanisms will help determine whether stress will have a net positive or negative effect.

3 What is your stress tolerance threshold? If you've had difficulties coping with stress in the past, you'll need to be proactive and plan how you'll manage the stress of the preclinical years.

4 One effective coping strategy is problem-focused coping, in which efforts are made to solve or manage the problem causing the distress. This coping strategy is most effective in situations where you have at least some degree of control. The steps involved in problem-focused coping include:[30]

- Take responsibility for solving the problem
- Seek and obtain accurate information
- Utilize available resources for dependable advice and help
- Develop a reasonable action plan
- Follow through on the action plan
- Maintain optimism in one's capacity to solve the problem

5 Emotion-focused coping is another effective strategy. Some stressful situations are mostly, if not completely, out of your control. With these types of stressors, your only option may be to manage the emotional response that is associated with the stressful situation. This is called emotion-focused coping. Examples include seeking support and assistance from members of your support group, venting emotions with classmates, reframing of thoughts, utilizing humor when dealing with stressful situations, incorporating relaxation routines, and engaging in physical exercise.

6 Coping strategies that involve avoidance have been shown to be harmful to emotional and physical health. Examples include the denial or suppression of feelings or thoughts, or actual disengagement. Students who utilize these maladaptive coping strategies over the long term may be at higher risk for the development of depression and anxiety. Other maladaptive strategies include:

- Problem avoidance: not dealing with the problem situation, hoping that it'll simply go away
- Wishful thinking: hoping that the problem resolves on its own
- Social withdrawal: distancing oneself from the problem situation as well as those who might be able to help, such as friends or family
- Self-criticism: excessive preoccupation with one's inability to handle the problem situation
- Distraction: using food, entertainment, alcohol, or drugs to avoid dealing with the problem

7 As a new medical student, it's helpful to learn about how you typically cope with issues. In 1997, Charles Carver, a professor at the University of Miami, developed the brief COPE questionnaire, which can be used as a tool to help determine the coping strategies that you tend to use.[31] If your total scores are higher in the coping strategy categories of self-distraction, denial, substance abuse, or self-blame, you'll need to learn how to develop and use healthier and more effective coping skills. Dr. Julie Gentile, Director of Medical Student Mental Health Services at the Boonshoft School of Medicine at Wright State University, states that medical school "is a critical period in which to develop and utilize functional and effective coping strategies."[32]

To Move or Not To Move: Exercise in Medical School

Medical students recognize the importance of exercise in the maintenance of health. Most students also understand the power of regular exercise in reducing tension, aiding concentration, easing frustration, and increasing a sense of well-being.

1 Numerous studies support these benefits. Dimeo found that mood is improved with regular exercise, an effect that was seen even for people with major depression.[33]

2 Exercise has also been shown to be a protective factor, mitigating the negative impact of stressful life events on physical and psychological health.[34]

3 In a cross-sectional study of students at a single medical school, approximately 77% suffered some degree of anxiety. Anxiety symptoms were considerably less common in students exercising at least 30 minutes three times a week.[35]

4 In a study of over 40,000 college students, researchers found a reduction in the risk of hopelessness, depression, and suicidal behavior among men and women engaged in physical activity.[36]

5 However, knowledge about the benefits of regular exercise does not necessarily lead to participation. In a survey of over 1,600 medical students from 16 schools, researchers found 61% of students met CDC recommendations regarding physical activity.[37] While this demonstrates that medical students are more active than adults of the same age in the general population, nearly 40% of students are not meeting the recommendations. These students often report that the demands of medical education impede their ability to participate in regular exercise. Similar findings have been reported in single-school studies. In a study of West Virginia medical students, over 50% of second-year medical students reported no significant exercise.[38] Only 45% of New York Medical College students reported exercising 30 – 60 minutes at least 5 days per week.[39]

6 No matter how busy you are, there are numerous compelling reasons to take the time and make the effort to exercise regularly. Incorporating exercise as part of your routine can help alleviate stress and improve your mental well-being. Research has shown that students who exercise regularly have less short-term and long-term stress, with fewer days of "bad mental health," than those who do not follow physical activity guidelines.[37]

7 Students often find that exercising with classmates helps. Researchers have noted increased adherence to CDC physical activity recommendations when students exercise with classmates.[37]

8 Many students feel compelled to put off exercise when under particularly high stress, such as just before an exam. However, this is precisely the time when students need exercise the most. Exercise helps students remain maximally productive. Even short intervals of exercise can significantly lower stress levels.

9 Many schools emphasize the importance of exercise and encourage students to incorporate exercise into their routine. At the Vanderbilt University School of Medicine, students are placed in one of four colleges. Each college competes against one another in the College Cup.[40] The competition includes athletic events, such as basketball, a 5K walk/run, track, and swimming. Nonathletic events are also included, such as Iron Chef and Trivia Challenge. Widely popular among Vanderbilt students, the College Cup is just one of many activities and events instituted by the school to encourage student wellness.

10 A lack of physical activity has become a national health issue. Physicians who exercise themselves are more likely to counsel patients about exercise and diet.[41]

Alcohol and Drug Use Among Medical Students: 5 Surprising Statistics

Faced with the stressors of medical school, students may turn to alcohol and sometimes even drugs. "I just need these two glasses of wine every night to help me relax and unwind from my stressful day." The use of alcohol or drugs is clearly a maladaptive way of managing stress. These habits are difficult to break and may increase the risk of substance abuse following graduation. They're certainly a risky habit in clinical practice, when stress levels are further increased. Substance abuse has destroyed the personal and professional lives of many physicians. Substance abuse may lead to physician impairment, defined by the AMA as a physician who is "unable to practice medicine with reasonable skill and safety to patients because of physical or mental illness…or excessive use or abuse of drugs including alcohol."[42] It is estimated that 15% of physicians will become impaired at some point in their medical career.

1 In a 2009 survey of over 2,700 medical students at 36 US medical schools, 86% reported consuming alcohol. Twenty percent reported binging on a monthly basis. Eighteen percent were identified as having at-risk drinking.[43]

2 Eighteen percent of graduating medical students in 1996 drank alcohol more frequently than three times a week, with 21% binging at least once in the preceding 30 days. Of note, 18% and 11% of women and men, respectively, indicated an increase in their drinking while in medical school.[44]

3 Baldwin and colleagues surveyed over 2,000 senior medical students at 23 medical schools regarding substance use in the last 30 days. The reported incidence of marijuana use was 10%, cocaine 2.8%, tranquilizers 2.3%, heroin/opiates 1.1%, psychedelics 0.7%, amphetamine 0.3%, and barbiturates 0.2%.[45]

4 In a more recent study performed at one medical school, the use of club drugs by students was assessed.[46] Using an anonymous questionnaire, researchers found a 16.8% prevalence of club drug use of any type, with MDMA and cocaine most commonly used. The other drugs used by students in this study were LSD, ketamine, Ecstasy, methamphetamine, rohypnol, and dextromethorphan.

5 Using the Michigan Alcohol Screening Test, researchers at a Southeastern US medical school found that 12% of students had scores indicating early or middle problem drinking.[47] One percent of students were found to be problem drinkers.

Feeling Sleepy: 4 Reasons Not to Fight It

Sleep deprivation is a well-recognized problem during the clinical years of med school and residency. However, changes in sleep habits may begin during the first year of medical school. In the preclinical years, students frequently stay up late or wake up early to study. By the end of the first semester, Ball found that over 50% of students were "staying up late to study, waking up early to study, taking daytime naps, and sleeping in places other than the bed..." Not uncommonly, students "pull all-nighters" before exams.[48]

When second-year medical students at the Northwestern University Feinberg School of Medicine were asked to identify a personal health behavior to change, 15% chose sleep among a group of behaviors that included exercise, nutrition, personal habits/hygiene, and study/work habits. After setting a goal and tracking progress, some students were successful in improving their sleep hygiene.[49] Below, we offer reasons why sleep quantity and quality are important issues for all medical students.

1 Inadequate or insufficient sleep can negatively impact academic performance. The consequences include decreased attention, difficulty in thinking, deficits in recent memory, learning impairment, sensitivity to criticism, and increase in errors on tasks. Dr. Lawrence Epstein, Instructor of Medicine at Harvard Medical School and Past President of the American Academy of Sleep Medicine, states that "recent studies have shown that adequate sleep is essential to feeling awake and alert, maintaining good health and working at peak performance. After two weeks of sleeping six hours or less a night, students feel as bad and perform as poorly as someone who has gone without sleep for 48 hours."[50]

2 In a survey of third-year students performed before the start of clerkships, burnout was common, affecting 71% of students.[51] The authors found that "burnt out students were significantly more likely to suffer from sleep deprivation."

3 To determine the effect of sleep deprivation on student cognitive function, researchers administered cognitive function tests before and

after on-call duty during an obstetrics and gynecology clerkship. Cognitive function scores were found to decrease after on-call duty.[52]

4 In a recent study, Dr. Papp, Director of the Center for the Advancement of Medical Learning at Case Western University, and colleagues conducted focus groups with approximately 150 residents at five U.S. academic health centers.[53] The group found a possible relationship between resident well-being and professionalism. In particular, sleep loss and fatigue were reported as having adverse effects on professionalism.

Keeping Your Spirits Up: 14 Highest Rated Uplifts in Medical School

In a focus group session of students at the West Virginia University School of Medicine, students were asked about their life priorities.[54] Highest ranked was family and friends, followed by healthy lifestyle. While there were a number of barriers to these life priorities, the greatest was lack of time. Other barriers included stress, conflicting priorities, lack of energy, high expectations for self, loss of control over their lives, and losing perspective of what's really important.

Given the time demands of med school, it's not surprising that many preclinical students feel that they're unable to participate in enjoyable and meaningful hobbies and activities that had previously been a major part of their lives. Dr. Phyllis Carr, Associate Dean for Student Affairs at Boston University School of Medicine, encourages students not to lose track of their personal pursuits and hobbies.[55] At a recent white coat ceremony at the Vanderbilt University School of Medicine, Dr. Steven Gabbe, Dean of the medical school, offered some important lessons for students. "Manage your time carefully and find the time to do those activities that bring joy to your life."[56]

We've included below the results of a survey done by Wolf of graduating medical students at a single medical school.[28] Students were asked to rate "uplifts", defined as a pleasant, happy, or satisfying experience during medical school. Rated most uplifting by students was recreation and entertainment, again emphasizing the importance of keeping up with the things you enjoy.

1 Recreation and entertainment

2 Good examination performance

3 Rest and relaxation

4 Sex

5 Time with friends: Medical school is difficult, and students whose support group includes classmates find medical school to be less difficult, and certainly less lonely. No one will better understand what you're going through than your classmates. In the process of making new connections and nurturing these relationships, students are able to develop a support network. As one student from the University of Washington stated, "It is absolutely true that the hardest part of medical school is the social adjustment... Make lots of friends. Life is much easier when you have a strong support group." Another student emphasized the importance of keeping up with your old friends. "If you have friends in the area that are not in med school, make sure to spend time with them! While your classmates may end up being some of your best friends, it's a really nice breather to 'get away from it all' with non-school friends."[57]

6 Time with family: "In order to reach your goal of becoming a doctor, you'll need to have a support group," says Dr. Hamilton, Dean of Multicultural Affairs at the University of Pennsylvania School of Medicine.[58] "Even the most capable students need a strong support system." For many students, family will play an integral role. Having family to support and care for you as you handle the challenges of medical school can be invaluable.

7 Improvement in personal physical health

8 Cooperative patients

9 Good relationships with peers: Once you've established a support group, do your part to maintain and nurture these relationships. Medical school will challenge your ability to do so. While students recognize the importance of socializing, the demands of school may make it difficult to put this into practice. In fact, studies have shown a decrease in socializing in medical school.[48]

10 Relationship with parents

11 Improvement in personal psychological health: Maintaining balance between medical school and your social and personal life is clearly important, with one study showing that insufficient or inadequate social activity was associated with a decline in psychological health.[59] Another study revealed that "strong social ties was the factor most positively related to better health and life satisfaction" among a group of first-year medical students.[60]

12 Improvement in sleeping habits

13 Having time alone

14 Good relationships with teachers

Advice for your Loved Ones: 13 Important Tips

The Indiana University School of Medicine instituted a Family Day program to educate families and friends of new students about the challenges of medical school. In surveys performed before and after the program, researchers found significant improvement in understanding of medical school culture, factors contributing to stress, and importance of support for medical student well-being.[61] The authors concluded that "the inclusion of family members and other loved ones in pre-matriculation educational programs may serve to mitigate the stress associated with medical school by enhancing the students' social support systems."

Loved ones who aren't in the medical field may not truly understand the challenges that await students. It's important that you take the time to communicate the magnitude of the challenge. Once they have some awareness and a better understanding of your situation, they'll be in a better position to provide much-needed support. While this book is written for a medical school audience, this particular section is written for the important individuals who support medical students and enable their success: family, loved ones, and friends.

1 Medical school is incredibly challenging. From day one until graduation, medical students experience tremendous highs and lows. At times, and perhaps more so during the first year, your loved one may wonder if he or she made the right choice to pursue a career in medicine. Your unwavering support will be critical.

2 Students entering medical school have generally and consistently earned high grades, sometimes with relatively little effort compared to their peers. This is likely to change in medical school, where the volume of information forces students to study longer and harder than they ever did before. As a consequence, students won't be able to spend as much time with their family and friends as they did in the past.

3 With so many excellent students in the class, it's not surprising that many students soon feel they're simply average. At schools where grading is on an honors/pass/fail system, or its equivalent, only 10 to

20% of students will achieve an honors grade in each course. While there's no shame in earning a pass grade in a course, especially if 80 to 90% of the class is doing the same, this can be a major blow to students' egos. Family and friends serve as an important support network for students, and they can lessen the impact of these new truths. Remind students how much they've accomplished, and emphasize how proud you are that they're working so hard to accomplish such an important goal.

4 As a family member or friend, you'll understandably want to see your student as often as you have in the past. However, this may not be possible. Although students would like to continue the same enjoyable activities, their workload often interferes. This shouldn't stop you from including them in activities and plans. However, if they're unable to join you, don't express disappointment or frustration. They have enough on their mind, and guilt doesn't help.

5 If you've been accustomed to spending significant time together on weekends, realize that this will change. You'll no longer have the luxury of spending the entire weekend together. Doing so places students significantly behind in their studies, and adds to the stress. A better approach is to plan together in advance to identify an evening, afternoon, or a day that can be spent together.

6 At many schools, the weekend following exams is often free for students. It may be more realistic for you to spend considerable time together on this "golden weekend." As always, discussing the schedule well in advance will help avoid disappointment.

7 When family or loved ones don't see medical students as often as they once did, they sometimes start to question their time management skills. Please refrain from passing judgment, and instead offer assistance whenever possible with students' non-academic responsibilities.

8 Provide as much lead time as possible when scheduling or communicating important family activities. Students may need significant advance notice if they're going to be able to participate.

9 Don't be surprised if your medical student expresses concerns that you've rarely heard in his or her prior academic pursuits. While this can be unsettling, your role is to listen and offer encouragement.

10 Although you may feel powerless in your ability to help with specific issues, the fact that you are there, offering unconditional support, is incredibly meaningful. While parents or loved ones may be tempted to rush in and fix things, you should avoid dispensing advice unless specifically requested to do so. In many instances, students simply need to know that you're there to listen, and the act of venting is often enough to make them feel better.

11 There are many ways to offer words of encouragement, support, or praise. A voicemail, a personal note slipped into a book bag, or a quick positive email are all simple yet uplifting gestures.

12 Sending a care package, cooking a favorite meal, doing laundry, and running errands are other ways to express love and support.

13 Medical school exams are typically grouped, and take place over the course of a few days. Therefore, the week prior to exams tends to be very stressful. Step up your efforts to support your student during these times.

Top 10 Sources of Conflict Cited by Spouses of Physicians

1 Lack of time for fun, family, and self

2 Lack of intimacy

3 Money management

4 Frequency of sexual relations

5 Finances

6 Lack of shared responsibilities for children and work around the home

7 Tension in the home

8 Amount of time away from home at work

9 Philosophy of child rearing

10 Quality of sexual relations

From Gabbard G, Menninger R, Coyne L. Sources of conflict in the medical marriage. *Am J Psychiatry* 1987; 144: 567-72.

Words of Wisdom for Married Medical Students

The 1995 AAMC graduation questionnaire revealed that 30% of graduating allopathic medical students were married.[62] Another 14% were either engaged or had partners. In a 2003-2004 survey of osteopathic medical students, 45% of senior students were married.[63] Maintaining a healthy marriage requires work, and the rigors and demands of medical school can present a couple with significant challenges. In the article "Balancing personal and professional life for the medical family," Jennifer West writes that "prioritization, effective time management, focus on communication, making small changes, and taking a proactive role in life are small steps that can promote and support a balanced life."[64] In this section, we share information for married medical students.

1 James Wallace, a student at the Medical College of Georgia, is married with children. He makes it a point to contact his wife during the school day, even if it's for a brief moment. "The hours can be pretty bad but you have to make sure you have constant contact, taking time just to send a text to your wife and when you get a moment to call your kids."[65]

2 Dr. Wayne Sotile is the Director of Psychological Services for the Wake Forest University Healthy Exercise and Lifestyles Program, and has counseled over 700 physicians. He reminds married professionals to protect communication-generating rituals. "Every couple starts out with a wonderful set of rituals that create time and space for them to give undivided attention to each other...Some develop the habit of setting aside 20 minutes each evening to sit and chat in a quiet room. Others make mealtime a time to sit at the table for an extra 15 minutes, just to touch base. Still others protect their weekly walks...It doesn't matter what you do, just do it!"[66]

3 Drs. Linda and Robert Miles are the authors of *The New Marriage: Transcending the Happily –Ever-After Myth*. Based on the research of Dr. John Gottman, they've identified four factors that can ruin a marriage – criticism, contempt, defensiveness, and stone-walling.[67]

4 At a meeting of the Vanderbilt House Staff Alliance, Dr. John Tarpley, Professor of Surgery, and his wife lectured about the challenges of a medical marriage. They have five principles for a successful marriage – forgiveness, faithfulness, fiscal responsibility, fair fighting, and food. "If you are honest and realistic there will be some low places. And if you work together these low places can lead to a stronger union and end up, in retrospect, being highlights and opportunities to improve."[68]

5 Martina Esisi writes about the importance of friendship between partners in a medical marriage. "Friendship is vital in a healthy marriage, and friendships are nurtured through shared quality time. It is therefore important to be able to create that time, by setting strict boundaries between work and family time. It is important to avoid bringing work home, to have good holidays, and to have a range of interests outside of medicine."[69]

6 In an orientation given to families of new medical students, Dr. Suzanne Kunkle reminds students to remember that "your spouse is following your dream. Show regular appreciation for all that is done to support you." As you talk about your day, "be open rather than defensive if your partner complains about his/her day. Be curious, ask questions, listen and ask how can I help?"[70]

7 "Respect your own mind, body, and spirit," says Dr. Wayne Sotile. "You cannot have a healthy marriage unless you are healthy…This can lead to misery at home and at work."[66]

8 "Acknowledge the good," writes Dr. J. Lebron McBride, Director of Behavior Medicine at Floyd Medical Center. "It is human tendency to take the significant people in our lives for granted. For example, how often have you thought something positive about your partner but somehow failed to say it out loud? Begin affirming the good you see in your partner. It will make him or her feel valued and will help you to become more positive yourself."[71]

9 "You must learn to ignore minor irritations if you expect any peace and harmony," says Barbara Linney. "It doesn't matter that I wipe up spills and he walks through them, that my closet is messy and his is neat, that I leave my shoes anywhere and he always puts his away, that we don't agree on the management of the toilet seat."[72]

10 As a Clinical Professor of Psychiatry and specialist in physician health, Dr. Michael Myers has extensive experience counseling in this area. He urges couples to seek therapy if there is unrelenting strain in the relationship. "Couples therapy is not only of proven value as an intervention, it can also be a comforting experience."[73]

Words of Wisdom for Medical Student Spouses

The 1995 AAMC graduation questionnaire revealed that 30% of graduating allopathic medical students were married.[62] Another 14% were either engaged or had partners. In a 2003-2004 survey of osteopathic medical students, 45% of senior students were married.[63] Maintaining a healthy marriage requires work, and the rigors and demands of medical school can present a couple with significant challenges. "Spouses often feel taken for granted. Students often feel torn between academic performance and the ability to be a contributing member of the couple and family," says Dr. Lynn Martin, Director of Educational Support Services at Des Moines University.[74] In this section, we share words of wisdom for medical student spouses from those who have walked in their shoes.

1 Learn what medical school actually involves. In the book *Living with Medicine: A Family Guide*, author Deborah McManus encourages spouses to read the student handbook, books written for students about medical school, and resources developed specifically for spouses in medicine.[75]

2 "Communication is important in any relationship, but during medical school, it takes on a special significance" writes McManus.[75] The general rules for communication in marriage apply even more strongly in medical marriages. Raise issues as early as possible, and maintain open lines of communication. Given the complexities of medical education, though, it becomes even more important to pay close attention to timing.

3 Develop independent interests and hobbies. Spouses should consider how they'll spend their time while their medical student is away at class or studying. Have they identified activities or pursuits that will lead to their own personal or professional growth? The School of Medicine at the University of North Carolina offers the following advice: "Because you may not be able to spend as much quality time with your spouse, you may find it helpful to become involved with your own personal activities. Church groups, volunteer activities, and community classes (such as those offered at the YMCA) are easy ways to meet new people and do great things. Also, if you would like to learn more about the field of medicine and gain an understanding of your spouse's new life, UNC Hospitals offer many volunteer opportunities."[76]

4 Maintain your sense of humor. "Sometimes when my medical student and I were at our lowest, one of us would see the absurdity of the situation, or think of a dumb pun, and we would share a laugh and things wouldn't look quite so bad," writes Deborah McManus.[75]

5 Join a support group. Many schools have organizations for medical students and their spouses. Through these organizations, you'll find that you're not alone in what you're experiencing and feeling. Listening to others' stories and sharing your own may help. An online resource that offers support and understanding is the International Medical Spouse Network. If you're having difficulty locating a group, visit the AMA Alliance website for a list of groups and organizations.

6 Connect throughout the day. Kristen Match, author of *Surviving Residency: A Medical Spouse Guide to Embracing The Training Years*, writes that "touching base throughout the day will help you both to maintain an emotional connection to each other."[77]

7 Although time spent with your loved one may be lacking in quantity, make every moment count. Even small amounts of time can make a difference if you're both engaged.

234 **SUCCESS IN MEDICAL SCHOOL**

References

[1]Medscape. Available at: http://www.medscape/viewarticle/457429. Accessed February 12, 2012.

[2]Fahrenkopf A, Sectish T, Barger L, Sharek P, Lewin D, Chiang V, Edwards S, Wiedermann B, Landrigan C. Rates of medication errors among depressed and burnt out residents: prospective cohort study. *BMJ* 2008; 336(7642): 488-91.

[3]Dyrbye L, Thomas M, Huntington J, Lawson K, Novotny P, Sloan J, Shanafelt T. Personal life events and medical student burnout: a multicenter study. *Acad Med* 2006; 81 (4): 374-84.

[4]Compton M, Carrera J, Frank E. Stress and depressive symptoms/dysphoria among US medical students: results from a large, nationally representative survey. *J Nerv Ment Dis* 2008; 196(12): 891-7.

[5]Goebert D, Thompson D, Takeshita J, Beach C, Bryson P, Ephgrave K, Kent A, Kunkel M, Schecter J, Tate J. Depressive symptoms in medical students and residents: a multischool study. *Acad Med* 2009; 84(2): 236-41.

[6]Givens J, Tila J. Depressed medical students' use of mental health services and barriers. *Acad Med* 2002; 77(9): 918-21.

[7]Rosenthal J, Okie S. White coat, mood indigo – depression in medical school. *N Engl J Med* 2005; 353: 1085-8.

[8]Rosal M, Ockene I, Ockene J, Barrett S, Ma Y, Hebert J. A longitudinal study of students' depression at one medical school. *Acad Med* 1997; 72(6): 542-6.

[9]Wolf T, von Almen T, Faucett J, Randall H, Franklin F. Psychosocial changes during the first year of medical school. *Med Educ* 1991; 25(3): 174-81.

[10]Clark D, Zeldow P. Vicissitudes of depressed mood during four years of medical school. *JAMA* 1988; 260(17): 2521-8.

[11]Tekian A. Attrition rates of underrepresented minority students at the University of Illinois at Chicago College of Medicine, 1993–1997. *Acad Med* 1998; 73: 336–338.

[12]Stetto J, Gackstetter G, Cruess D, Hooper T. Variables associated with attrition from Uniformed Services University of the Health Sciences Medical School. *Mil Med* 2004; 169: 102–107.

[13]Fogleman B, Vander Zwagg R. Demographic, situational, and scholastic factors in medical school attrition. *South Med* 1981; 74: 602–606.

[14]Garrison G, Mikesell C, Matthew D. Medical school graduation and attrition rates. *AAMC Analysis in Brief* April 2007; 7.

[15]Dyrbye L, Thomas M, Power D, Durning S, Moutier C, Massie F, Harper W, Eacker A, Szydlo D, Sloan J, Shanafelt T. Burnout and serious thoughts of dropping out of medical school: a mutli-institutional study. *Acad Med* 2010; 85(1): 94-102.

[16]Hojat M, Glaser K, Xu G, Veloski J, Christian E. Gender comparisons of medical students' psychosocial profiles. *Med Educ* 1999; 33: 342-49.

[17]Vitaliano P, Maiuro R, Russo J, Mitchell E. Medical student distress: a longitudinal study. *J Nerv Ment Dis* 1989; 177: 70-76.

[18]Richman J, Flaherty J. Gender differences in medical student distress: contributions of prior socialization and current role-related stress. *Soc Sci Med* 1990; 30: 777-87.

[19]Lloyd C, Gartrell N. Sex differences in medical student mental health. *Am J Psychiatry* 1981; 138: 1346-51.

[20]Schernhammer E, Colditz G. Suicide rates among physicians: a quantitative and gender assessment (meta-analysis). *Am J Psychiatry* 2004; 161: 2295-302.

[21]Dyrbye L, Thomas M, Massie F, Power D, Eacker A, Harper W, Durning S, Moutier C, Szydlo D, Novotny P, Sloan J, Shanafelt T. Burnout and suicidal ideation among U.S. medical students. *Ann Intern Med* 2008; 2: 149(5): 334-41.

[22]Crosby A, Cheltenham M, Sacks J. Incidence of suicidal ideation and behavior in the United States, 1994. *Suicide Life Threat Behav* 1999; 29: 131-40.

[23]Hays L, Cheever T, Patel P. Medical student suicide, 1989-1994. *Am J Psychiatry* 153 (4): 553-5.

[24]Association of American Medical Colleges. Available at: https://www.aamc.org/download/49146/data/counselingresponses.pdf. Accessed on October 24, 2011.

[25]AAMC Reporter. Available at: http://www.aamc.org/newsroom/reporter/dec08/mentalillness.htm. Accessed May 14, 2011.

[26]Desai S, Katta R. The Successful Match: Maintaining Your Emotional Well-Being During the Clinical Years of Medical School (article submitted to Student Doctor Network).

[27]AAMC Reporter. Available at: http://s3.amazonaws.com/zanran_storage/www.aamc.org/ContentPages/907501 1.pdf. Accessed August 12, 2011.

[28]Wolf T, Faucett J, Randall H, Balson P. Graduating medical students' ratings of stresses, pleasures, and coping strategies. *J Med Educ* 1988; 63(8): 636-42.

[29]Dunn L, Iglewicz A, Moutier C. A conceptual model of medical student well-being: promoting resilience and preventing burnout. *Acad Psychiatry* 2008; 32: 44-53.

[30]Carr A. Positive Psychology: The Science of Happiness and Human Strengths. New York: Brunner-Routledge; 2004.

[31]Carver C. You want to measure coping but your protocol's too long: consider the brief COPE. *International Journal of Behavioral Medicine* 1997; 4: 92-100.

[32]Gentile J, Roman B. Medical student mental health services; psychiatrists treating medical students. *Psychiatry* 2009; 6(5): 38-45.

[33]Dimeo F, Bauer M, Varahram I, Proest G, Halter U. Benefits from aerobic exercise in patients with major depression: a pilot study. *Br J Sports Med* 2001; 35: 114-17.

[34]Roth S, Holmes D. Influence of physical fitness in determining the impact of stressful life events on physical and psychological health. *Psychosomatic Medicine* 47(2): 164-73.

[35]Hussein E, Gabr A, Mohamed A, Hameed A. Physical exercise and anxiety among medical students at Ain Shams University. Presented at the 13th Annual International Ain Shams Medical Students' Congress, Feb 14-16, 2005.

[36]Taliaferro L, Rienzo B, Pigg R, Miller M, Dodd V. Associations between physical activity and reduced rates of hopelessness, depression, and suicidal behavior among college students. *Am Coll Health* 2009; 57(4): 427-36.

[37]Frank E, Tong E, Lobelo F, Carrera J, Duperly J. Physical activity levels and counseling practices of U.S. medical students. *Med Sci Sports Exerc* 2008; 40(3): 413-21.

[38]Troyer D, Ullrich I, Yeater R, Hopewell R. Physical activity and condition, dietary habits, and serum lipids in second-year medical students. *J Am Coll Nutr* 1990; 9:303-307.

[39]New York Medical College. Available at: http://www.nymc.edu/Clubs/quill_and_scope/volume2/yam.pdf. Accessed September 12, 2011.

[40]Drolet B, Rogdgers S. A comprehensive medical student wellness program – design and implementation at Vanderbilt School of Medicine. *Acad Med* 2010; 85(1): 103-110.

[41]Lobelo F, Duperly J, Frank E. Physical activity habits of doctors and medical students influence their counseling practices. *Br J Sports Med* 2009; 43 (2): 89-92.

[42]Krych R, Leath M, Nace E. Chemical dependence in physicians: identification and intervention. PHR CME course. Available at: http://www.texmed.org/Template.aspx?id=4760. Accessed on October 24, 2011.

[43]Shah A, Bazargan-Hejazi S, Lindstrom R, Wolf K. Prevalence of at-risk drinking among a national sample of medical students. *Subst Abus* 2009; 30(2): 141-9.

[44]Mangus R, Hawkins C, Miller M. Tobacco and alcohol use among 1996 medical school graduates. *JAMA* 1998; 280(13): 1192-1193, 1195.

[45]Baldwin D, Hughes P, Conard S, Storr C, Sheehan D. Substance use among senior medical students. A survey of 23 medical schools. *JAMA* 1991; 265(16): 2074-8.

[46]Horowitz A, Galanter M, Dermatis H, Franklin J. Use of an attitudes toward club drugs by medical students. *J Addict Dis* 2008; 27(4): 35-42.

[47]Ghodosara S, Davidson M, Reich M, Savoie C, Rodgers S. Assessing student mental health at the Vanderbilt University School of Medicine. *Acad Med* 2011; 86(1): 116-21.

[48]Ball S, Bax A. Self-care in medical education: effectiveness of health-habit interventions for first-year medical students. *Acad Med* 2002; 77(9): 911-7.

[49]Kushner R, Kessler S, McGahie W. Using behavior change plans to improve medical student self-care. *Acad Med* 2011; 86(7): 901-6.

[50]American Academy of Sleep Medicine. Available at: http://www.aasmnet.org/Articles.aspx?id=659. Accessed February 14, 2012.

[51]Mazurkiewicz R, Korenstein D, Fallar R, Ripp J. The prevalence and correlations of medical student burnout in the pre-clinical years: a cross-sectional study. *Psychol Health Med* 2011; July 25.

[52]Halbach M, Spann C, Egan G. Effect of sleep deprivation on medical resident and student cognitive function: a prospective study. *Am J Obstet Gynecol* 2003; 188(5): 1198-1201.

[53]Papp K, Stoller E, Sage P, Aikens J, Owens J, Avidan A, Phillips B, Rosen R, Strohl K. The effects of sleep loss and fatigue on resident physicians: a multi-institutional, mixed-method study. *Acad Med* 2004; 79: 394-406.

[54]Nuss M. Medical student perceptions of healthy lifestyles: a qualitative study. *Californian Journal of Health Promotion* 2004; 2(1): 127-134.
[55]AMSA. Available at: http://www.amsa.org. Accessed June 13, 2011.
[56]Vanderbilt University Medical Center Reporter. Available at: http://www.mc.vanderbilt.edu/reporter/index.html?ID=3462. Accessed February 14, 2012.
[57]University of Washington School of Medicine. Available at: http://uwmedicine.washington.edu/NR/rdonlyres/41AB4807-24F4-4944-A099-9A2D76ECA5E2/0/ManagingtheFirstYearofMedicalSchool.pdf. Accessed June 1, 2011.
[58]American Medical Association. Available at: http://www.ama-assn.org/ama/pub/about-ama/our-people/member-groups-sections/minority-affairs-consortium/transitioning-residency/getting-ready-medical-school-years-1.page. Accessed May 10, 2011.
[59]Aktekin M, Karaman T, Senol Y, Erdem S, Erengin H, Akaydin M. Anxiety, depression, and stressful life events among medical students: a prospective study in Antalya, Turkey. *Med Educ* 2001; 35(1): 12-7.
[60]Parkerson G, Broadhead W, Tse C. The health status and life satisfaction of first-year medical students. *Acad Med* 1990; 65(9): 586-8.
[61]Bell M, Smith P, Brokaw J, Cushing H. A Family Day program enhances knowledge about medical school culture and necessary supports. *BMC Med Educ* 2004; 4: 3.
[62]1995 AAMC Graduation Questionnaire. Available at: http://www.aamc.org.
[63]Osteopathic Medical Education in the United States. Available at: http://www.aacom.org/resources/bookstore/Documents/special-report.pdf. Accessed February 14, 2012.
[64]Balancing personal and professional life. Available at: http://www.amaalliance.org/site/files/625/41977/163960/354458/Balancing_Personal_and_Professional_Life_-_AMAAlli. Accessed February 14, 2012.
[65]Medical students balance school, clinicals, family, and second jobs. Available at: http://www.mysouthwestga.com/news/story.aspx?id=624061. Accessed February 14, 2012.
[66]Wayne and Mary Sotile. Available at: http://www.sotile.com/advice_articles.php?article=4. Accessed February 14, 2012.
[67]The Medical Marriage. Available at: http://www.amaalliance.org/site/files/625/41977/163960/332948/Marriage-JanFebToday.pdf. Accessed February 14, 2012.
[68]Vanderbilt University Medical Center Reporter. Available at: http://www.mc.vanderbilt.edu/reporter/index.html?ID=4397. Accessed February 14, 2012.
[69]BMJ Careers. Available at: http://careers.bmj.com/careers/advice/view-article.html?id=2191. Accessed February 14, 2012.
[70]Indiana University School of Medicine Understanding and Supporting Your Medical Student. Available at: http://alumni.iupui.edu/medicine/documents/Understanding%20and%20Supporting%20Your%20Medical%20Student.pdf. Accessed February 14, 2012.

[71]McBride J. 8 ways to improve your relationships. *Fam Pract Manag* 2003; 10(8): 80.

[72]Linney B. Medical marriages. *Physician Executive* 1999.

[73]Myers M. The well-being of physician relationships. *West J Med* 2001; 174: 30-33.

[74]DMU Magazine Fall/Winter 2010. Available at: http://www.dmu.edu/magazine/fall-2010/you-can-meld-marriage-and-medical-school/. Accessed June 10, 2011.

[75]Smith M. *Living with Medicine: A Family Guide*. American Psychiatric Publishing; 1987.

[76]University of North Carolina School of Medicine. Available at: http://www.med.unc.edu/md/orientation/first-year-resources/life-outside-of-school/information-for-spouses-and-families. Accessed February 14, 2012.

[77]Match K. *Surviving Residency: A Medical Spouse Guide to Embracing The Training Years*. iUniverse Publishing; 2011.

Chapter 12

Professionalism

What is professionalism, and why does it matter?

Consider the following observation made by a student:

Two doctors were down the hall from each other, and there were people around. One said to the other, "Did you hear about Mr. X?" And the other doctor said no, and he made a face like a dead face...sticking his tongue out, crossing his eyes, and tilting his head to the side. If anybody had noticed they wouldn't have been too happy with it.[1]

Students must be prepared to deal with issues of professionalism in their peers, in members of the healthcare team, and even in their teachers. Researchers found that exposure to unprofessional behavior began early in the medical education process and increased in each successive year. In Year 1 of medical school, 66% of students had "heard derogatory comments not in patient's presence" and 35% had "observed unethical conduct by residents or attending physicians."[2]

Why else does professionalism matter?

The vast majority of the students we meet have core values and a strong sense of personal integrity. Many therefore assume that issues of professionalism, while they may impact others around them, don't have any relevance to their own behavior. This is due to the common assumption that our core values regarding unethical behavior are stable over time. Studies of medical students contradict this assumption.

In one study, medical students were given a list of 11 unprofessional behaviors, and asked "Is the following behavior unprofessional for a medical student?"[3] Students were surveyed before matriculation and again six months into their first year of medical school. Researchers found that behaviors originally considered unprofessional rapidly became more acceptable. Medical students were also presented with four different scenarios, and asked "Must one do the following to be professional?" For the scenario "Report Cheating to a Professor or Administrator," 69% of students originally answered "yes." Six months into medical school, only 41% answered "yes." There are therefore two core reasons to focus on this field. If you're a medical student, you are likely to witness lapses in professionalism in patient care, and you need to be prepared to deal with those lapses and protect your patients. You also need to define and protect your own core values and personal integrity.

What is professionalism? The foundation of the medical profession rests upon the trust that patients place in their physicians. Professionalism focuses on this foundation of trust. Although it's been defined in various ways, the core values and elements agreed upon include honesty, integrity, compassion, empathy, ability to communicate effectively with patients, and respect for others. Professionalism is a hot topic in undergraduate medical education. A number of medical education organizations, including the American Board of Internal Medicine, the Association of American Medical Colleges, and the National Board of Medical Examiners, have established professionalism as a required competency across the spectrum of medical education. Medical schools, in turn, have made it a point to educate preclinical students.

Many students, when hearing about a curriculum on professionalism, have similar reactions. "I already hold these values. Why should any of this concern me?" The studies that we describe in this chapter provide a definitive answer to that question. Most students are surprised to learn that the stresses and challenges of medical school can affect attitude, behavior, and conduct. However, this conclusion is clearly supported by a number of studies.

Even though medical students may actually harm patients when they act unethically, such actions persist. In a survey of students at a single school, 13 to 24% admitted to cheating during the clinical years of medical school.[4] Examples included "recording tasks not performed" and "lying about having ordered tests." In another study, students were asked whether they had heard of or witnessed unethical behaviors on the part of their student colleagues.[5] In response, 21% had personal knowledge of students "reporting a pelvic examination as 'normal' during rounds when it had been inadvertently omitted from the physical examination."

As students, you are likely to witness lapses in professional behavior, and may witness outright unethical behavior and fraud. These issues affect every level of our profession, and therefore you have to be prepared. You must guard against lapses in your own behavior, and be prepared to deal with lapses in colleagues or supervisors. As physicians, our goal is to treat and protect the patient, and this can be challenging in the real world of clinical medicine.

In a survey, third-year students at the University of Texas Medical Branch at Galveston were asked to evaluate their physicians' professionalism.[6] Although this review of nearly 3,000 evaluation forms revealed significant praise for positive faculty role modeling, negative comments were not infrequent. The majority dealt with "issues of language use, inappropriate use of humor, disrespectful treatment of patients or colleagues, and apparent disinterest in teaching."

Although we think of physicians as highly compassionate and ethical individuals, ethical lapses can extend to the highest levels of our profession. In a stunning case of scientific fraud, Dr. Scott Reuben, a highly regarded anesthesiologist whose research has significantly impacted how physicians treat surgical patients for pain, was found to have fabricated results in over 20 published studies.[7] In some cases, he is alleged to have even invented patients.

Professionalism in Medical Students: 8 Reasons Why This Topic Is More Important Than You Might Believe

A number of medical education organizations, including the American Board of Internal Medicine, the Association of American Medical Colleges, and the National Board of Medical Examiners, have established professionalism as a required competency across the spectrum of medical education. Medical schools, in turn, have made it a point to educate preclinical students about professionalism.

1 A growing body of research shows that professionalism may affect the quality of care that physicians provide to their patients. Recently, studies have shown that many physicians develop burnout, defined as a syndrome of emotional exhaustion, depersonalization, and sense of low accomplishment. Physician burnout is associated with erosion in professionalism, and may lead to suboptimal care. In a survey of over 700 surgeons who reported making a major medical error over a period of three months, researchers found a strong relationship between major medical errors and the surgeon's degree of burnout.[8]

2 The ACGME document "Advancing education in medical professionalism" explores the ways in which professionalism, or lack thereof, can affect the patient-physician relationship.[9] Patients who perceive their physician as behaving professionally are more likely to be satisfied, follow through with treatment recommendations, stay with their doctor, and recommend him or her to others. In contrast, patients are more likely to bring legal action against unprofessional physicians.

3 Unprofessional behavior in medical school is a possible predictor of future disciplinary action. A particularly notable study, led by Dr. Maxine Papadakis, Associate Dean for Student Affairs at the UCSF School of Medicine, showed that 95% of disciplinary actions leveled against UCSF-graduated physicians by the California state medical board over a 10-year period were due to deficiencies of professionalism.[10] When compared with a control group, physicians disciplined by the board were twice as likely to have negative comments related to professionalism in their medical school records.

4 In a follow-up study, Dr. Papadakis and colleagues examined the medical school records of 235 graduates of three medical schools, all of whom had been disciplined by one of 40 state medical boards over a 13-year period. Similar results were found, with disciplined physicians being three times more likely than the control group to have had deficiencies in professionalism documented in medical school.[11]

5 A common assumption is that our core values regarding unethical behavior are stable over time. Studies of medical students contradict this assumption. In one study, medical students were given a list of 11 unprofessional behaviors, and asked "Is the following behavior unprofessional for a medical student?"[3] Students were surveyed before matriculation and again six months into their first year of medical school. Researchers found that behaviors originally considered unprofessional rapidly became more acceptable. Medical students were also presented with four different scenarios, and asked "Must one do the following to be professional?" For the scenario "Report Cheating to a Professor or Administrator," 69% of students originally answered "yes." Six months into medical school, only 41% answered "yes."

6 Some researchers have examined how lapses in professionalism during the preclinical years may relate to performance in the clinical years. In one study, certain student attitudes, such as a negative attitude towards a course, were found to be predictive of problems in future clinical performance.[12]

7 Is there a relationship between unprofessional behaviors in medical students and the type of behaviors for which physicians are sanctioned by state medical boards? Dr. Michael Ainsworth, Associate Dean for Regional Education at the University of Texas Medical Branch in Galveston, sought to answer this question through an analysis of unprofessional behavior at a single medical school.[13] Of the 110 lapses of professionalism documented, 40% occurred in the preclinical years. The behaviors included:

- Failure to fulfill responsibilities reliably
- Fails to accept responsibility for actions
- Abuses student privileges
- Does not function/interact appropriately within groups
- Insensitive to needs, feelings of others
- Uses disrespectful language
- Arrogant or abusive during stress

Dr. Ainsworth noted similarities between these unprofessional behaviors and the types of behaviors warranting physician sanctioning: failure to maintain medical records, failure to renew license/complete CME, abuses physician privileges, poor function with healthcare providers, arrogant/abusive with patients.

8 In 2005, Teherani published the results of a study seeking to identify the domains of unprofessional behavior in medical school associated with disciplinary action by a state medical board.[14] Three domains of unprofessional behavior were significantly associated with future disciplinary action: poor reliability and responsibility, poor initiative and motivation, and lack of self-improvement and adaptability.

Making the Most of Professionalism Instruction in Medical School: 13 Tips

Researchers have noted that first-year students "quickly grow weary of being talked to about professionalism."[3] At one medical school in the Pacific Northwest, "a substantial number of second-year medical students complained...about the professionalism curriculum, especially about overuse of the word 'professionalism' itself."[15] However, according to the results of these studies, there are compelling reasons for schools to continue their efforts in this area.

1 The challenge medical schools face is in how to educate students at a time when they are mostly in the classroom as opposed to the clinic or hospital setting. The techniques used by schools include case-based small group discussions, formal lectures in ethics and humanism, panels, faculty role modeling, shared reflections, required participation in charitable care and community service, and other didactic exercises.

2 Behaviors and attitudes expected of physicians by society are often introduced to students early in medical school. In fact, many schools address these issues during orientation or the white coat ceremony. Some schools ask that new students recite a class professionalism policy as a promise or oath. Approximately 90% of allopathic and osteopathic medical schools in the U.S. and Canada have a White Coat Ceremony to welcome their incoming students. "Students are given their first 'white coat', a much recognized symbol of physicianship. Said to represent altruism, good will, and purity, the white coat is placed on the student by a respected member of the profession."[16]

3 At a recent freshman orientation for University of Arkansas College of Medicine students, the school presented "skits depicting situations that raise ethical questions to help students visualize what they might have to face within the next four years...One scenario showed a group of residents violating patient confidentiality by loudly discussing cases in the cafeteria. Another showed a resident ordering a medical student to falsify a patient record."[17] In commenting on these scenarios, Dr. Richard Wheeler, Dean for Student and Academic Affairs, had this reminder for students. "There are no excuses for this type of behavior. The patient always comes first – before you, before your grades."

4 Professionalism has become a part of the grading process at most medical schools. For example, students at the University of Texas Medical Branch "receive a score on their ability to demonstrate professional behavior" in every class, according to Dr. Michael Ainsworth, Regional Dean for Medical Education.[18]

5 Medical students have traditionally learned about professionalism largely through observation of their residents and attending physicians in a clinical setting. Several decades ago, new medical students had little contact with patients during their first year. Over time, though, schools have made it a priority to introduce patient contact earlier in their education and on a more frequent basis. As a first and second-year student, you'll have many opportunities to observe the physician-patient relationship. Often, your preceptors will provide positive role models for professionalism. As one student remarked, "Watching their bedside manner is almost like watching a reverend speak on the pulpit."[1] As you gain more experience in the clinical setting, make a conscious effort to recognize these examples and learn from them, in order to incorporate and emulate those behaviors in your own patient interactions.

6 While many of your observations will be positive, you're also likely to observe physicians and educators demonstrating undesirable behavior and attitudes. In a qualitative study, researchers at the University of Washington learned that preclinical students often witness unprofessional behavior in the classroom. Lecturers were found to belittle students, tell vulgar jokes, and make disrespectful comments about patients.[1] This is seen in the clinical setting as well. Consider the following observation made by a student:

Two doctors were down the hall from each other, and there were people around. One said to the other, "Did you hear about Mr. X?" And the other doctor said no, and he made a face like a dead face...sticking his tongue out, crossing his eyes, and tilting his head to the side. If anybody had noticed they wouldn't have been too happy with it.[1]

7 In fact, a number of studies have shown that supervising physicians are not always the best role models. In a survey of senior clerks at three Canadian medical schools, only 53% agreed that their teachers are "good role models in teaching the patient-doctor relationship."[19] Only 52% felt that their teachers "are concerned about the overall well-being of patients not just their presenting complaints." Just 25% agreed "that most of their teachers are concerned about how patients adapt psychologically to their illnesses."

8 In another survey, third-year students at University of Texas Medical Branch at Galveston were asked to evaluate their physicians' professionalism. Although this review of nearly 3,000 evaluation forms revealed significant praise for positive faculty role modeling, negative comments were not infrequent. The majority dealt with "issues of language use, inappropriate use of humor, disrespectful treatment of patients or colleagues, and apparent disinterest in teaching."[6]

9 Student exposure or participation in unethical situations was further examined in a study done at Wake Forest University School of Medicine. Researchers found that exposure to unprofessional behavior began early in the medical education process and increased in each successive year. In Year 1 of medical school, 66% of students had "heard derogatory comments not in patient's presence" and 35% had "observed unethical conduct by residents or attending physicians."[2]

10 As important as it is to identify examples of positive role models, it is equally important to note negative role modeling. These are, of course, the behaviors and attitudes you want to avoid at all costs. The Ethics in Medicine website established by the University of Washington School of Medicine states it succinctly: unprofessional behaviors and actions should be viewed "as a negative lesson in how NOT to be a physician."[20]

11 While role modeling is important in the teaching of professionalism, research has shown that, in and of itself, role modeling may not be enough. In a review of professionalism in medical education, Drs. David Stern and Maxine Papadakis wrote that "role modeling must be combined with reflection on the action to truly teach professionalism."[21]

12 Make a habit of reviewing the situations that you encounter every day, particularly those that challenge professionalism. Did the student or faculty member handle themselves in a professional manner? If not, what could he or she have done differently? Then consider how you would respond to the same situation. This type of hypothetical exercise can help you prepare for your own challenging encounters. To help you reflect on the situation, Stark offered the following suggestions:[22]

- Describe the incident in your own words
- Illustrate the ways in which the incident challenged your values, beliefs or understanding
- Describe which learning resources you used to increase your understanding of the issues you described. Which were useful and which were not?
- Describe how the situation may have been handled differently
- What did you learn personally from this incident?
- What future learning do you plan to do around this incident?

13 In a recent study, residents described well-being "as a balance among multiple parts of their personal and professional lives: family, friends, physical health, mental health, spiritual health, financial security, and professional satisfaction."[23] Through interviews with these residents, researchers sought to explore how sense of well-being affects relationships with patients, interactions with colleagues, and performance in patient care. When residents had a better sense of well-being, they reported a greater capacity to relate to patients and interact with colleagues. In fact, research has suggested that enhanced personal well-being may lead physicians to deliver more compassionate care to their patients.[24-26] However, physicians often don't recognize the relationship between their own sense of well-being and the care they provide to patients. In one survey, residents were asked to list attributes associated with professionalism. Among the 28 reported characteristics, "balance between personal and professional life" was listed last among the group.[27] In Chapter 11, we discuss the importance of balance in medical school and review the ways in which you can maintain balance despite the many challenges.

Cheating in Medical School: Statistics and Consequences

Although medical schools often have honor codes or codes of academic honesty, studies have shown that cheating is common.

1 Nearly 25% of medical students admitted to cheating at one medical school.[4]

2 A more recent study of nearly 2,500 second-year medical students revealed that 29.7% agreed with the statement that "cheating is a normal outgrowth of the competitive nature of medical school."[28] Approximately 32% of students agreed with the statement "Not a single exam goes by without someone cheating on it."

3 In another study, 21.8% of medical students had witnessed another student copying on an examination.[3] Approximately 19% had "given permission to let another student copy" work or exam answers.

4 In 1997, the National Board of Medical Examiners placed the USMLE scores of over 20,000 medical students on hold while investigating alleged cheating on the test. The NBME president stated that "some examinees could have had access to the exam before the administration of the test."[29]

5 Some students, who find cheating acceptable on exams, insist that they would never carry over such behavior to patient care. However, the literature does show that students also engage in unethical behavior while taking care of patients. In a survey of students at The Johns Hopkins University School of Medicine, 13 to 24% admitted to cheating during the clinical years of medical school.[4] Examples included "recording tasks not performed" and "lying about having ordered tests." In another study performed at the University of New Mexico School of Medicine, students were asked whether they had heard of or witnessed unethical behaviors on the part of their student colleagues.[5] In response, 21% had personal knowledge of students "reporting a pelvic examination as 'normal' during rounds when it had been inadvertently omitted from the physical examination." Another 35% had personal knowledge of students "reporting a lab test or x-ray as 'normal' when in actual fact there had been no attempt to obtain the information."

6 There are a number of reasons why students are tempted to cheat on an exam or to plagiarize a paper. Some justify their cheating because they feel unprepared, lack confidence in their own abilities, or because "everyone else does it." No matter what self-justification a student can find, though, these choices ultimately come down to core values and personal integrity. With every choice you make, you have the decision: you're either an individual with the highest personal integrity, or you're not.

7 The consequences of engaging in questionable behavior can be severe, including reprimands, suspensions, or expulsions. In some cases, students have failed a course or been forced to repeat an entire year. We also know of students who have had a permanent notation attached to their academic record. Such information in a residency application is certainly viewed as a red flag, and can potentially jeopardize your career.

A recent investigation was launched at a Northeastern US medical school after administrators were notified that students may have engaged in unauthorized collaboration on a quiz. Possible consequences included dismissal or other disciplinary actions.[30]

8 In Webster's dictionary, the word *plagiarize* means "to steal and pass off (the ideas or words of another) as one's own."[31] Examples of plagiarism include:

- Reprinting or copying a direct quote without placing the material in quotes or listing its source
- Paraphrasing information from another source without acknowledgement
- Inadequate citation or crediting of the source

Although plagiarism isn't a new problem, it's become much easier now that information is readily and easily available on the Internet. Studies of college students have shown that plagiarism is quite common. While studies of medical students are lacking, anecdotal stories from our medical school colleagues suggests that plagiarism is not unusual. Some schools have established professionalism policies, which include plagiarism. In these statements, schools make it clear that students must understand the meaning of plagiarism, recognize the difference between plagiarism and paraphrasing, and learn how to appropriately acknowledge material used from other sources.

9 Famous Cases of Medical Students and Physicians Behaving Badly

1 In 1998, an article in *The Lancet* described how eight of 12 children developed autism within days of receiving the MMR vaccine.[32] The effect of the report was tremendous, leading to a decline in the rate of inoculation from 92% to below 80%. This led to an increase in confirmed cases of measles in England and Wales from 56 in 1998 to over 1,300 cases in 2008. Two children died of their illness. Recently, evidence was uncovered that suggested that the research group, led by Dr. Andrew Wakefield, had manipulated the data.[33]

2 A recent article in *The New York Times* alleged that Dr. Timothy Kuklo, a former surgeon at the Walter Reed Army Medical Center, falsified information pertaining to the number of soldiers he successfully treated with Infuse.[34] According to the article, Dr. Kuklo performed experiments on soldiers without approval and, in an article submitted to *The Journal of Bone and Joint Surgery*, falsified the signatures of co-authors. Dr. Kuklo is a paid consultant for Medtronic, the manufacturer of Infuse. The study was later retracted by the journal.

3 In another highly publicized case, the journal *Sleep* retracted a 2003 article written by Dr. Robert Fogel, a former faculty member at Harvard Medical School, after he admitted to altering numbers and fabricating anatomic details.[35] The fraud came to light when Dr. Fogel admitted his transgressions to his former supervisor, Dr. David White. Dr. White stated that Dr. Fogel "wanted to have the data come out to meet the hypothesis. It wasn't coming out that way, so he made it come out that way."

4 In another stunning case of scientific fraud, Dr. Scott Reuben, a highly regarded anesthesiologist whose research has significantly impacted how physicians treat surgical patients for pain, was found to have fabricated results in over 20 published studies.[36] In some cases, he is alleged to have even invented patients. Dr. Steven Shafer, editor of the journal *Anesthesia and Analgesia*, said, "This would be the largest research fraud in anesthesia. Doctors have been using his findings very widely. His findings had a huge impact on the field."

5 The American Board of Internal Medicine suspended or revoked the status of 139 physicians after discovering that these doctors had shared test items with the Arora Board Review, a New Jersey-based test preparation course. The Board found that many of the questions posted on the company's website were taken directly from the actual exam. Dr. Christine Cassel, President of ABIM, said that the offenders would face consequences. "Many hospitals, medical groups, and health plans require or strongly prefer that physicians be board certified..."[37]

6 Medicare fraud is a major problem. A recent federal bust led to criminal charges against 91 individuals, including ten physicians. Medicare was billed 295 million dollars for these false claims. In one scam, a physician billed Medicare for thousands of psychotherapy sessions that never took place. In another scam, several physicians referred patients for physical therapy and other services when these services were not required. Patients were recruited through kickbacks.[38]

7 In an elaborate scheme, two men from British Columbia were caught and now face criminal charges for theft of data from the Medical College Admissions Test.[39] While taking the exam, one man transmitted images of computerized test questions to his co-conspirator using a pinhole camera and wireless technology. The other had hired several MCAT tutors to answer the questions. When he left the room to transmit the answers back to the examinee, the tutors became suspicious.

8 After a patient was left paralyzed following spine surgery, an orthopedic surgeon knew that he had failed to follow the standard of care, and faced a malpractice suit.[40] Through a middleman, the surgeon tried to cut a deal with the patient's attorney. For dropping the case, the middleman would refer personal injury cases to the patient's attorney. The FBI uncovered the plot, and the doctor was charged with fraud and conspiracy.

9 In an analysis of residency applications to programs at the Brigham and Women's Hospital, researchers found evidence of plagiarism in over 5% of personal statements.[41]

References

[1]Baernstein A, Oelschlager A, Chang T, Wenrich M. Learning professionalism: perspectives of preclinical medical students. *Acad Med* 2009; 84(5): 574-81.

[2]Satterwhite W, Satterwhite R, Enarson C. Medical students' perceptions of unethical conduct at one medical school. *Acad Med* 1998; 73(5): 529-531.

[3]Humphrey H, Smith K, Reddy S, Scott D, Madara J, Arora V. Promoting an environment of professionalism: The University of Chicago "Roadmap." *Acad Med* 2007; 82(11): 1098-1107.

[4]Dans P. Self-reported cheating by students at one medical school. *Acad Med* 1996; 71 (1, suppl): S70-72.

[5]Anderson R, Obenshain S. Cheating by students: findings, reflections, and remedies. *Acad Med* 1994; 69(5): 323-332.

[6]Szauter K, Turner H. Using students' perceptions of internal medicine teachers' professionalism. *Acad Med* 2001; 76(5): 575-6.

[7]Kowalczyk L. Doctor accused of faking studies. *The Boston Globe*; March 11, 2009.

[8]Shanafelt T, Balch C, Bechamps G, Russell T, Dyrbye L, Satele D, Collicott P, Novotny P, Sloan J, Freischlag J. Burnout and medical errors among American surgeons. *Ann Surg* 2010; 251(6): 995-1000.

[9]Advancing education in medical professionalism: An educational resource from the ACGME Outcome Project. Available at: http://www.acgme.org/outcome/implement/profm_resource.pdf. Accessed June 12, 2011.

[10]Papadakis M, Hodgson C, Teherani A, Kohatsu N. Unprofessional behavior in medical school is associated with subsequent disciplinary action by a state medical board. *Acad Med* 2004; 79(3): 244-9.

[11]Papadakis M, Teherani A, Banach M, Knettler R, Rattner S, Stern D, Veloski J, Hodgson C. Disciplinary action by medical boards and prior behavior in medical school. *N Engl J Med* 2005; 353(25): 2673-82.

[12]Murden R, Way D, Hudson A, Westman J. Professionalism deficiencies in a first-quarter doctor-patient relationships course predict poor clinical performance in medical school. *Acad Med* 2004; 79(10 Suppl): S46-8.

[13]Ainsworth M, Szauter K. Medical student professionalism: are we measuring the right behaviors? A comparison of professional lapses by students and physicians. *Acad Med* 2006; 81(10 Suppl): S83-6.

[14]Teherani A, Hodgson C, Banach M, Papadakis M. Domains of unprofessional behavior during medical school associated with future disciplinary action by a state medical board. *Acad Med* 2005; 80(10 Suppl): S17-20.

[15]Goldstein E, Maestas R, Fryer-Edwards K, Wenrich M, Oelschlager A, Baernstein A, Kimball H. Professionalism in medical education: an institutional challenge. *Acad Med* 2006; 81(10): 871-6.

[16]Lazarus C. Elevating humanism through formal recognition programs. *Academic Physician & Scientist* 2008; September.

[17]University of Arkansas for Medical Sciences. Available at: http://www.uams.edu/info/pdfs/dose.pdf. Accessed July 5, 2011.

[18]Thomson P. Jamming the intangible into students. *The New Physician* 2006; 55 (1).

[19]Beaudoin C, Maheux B, Cote L, Des Marchais J, Jean P, Berkson L. Clinical teachers as humanistic caregivers and educators: perceptions of senior clerks and second-year residents. *CMAJ* 1998; 159(7): 765-9.

[20]University of Washington School of Medicine. Available at: http://depts.washington.edu/bioethx/topics/student.html#ques3. Accessed May 10, 2011.

[21]Stern D, Papadakis M. The developing physician – becoming a professional. *N Engl J Med* 2006; 355(17): 1794-9.

[22]Stark P, Roberts C, Newble D, Bax N. Discovering professionalism through guided reflection. *Med Teach* 2006; 28(1): e25-31.

[23]Ratanawongsa N, Wright S, Carrese J. Well-being in residency: effects on relationships with patients, interactions with colleagues, performance, and motivation. *Patient Educ Couns* 2008; 72(2): 194-200.

[24]Shanafelt T, Sloan J, Habermann T. The well-being of physicians. *Am J Med* 2003; 114: 513-519

[25]Shanafelt T, West C, Zhao X, Novotny P, Kolars J, Habermann T, Sloan J. Relationship between increased personal well-being and enhanced empathy among internal medicine residents. *J Gen Intern Med* 2005; 559-564.

[26]Thomas M, Dyrbye L, Huntington J, Lawson K, Novotny P, Sloan J, Shanafelt T. How do distress and well-being relate to medical student empathy? A multicenter study. *J Gen Intern Med* 2007; 22: 177-183.

[27]Brownell A, Cote L. Senior residents' views on the meaning of professionalism and how they learn about it. *Acad Med* 2001; 76: 734-737.

[28]Baldwin D, Daugherty S, Beverley D, Rowley B, Schwarz M. Cheating in medical school: a survey of second year students at 31 schools. *Acad Med* 1996; 71: 267-273.

[29]Cizek G. Cheating on Tests: How to do it, detect it, and prevent it. Lawrence Erlbaum Associates; Mahwah, NJ, 1999.

[30]Upstate medical students may be disciplined if investigation shows they cheated on quizzes. Available at: http://www.syracuse.com/news/index/ssf/2011/03/upstate_medical_students_may_b/978/comments-2.html. Accessed February 14, 2012.

[31]*Merriam-Webster's Collegiate Directory 11th ed.*

[32]Wakefield A, Murch S, Anthony A, Linnell J, Casson D, Malik M, Berelowitz M, Dhillon A, Thomson M, Harvey P, Valentine A, Davies S, Walker-Smith J. Ileal-lymphoid-nodular hyperplasia, non-specific colitis, and pervasive developmental disorder in children. *Lancet* 351(9103): 637-41.

[33]The Editors of the Lancet (February 2010). Retraction – ileal-lymphoid-nodular hyperplasia, non-specific colitis, and pervasive developmental disorder in children. *Lancet* 375(9713): 445.

[34]Wilson D, Meier B. Army disputes doctor's claim in study of injured. *The New York Times*; May 13, 2009.

[35]Mirviss L. Erstwhile medical school professor falsified sleep study data. *The Harvard Crimson*; April 9, 2009.

[36]Kowalczyk L. Doctor accused of faking studies. *The Boston Globe*; March 11, 2009.

[37]Health Leaders Media. Available at: http://www.healthleadersmedia.com/content/PHY-252334/Doctors-Caught-Cheating-on-ABIM-Certification-Exam. Accessed February 14, 2012.

[38]Medscape. Available at: http://www.medscape.com/viewarticle/749378. Accessed June 12, 2011.

[39]CBC. Available at: http://www.cbc.ca/news/Canada/british-columbia/story/2011/05/31/bc-high-tech-mcat-scam.html. Accessed September 4, 2011.

[40]USC Annenberg School for Communication and Journalism. Available at: http://www.reportingonhealth.org/blogs/doctors-behaving-badly-doctor%E2%80%99s-underhanded-deal-undone-fbi. Accessed February 14, 2012.

[41]Segal S, Gelfand B, Hurwitz S, Berkowitz L, Ashley S, Nadel E, Katz J. Plagiarism in residency application essays. *Ann Intern Med* 2010; 153(2): 112-20.

Chapter 13

First Summer in Medical School

10 Ways to Spend Your First Summer in Medical School

What should you do with the summer between your first and second year? This will probably be your last "free summer", and it's an important decision. As you progress through first year, you'll hear conflicting advice. "You have to do research. That's what residency programs want to see." "Use that time to study hard for the boards." "Don't do anything medical. After all, it's your last summer."

1 In a survey of the class of 2010 at the University of Michigan Medical School, performed after starting second year, 62% of the class indicated that they had spent their summer performing research.[1] Of those who chose not to do research, summer activities were split between physician shadowing, community health projects, international medical experience, teaching/tutoring (Kaplan, Princeton Review), and AMSA programs in health policy/leadership. A number of students also chose activities entirely unrelated to medicine. Students are often under the impression that research is essential to match well. However, surveys of residency program directors in most fields have shown that research is far less important in the residency selection process than other factors. While med school research in general is not highly valued relative to other academic selection criteria, the most competitive specialties do place greater importance on research experience. These residency programs are particularly impressed by published medical school research. In a survey of residency program directors, while published medical school research was next to last in overall importance, the most competitive specialties, like plastic surgery and radiation oncology, did rank it highly.[2]

2 In a survey of University of Texas Southwestern (UTSW) medical students, 14% reported participation in a summer preceptorship (physician shadowing) program.[3] You can arrange a shadowing experience through a formal program offered by your school or department of interest, a national organization, or informally through networking at your school and in the community. Student organizations may also provide summer shadowing opportunities.

3 Nine percent of UTSW students spent their first summer in medical school traveling. Dr. Suzanne Sarfaty, Assistant Dean of Academic Affairs at Boston University School of Medicine, offers the following advice.[4] "It is more important that you use the time in a way that is meaningful for you and enables you to get a better perspective on what you want to do with your future. You may decide to work on a community service project, travel, visit family, or read those novels you have been saving for a rainy day."

4 International health programs are another great way to spend the summer. Columbia University medical students can take part in a variety of international health programs. Summer experiences are available in Ethiopia, Tanzania, Israel, and the Dominican Republic. Your school may also have an office dedicated to international health experiences. Some schools, like the Chicago Medical School at Rosalind Franklin University, have an International Health Interest Group. These groups may have a list of international health opportunities based on the experiences of previous students and faculty. National organizations such as Doctors without Borders, the US Agency for International Development, and the International Rescue Committee may offer summer internships. AMSA has an extensive directory of international health opportunities at its website. Another useful resource is the International Health Medical Education Consortium website. Once you've targeted some programs, communicate with other students who have completed the elective. A frank discussion of the pros and cons can help you make an informed decision.

6 Develop your teaching skills. Training Tomorrow's Teachers Today is a five-day summer program held at George Washington University.[5] The program is a joint effort of George Washington University and AMSA. "At T4, students can expect to learn skills that will help them develop effective teaching methods, be a good bedside teacher during residency, become a stronger leader, and prepare for a successful career in academic medicine." Kaplan and Princeton Review often have teaching positions for medical students. Medical schools have summer courses for health professions students, and opportunities to teach may be available in the basic sciences. Prematriculation programs for incoming medical students often include medical students in a teaching or mentoring role.

7 Summer programs in Complementary and Alternative Medicine are available for interested medical students. Bastyr University's program involves education in Chinese medicine, whole foods nutrition, and naturopathic medicine.

8 Further your leadership skills through such programs as the Garcia Leadership and Advocacy Seminar, sponsored by the Latino Medical Student Association.[6] The program is "designed to cultivate and develop the leadership, organizational, and advocacy skills of recognized Latino medical student leaders from across the United States." Other leadership programs include AMSA's Leadership Institute and the Paul Ambrose Health Care for All Leadership Institute.

9 Learn about the impact of chronic illness on children through service-learning activities at summer camps. Indiana University medical students have been volunteering at Camp Boggy Creek Gang in Florida. The camp experience allows students to interact with children with chronic disease, including cancer, hemophilia, and paralysis, in a non-medical setting.

10 Immerse yourself in a foreign language. Some language immersion institutes, such as the Adventure Education Center in Costa Rica, offer Medical Spanish programs for health care professionals.

References

[1] University of Michigan Medical School Code Blue: A Guide to the M1/M2 Years. Available at: http://www.med.umich.edu/medstudents/siteParts/codeblue.pdf. Accessed February 15, 2012.

[2] Green M, Jones P, Thomas J. Selection criteria for residency: results of a national program directors survey. *Acad Med* 2009; 84(3): 362-7.

[3] AMSA's Unofficial Guide to UT Southwestern 2008-2009. Available at: http://www.southwesternstudents.com/AMSAUnofficialGuidetoUTSW.pdf. Accessed October 22, 2011.

[4] Boston University School of Medicine. Available at: http://www.bumc.bu.edu/enrichment/planningsummer/common-myths-realities-of-planning-your-summer/. Accessed February 15, 2012.

[5] AMSA Training Tomorrow's Teachers Today. Available at: http://www.amsa.org/AMSA/Homepage/EducationCareerDevelopment/AMSA Academy/T4.aspx. Accessed February 15, 2012.

[6] Garcia Leadership and Advocacy Seminar. Available at: http://lmsa.net/national-conference/glas. Accessed February 15, 2012.

Chapter 14

International Health Experiences

10 Benefits of an International Health Experience

In 1979, approximately 6% of graduating medical students reported participation in a clinical overseas elective.[1] In 2007, nearly thirty years later, over 27% of all medical students in the U.S. had taken part in an international health experience.[2]

1 Medical students returning from an international health elective describe seeing diseases that are rarely encountered in the U.S. Because the developing world often has fewer resources in terms of imaging and laboratory services, students have to rely heavily on history and physical exam skills to reach a diagnosis. Research indicates that such experiences can improve physical exam skills.[3]

2 International health experiences often provide exposure to underserved populations, social determinants of health, and health inequities. In one study of students following an overseas rotation, researchers found that 100% of respondents had greater awareness of public health issues.[4]

3 Following such experiences, medical students are more likely to remain involved in volunteerism and continue their work with underserved populations both in the U.S. and abroad.[5, 6]

4 Exposure to different cultures helps produce more culturally competent physicians. Medical students who participated in an

International Acupuncture Elective in China gained a better understanding of the importance of culture in the delivery of health care.[7]

5 The domestic patient population is becoming even more diverse, with immigration and travel bringing diseases that are endemic to other parts of the world to the United States. International health experiences serve to familiarize doctors with the evaluation and management of medical issues that are relatively uncommon in the developed world. "As a student on the infectious disease ward of Hospital Clinic in Sao Paulo, Brazil, I met my first patients with scrofula, Chagas disease, and Leishmaniasis. While these diseases are still rare in the US, I feel well equipped to treat patients who are recent immigrants or who have recently returned from abroad."[8]

6 You may inspire others. Following an 8-week field experience in a developing country, 96% of students reported that they recommended international health experiences to other students.[9] In another study, 48% of students who had completed an international health experience had given talks in international health and 33% had developed overseas electives for other physicians.[10]

7 You may look at patients differently. Students in a Global Multiculturalism Track, which included an international health experience, were found to have a higher degree of compassion toward neglectful patients and more respect overall for patients when compared to non-Track classmates.[11]

8 You may practice more cost-effective medicine. Following an international elective, 100% of medical students reported less dependence on the laboratory.[12]

9 You may be spurred to learn a new language. Preclinical students who completed a six-week international health experience reported a perceived need to know another language.[13]

10 Your experience may have an influence on career choice and further training. Medical students who participated in a field experience in a developing country were surveyed 4-7 years after the elective. Sixty-seven percent felt that the experience had influenced their careers. Seventy-four percent were in primary care, a percentage substantially higher than the comparison group.[14] Twenty-nine percent had an MPH (Master of Public Health) or were in the midst of training for the degree.

10 Important Safety Tips for International Health Experiences

Planning for your personal safety abroad is important, and some necessary precautions should be taken. Highlighting this fact was a study of Australian medical students. Sixty-four percent of students participating in an overseas elective experienced a health problem.[15]

1 Visit the U.S. Department of State travel information website for travel recommendations.[16] In particular, take note of any travel warnings related to the country you have in mind. Avoid scheduling electives in politically unstable countries at the time of elections.

2 Register with the local U.S. Embassy or consulate as a precaution.

3 Visit the CDC and WHO websites. Both organizations have travel sections with key information about vaccination and chemoprophylaxis prior to travel. These recommendations are specific to each country.

4 See a physician specializing in travel medicine 6 weeks before travel. Bring your immunization record with you. Determine if you need any vaccines or medications.

5 Obtain a post-exposure prophylaxis (PEP) kit for HIV. In the event you're exposed to contaminated or potentially contaminated blood, you can take the short-term anti-retroviral medications in the kit. Kits for hepatitis B are also available, but you may not need to utilize those if you've been vaccinated and have demonstrated immunity. If you won't be bringing a PEP kit, determine in advance how you would secure prophylactic anti-retroviral therapy.

6 Call your medical insurance provider to see if your coverage extends outside the U.S. If no coverage is provided, buy short-term travel insurance to cover for medical emergencies. Make sure your policy includes medical evacuation. A list of insurance companies providing coverage overseas is available at the U.S. Department of State website.

7 Make a copy of your passport, visa, driver's license, and insurance card. Leave a copy at home with a family member. Take a copy with you to your overseas destination, and keep it in a safe location separate from the original documents.

8 Find out before travel about the availability of gloves and safety glasses. If these items won't be provided, bring your own.

9 Take the same precautions with food and drink as you would in regular travel to foreign countries.

10 Some countries require visitors to register with the local police. If this isn't required, consider meeting with government and law officials in the area in case you later require their assistance.

References

[1]Association of American Medical Colleges. Medical Student Graduation Questionnaire. Washington, DC: AAMC; 1979.

[2]Association of American Medical Colleges. Medical Student Graduation Questionnaire. Washington, DC: AAMC; 2007.

[3]Thompson M, Huntington M, Hunt D, Pinsky L, Brodie J. Educational effects of international health electives on U.S. and Canadian medical students and residents: a literature review. *Acad Med* 2003; 78(3): 342-7.

[4]Bissonette R, Route C. the educational effect of clinical rotations in nonindustrialized countries. *Fam Med* 1994; 26: 226-31.

[5]Smith J, Weaver D. Capturing medical students' idealism. *Ann Fam Med* 2006; 4 (Suppl 1): S32-7.

[6]Ramsey A, Haq C, Gjerde C, Rothenberg D. Career influence of an international health experience during medical school. *Fam Med* 2004; 36(6): 412-6.

[7] Mao J, Wax J, Barg F, Margo K, Walrath D. A gain in cultural competence through an international acupuncture elective. *Fam Med* 2007; 39(1): 16-8.

[8]Grudzen C, Legome E. Loss of international medical experiences: knowledge, attitudes, and skills at risk. *BMC Med Educ* 2007; 7: 47.

[9]Haq C, Rothenberg D, Gjerde C, et al. New world views: preparing physicians in training for global health work. *Fam Med* 2000; 32(8): 566-72.

[10]Ramsey A, Haq C, Gjerde G, Rothenberg D. Career influences of an international health experience during medical school. *Fam Med* 2004; 36(6): 412-6.

[11]Godkin M, Savageau J. The effect of a global multiculturalism track on cultural competence of preclinical medical students. *Fam Med* 2001; 33(3): 178-86.

[12]Esfandiari A, Wilkerson L, Gill G. An international health/tropical medicine elective. *Acad Med* 2001; 76(5): 516.

[13]Godkin M, Savageau J. The effect of medical students' international experiences on attitudes toward serving underserved multicultural populations. *Fam Med* 2003; 35(4): 273-8.

[14]Ramsey A, Haq C, Gjerde G, Rothenberg D. Career influences of an international health experience during medical school. *Fam Med* 2004; 36(6): 412-6.

[15]Goldsmith J, Bettiol S, Sharples N. A preliminary study on travel health issues of medical students undertaking electives. *J Travel Med* 2003; 10(3): 160-3).

[16]United States Department of State. Available at: http://travel.state.gov/. Accessed February 15, 2012.

Chapter 15

Teaching

Teaching in Medical School: 10 Ways for Students to get Involved

The word "doctor," in Latin, means "to teach." Physicians are involved in teaching students, residents, colleagues, and other health care professionals. When discussing diagnosis and treatment, we teach patients. As future physicians, students recognize that they will be teachers, and surveys have shown that medical students are interested in teaching. Medical schools have responded by utilizing students as teachers.[1,2] Below we describe ways in which students can become involved in education and teaching.

1 As a second-, third-, or fourth-year medical student, you may be able to tutor underclassmen experiencing academic difficulty. Multiple studies have demonstrated success with this approach.[3,4] The University of Cincinnati School of Medicine has a well-established Peer Tutoring Program, and nearly the entire freshman class signs up for group tutoring. Individual tutoring is also available.[5] Recipients of near-peer and peer teaching feel that such teaching supplements faculty instruction. "The thing with peer teaching is that because they're not experts, they have a better understanding of what the basics are. When you're an expert like the faculty what you think is basic is no longer basic," remarked one student.[6]

2 Junior and senior medical students have taught physical diagnosis to first- and second-year students.[7] In one study, performance of first-year medical students in a Physical Examination Module with fourth-year student preceptors was compared to students with faculty preceptors. Both student groups fared equally well on the written final and standardized patient practical examinations.[8]

3 Opportunities to teach high school students may be available. At the Alpert Medical School at Brown University, introduction to medicine courses are held in the summer for high school students. The Office of Summer and Continuing Studies has funded teaching assistant positions for these courses.

4 Middle school children can also benefit from medical student teaching. For one Wednesday a month, a group of medical students at the University of Kansas teach science to more than 600 students at Argentine Middle School in Kansas City through the Students in Schools program. The program was founded by second-year medical student Justin Hoskins, a former substitute teacher. KU medical students "teach a science lesson relating to a part of the human body or a human health concern. The lesson also includes healthy life choices that can help prevent related health problems."[9]

5 Many medical schools have student groups focused on tutoring and teaching elementary school children. At the Temple University School of Medicine, students tutor 4th and 5th grade children at a local elementary school through the Big Friends program.

6 At the University of Texas Health Science Center in San Antonio, teaching assistant opportunities are available in a number of basic science courses, including gross anatomy, histology, physiology, microbiology, biochemistry, neuroscience, pathology, and pharmacology. Serving as a teaching assistant is one of the requirements for the school's MD with Distinction in Medical Education Program. The program provides students "with an opportunity to spend part of their medical school career participating in activities focused on different components of teaching and educational research."[10] Teaching assistant positions are offered at many U.S. medical schools.

7 Medical students often participate in study groups during basic science courses, which provide informal teaching opportunities. In one survey, 63% of students reported involvement in study groups.[11] In another survey exploring the benefits of study groups, the authors found that "effective study groups are supportive, socially cohesive groups who generate mutual trust and loyalty, and self- and co-regulate their learning by giving and receiving explanations and summaries and motivating individual study."[12]

8 Medical students have functioned as standardized patients (SPs). One study showed enhanced communication skills in an SP exam among students who had been trained to be SPs.[13]

9 You may be able to participate in course design. At the University of Arkansas for Medical Sciences, a vital signs module was created by a senior medical student. Senior medical student volunteers were recruited to be small group facilitators for teaching vital signs measurement to basic science students.[14]

10 In a 2008 survey of U.S. medical schools, although all reported utilizing students as teachers, only 44% had formal teaching skills programs.[2] Some schools have established formal teaching electives or workshops. At the Mt. Sinai School of Medicine, students can take the elective Becoming a Medical Teacher. This course provides "a comprehensive foundation for learning the principles of practical clinical and classroom teaching techniques...this class provides students with formal training to help them excel as clinical teachers."[15] AMSA has a Medical Education Leadership Institute which offers Training Tomorrows Teachers Today (T4), an intensive week-long experience in which students are equipped with practical teaching and leadership skills. Your participation in formal teaching skills instruction may fill a void in your future training. In one survey, the percentage of residency programs offering such instruction to residents varied from 31% in surgery to 80% in pediatrics.[16]

References

[1]Bing-You R, Sproul M. Medical students' perceptions of themselves and residents as teachers. *Med Teach* 1992; 14(2/3): 133–8.

[2]Soriano R, Greenberg L, Coplit L, Cichoskikelly E, Kosowicz L, Newman L, Pasquale S, Pretorius R, Rosen J, Saks N, Blatt B. Teaching medical students how to teach: a national survey of students-as-teachers programs in US medical schools. Available at: https://www.aamc.org/download/154610/data/rime_poste_40.pdf. Accessed February 8, 2012.

[3]Trevino F, Eiland D. Evaluation of a basic science, peer tutorial program for first- and second-year medical students. *J Med Educ* 1980; 55(11): 952-3.

[4]Walker-Bartnick L, Berger J, Kappelman M. A model for peer tutoring in the medical school setting. *J Med Educ* 1984; 59(4): 309-15.

[5] University of Cincinnati School of Medicine. Available at: http://www.med.uc.edu/StudentServices/AcademicSupport/PeertoPeer.aspx. Accessed February 2, 2012.

[6]Lockspeiser T, O'Sullivan P, Teherani A, Muller J. Understanding the experience of being taught by peers: the value of social and cognitive congruence. *Adv Health Sci Educ* 2008; 13: 361-72.

[7]Rund D, Jocoby K, Dahl M, Holman H. Clinical learning without prerequisites: students as clinical teachers. *J Med Educ* 1977; 52(6): 520-2.

[8]Haist S, Wilson J, Fosson S, Brigham N. Are fourth-year medical studnts effective teachers of the physical examination to first-year medical students? *J Gen Intern Med* 1997; 12(3): 177-81.

[9]University of Kansas School of Medicine. Available at: http://www.kumc.edu/news-listing-page/ku-school-of-medicine-students-share-the-joy-of-science-with-kck-middle-schoolers.html. Accessed February 13, 2012.

[10]University of Texas Health Science Center at San Antonio. Available at: http://som.uthscsa.edu/AcademicEnhancement/mddistinctionmedical.asp. Accessed February 15, 2012.

[11]Zhang J, Peterson R, Ozolins I. Student approaches for learning in medicine: what does it tell us about the informal curriculum? *BMC Med Educ* 2011; 11: 87.

[12]Hendry G, Hyde S, Davy P. Independent student study groups. *Med Educ* 2005; 39(7): 672-9.

[13]Sasson V, Blatt D, Kallenbert G, Delaney M, White F. "Teach 1, do 1…better": Superior communication skills in senior medical students serving as standardized patient-examiners for their junior peers. *Acad Med* 1999; 74: 932-7.

[14]Dwyer R, Deloney L, Cantrell M, Graham C. The first clinical skill: students teach students to take vital signs. *Med Educ Online* 2002; 7: 9.

[15]Mt. Sinai School of Medicine. Available at: http://www.mssm.edu/education/institute-for-medical-education/programs-courses-and-events/students-as-teachers. Accessed February 23, 2012.

[16]Morrison E, Friedland J, Boker J, et al. Residents-as-teachers training in U.S. residency programs and offices of graduate medical education. *Acad Med* 2001; 76 (10 Suppl): S1-4.

Chapter 16

Writing Awards

11 Writing Awards for Medical Students

1 The Alpha Omega Alpha Honor Medical Society presents the Helen H. Glaser Student Essay Award to medical students who have written excellent and thoughtful compositions addressing nontechnical topics in medicine. You need not be a member to apply for the award.

2 Unpublished essays written on a medical historical topic may be submitted for the American Association for the History of Medicine William Osler Medal Essay Contest. The competition is open to osteopathic and allopathic medical students in the U.S. and Canada. The award is presented to the winner at the annual AAHM meeting.

3 Medical student members of the American College of Physicians may submit an abstract to the American College of Physicians Medical Student Abstract Competition. The abstract can highlight a research project, community service program, or an interesting patient case. The winners receive an expense-paid trip to the College's Annual Session where they give oral presentations of their work.

4 Virtual Mentor invites students to submit essays for the John Conley Ethics Essay Contest. Essays should address the medical ethics or professionalism question chosen as the year's topic. The author of the winning essay receives a monetary award, and the essay is published in Virtual Mentor.

5 Three awards are available through the Arnold P. Gold – Francis A. Velay Humanism in Medicine Essay Contest. The focus of the essay is on "How Patients Teach Their Doctors about Humanism in Medicine."

6 The History Committee of the Massachusetts Medical Society sponsors the Annual Medical Student Essay Contest.

7 Original, unpublished poetry can be submitted to the Michael E. DeBakey Medical Student Poetry Award competition.

8 The Alpha Omega Alpha Pharos Poetry Competition awards several monetary prizes for poetry on medical subjects. All medical students at schools with an active AOA chapter are eligible to enter the competition.

9 The Student Essay Prize in the History of Medicine and Public Health is offered by the New York Academy of Medicine, and is open to medical students. The winning essay brings the author a monetary award. The essay is also considered for publication in the *Journal of Urban Health*.

10 The Northeastern Ohio Universities College of Medicine William Carlos Williams Poetry Competition is open to both allopathic and osteopathic medical students. Authors of the winning poems receive a stipend and support for travel to present their poems. The winning poems are also reviewed by the editors of the *Journal of Medical Humanities* for consideration of publication.

11 The Stanley M. Kaplan Medical Student Essay Contest honors original written work focusing on important problems in psychiatry.

Chapter 17

Choosing A Specialty

Choosing a Specialty: 15 Points to Consider

In a survey of 942 medical students attending 15 U.S. medical schools, researchers surveyed participants at freshman orientation, start of clerkships, and fourth year.[1] At each point, students were asked to name the specialty they were most interested in pursuing as a career. Notable findings included:

• At freshman orientation, pediatrics (20%) and surgery (18%) were the most common choices. Eight percent of freshman students reported general internal medicine as their initial specialty choice.

• 19% were undecided on specialty choice.

• When students were surveyed at the beginning of clerkships and in the fourth year of med school, researchers found that most students had changed their specialty choice. This was irrespective of their initial freshman choice.

In their conclusion, the authors wrote that "consistent with earlier reports, only 20-45% of medical students ultimately choose the specialty that they had been initially most interested in."

1 Specialties have been divided into person-oriented and technique-oriented fields, based on whether there is more of an orientation towards people or techniques and instruments. Person-oriented specialties include family practice, internal medicine, pediatrics, obstetrics/gynecology, psychiatry, and physical medicine and rehabilitation. Technique-oriented specialties include anesthesiology,

dermatology, pathology, radiology, emergency medicine, surgery, and otolaryngology. In one study, 349 first-year students were surveyed. Among students who indicated a preference for a person-oriented specialty, approximately 70% were found to enter one of these specialties.[2] However, only about 50% of those with a stated preference for a technique-oriented specialty in their first year ultimately entered one of those fields.

2 Your initial interest in a particular specialty may originate during the basic science years. In some cases, students find the subject matter in a course fascinating, and this leads them to further explore the specialty. Radiologists will often tell you that their enjoyment of anatomy led them to initially consider the specialty. Dr. Falk, a graduate of the Medical College of Wisconsin and a practicing diagnostic radiologist, describes the influence of anatomy on his specialty choice. "I would have to say that the most influential medical school course for me was anatomy, and in particular, neuroanatomy. I remember being amazed that something as complex as the human body could ever develop and function the way that it does. I have fond memories of the hours in the gross anatomy lab with my lab partners, struggling to dissect out and learn all of those structures. My interest in anatomy led to my ultimate career choice in radiology and subsequent neuroradiology fellowship."[3] Anesthesiologists point to coursework in pharmacology as stimulating their interest in the field. Dr. Jerry Reves, Vice President for Medical Affairs and Dean of the Medical University of South Carolina, writes that "the knowledge base required to practice Anesthesiology is primarily in the two general realms of physiology and pharmacology. Medical students who find these subjects of great interest will love anesthesiology because it is the practice of clinical physiology and pharmacology."[4]

3 Whatever field of medicine you choose, be prepared for negative feedback. Bashing of specialties is common, and some students have changed their career choices based on the comments of others. In a study of UCSF medical students, 95% of students considering a career in family medicine had received negative feedback about the specialty by their fourth year.[5] Hunt found that no specialty is immune from bashing, and that 76% of students experienced badmouthing of their specialty choices.[6] Negative comments can come not only from practicing physicians in other specialties, but also residents and students. In fact, one study found that the most frequent source of badmouthing was students.[7] Researchers have also looked at the effects of these negative comments, and have found that bashing of specialties can lead to a change in career choice.[8] In Hunt's study of over 1,100 students, negative comments led 17% of students to change their career choice. A more recent study showed that 67% of students received non-constructive criticism of their preferred specialty choice.[9] Most respondents (79%) believed that bashing was unprofessional.

4 Fit with personality, skills, and interests is the most important factor used to determine specialty choice. You can begin to explore fit during the basic science years. In a recent survey of graduating medical students, approximately 97% reported that fit with personality, skills, and interests was moderately or strongly influential in choosing which specialty to pursue as a career.[10] No other factor was given as much importance.

5 While many students wait until the clinical years to assess fit, this approach can be problematic. At most schools, students are required to rotate through the major or core specialties (internal medicine, general surgery, pediatrics, psychiatry, family medicine, obstetrics & gynecology) before pursuing clerkships in other fields. After completing these core rotations during the third year, students aren't left with much time. Most have two to three months of elective time to explore other specialties before they need to decide, since residency applications are typically submitted in September of the fourth year. In one study of medical students, 26.2% were unsure of their specialty choice at matriculation.[11] A similar proportion remained undecided at graduation.

6 Determining your fit for a specialty based on clinical exposure during rotations isn't always straightforward. Your rotation experience may be affected by the nature of your relationship with the attending or residents, the setting in which you rotate, and the extent and type of your responsibilities. This can make it difficult to accurately evaluate the specialty as a career choice.

7 Dr. Daniel Egan, Associate Director of the Emergency Medicine program at St. Luke's Roosevelt Hospital, reminds students that "what happens during your medical school rotation is quite different from everyday life in that specialty. For example, in the world of internal medicine, many practitioners spend most of their time in the outpatient setting, forming long-term relationships with their patients. For a surgeon, not every day is spent in the operating room as it is when you are the student. In obstetrics, the labor floor and postpartum evaluations are only a small part of the practice. It is clear that what you see as a student will help you understand what it will be like as a resident in that specialty. But one could argue that even residency may not perfectly emulate a long-term career in that specialty."[12]

8 During the preclinical years, one way to assess fit for specialties is by completing personality-type inventories. The premise of this approach is that people are most satisfied professionally when there is a good match between their specialty choice and their values, skills, and interests. Commonly used assessment methods include the AAMC Careers in Medicine program and the Glaxo Wellcome Pathway Evaluation Program. The AAMC Careers in Medicine (CiM) is a structured program designed to help students gain a better understanding of their personality, values, skills, and interests. The program also allows for exploration of different specialties. The AAMC writes that "as you work through the CiM program, you'll gain the tools to make an informed decision, based on guided self-reflection and the information you'll gather about many career options available to you."[13] The Glaxo Wellcome Pathway Evaluation Program, which has been designed to help students make informed specialty decisions, includes self-assessment exercises, an interactive workshop, and a specialty profile book. Many schools offer this program. If not, you can speak with your dean. For more information, contact Glaxo Wellcome at 1-800-444-PATH.

9 The Medical Specialty Aptitude Test is an online test developed by the University of Virginia School of Medicine.[14] It is based on content and material from the book *How to Choose a Medical Specialty*, by Anita Taylor. The website indicates that "you will be asked to rate your tendencies compared to the tendencies of physicians in each specialty.

The higher your score for a given specialty, the more similar you are to the physicians in that specialty."

10 Students often point to mentors and role models as being influential in choosing a specialty. In a survey of third- and fourth-year medical students at UCSF, 96% of all participants rated mentors as important or very important.[15] Unfortunately, recognizing the value of a mentoring relationship is a far cry from developing such a relationship. Although 96% of the participants rated mentors as important, only 36% actually reported having a mentor.

11 Shadowing physicians in different specialties may be enlightening, as Dr. Alfredo Quinones-Hinojosa, a neurosurgeon at the Johns Hopkins University School of Medicine, writes:[16]

"I'll never forget the day. It was as if a light switched on for me. In 1997, I was just finishing my second year in medical school and the Chairman of Neurosurgery at Brigham and Women's Hospital invited me into the operating room with him. During the surgery I saw this brain exposed to us, and it was so exciting to me. The brain is so intricate and complicated yet so fragile when removed from its protective skull. I would spend my Friday nights in the library reading about the brain and neurosciences. I just fell in love with the brain."

12 If you're interested in a particular specialty or specialties, take advantage of opportunities to learn about these fields during the basic science years. Research has shown that your efforts can increase the certainty of your choice.[17] There are a number of ways to learn more about a specialty during the preclinical years:

- Identify and work with a mentor
- Volunteer for clinical experiences (such as shadowing)
- Perform specialty-specific research
- Meet and speak with as many physicians as you can in your specialties of interest
- Attend local and national specialty organization meetings.

If you can make an informed decision, you significantly decrease your chances of having to switch specialties during residency, a process that can be uncomfortable, awkward, and certainly stressful. According to Gwen Garrison, Director of Student and Applicant Services at the AAMC, 30% of residents "either switch from their intended specialty after a transitional or preliminary year or switch outright during their specialty residency."[18] Dr. George Blackall, Director of Student Development at Penn State University College of Medicine, offers some reasons why residents switch. "Residents primarily switch because they a) realize their initial choice is not as interesting as another specialty, or b) desire a different lifestyle, level of flexibility, or income."[18]

13 Lifestyle considerations are an important issue for students in their decision-making process. Speak with physicians in different specialties to learn more. In the 2010 AAMC Medical School Graduation Questionnaire, over 11,000 graduating students were asked, "How influential was work/life balance in helping you choose your specialty?"[10] Over 70% of respondents reported work/life balance as being either moderately or strongly influential in their decision-making process. Only fit with personality/interests/skills and role model influences were given greater importance. Dr. Robert Cerfolio, a chest surgeon at the University of Alabama at Birmingham School of Medicine, writes that "medical students today are not just book-smart, they are life-smart. They want to work hard and play hard. Priorities have changed and the doctors of today are different from those of yesterday. They should be – hasn't everything else changed? The importance placed on being able to do things after the work-day is over is higher now than ever. We have listened to our parents, we have taken their advice. We realize and agree that there are more important things in life than just work."[19]

14 In 1989, Schwartz introduced the term *controllable lifestyle* to refer to "specialties that offer regular and predictable hours." These specialties are often characterized by fewer hours spent at work and less frequent on-call duties, allowing for greater personal time and flexibility to pursue other activities. When the influence of controllable lifestyle and other factors used in the decision-making process was quantified in a recent study, researchers found that controllable lifestyle was the most important factor.[21] In their conclusion, the authors wrote that "perception of controllable lifestyle accounts for most of the variability in recent changing patterns in the specialty choices of graduating US medical students." Specialties that are generally felt to offer a controllable lifestyle include anesthesiology, dermatology, neurology, ophthalmology, otolaryngology, pathology, psychiatry, and radiology. Specialties that are generally felt to offer a less-controllable lifestyle include family medicine, internal medicine, general surgery, obstetrics and gynecology, orthopedic surgery, pediatrics, and urology. It's important to note that within each of these specialties, though, there's a large degree of variability in practice settings and therefore in the degree of control accorded to physicians. An internist practicing as a solo practitioner has frequent on-call responsibilities. A hospitalist or an internist working for a large group will experience a significantly different work setting.

15 To learn about physician lifestyles in different specialties and in different practice settings, ask questions. That's the advice Dr. Daniel Egan, Associate Director of the Emergency Medicine Residency Program at St. Luke's Roosevelt, offers to medical students. "Ask questions not only about the specialty itself but about life outside of work... Try to get a sense of what life is like once residency is over. Residents have a unique perspective on things that may be somewhat limited to the lifestyle they experience during training. These are important issues to understand, as you will spend several years of your life in that role, but the rest of your life involves many more years after residency training."[12]

Anesthesiology: 10 Ways to Explore the Specialty as a Preclinical Student

Dr. Emery Neal Brown is Professor of Anesthesiology at Harvard Medical School. He reflects on why he found anesthesiology so appealing as a medical student. "I enjoyed my anesthesia rotation at medical school. I could see that it was very fast-paced and that you had to make important decisions quickly. That appealed. Plus: the regular hours. I saw myself doing research, as well as working with patients. You need a predictable schedule — which anesthesiologists have — to manage both. It's also a very important piece of modern medicine. If you think about what occurs when we do surgery, it's a very traumatic insult to the body. You're cutting people open, removing organs or possibly even transplanting them. The anesthesiologist puts people into a condition where they can tolerate such extreme assaults."[22]

Anesthesiology is a moderately competitive specialty. In the 2011 NRMP Match, there were approximately 1,400 available residency positions. In 2010, there were 5,443 total residents training in 131 allopathic anesthesiology residency programs.[23] Seventy-nine percent were U.S. MDs, 12.5% were IMGs, 8.1% were osteopathic graduates, and 0.2% were Canadian graduates. There are also 12 osteopathic residency programs offering positions through the AOA Match.

At most schools, anesthesiology is not a required or core rotation. Dr. Sharon Lin, Assistant Professor in the Department of Anesthesiology at the University of California – Irvine, recently surveyed 44 schools, and found that anesthesiology is an elective rotation in 66% of schools.[24] For most students, this means that unless you attend a school with a flexible clerkship curriculum, you won't be able to rotate through the specialty until the beginning of your fourth year. However, there are a number of opportunities to explore the field as a preclinical student.

1 Dr. William McDade, Associate Dean of Multicultural Affairs at the University of Chicago Pritzker School of Medicine, offers an excellent overview of the specialty at the AMA website.[25]

2 The American Society of Anesthesiology (ASA) Medical Student Component is developing a Mentor program for students in the areas of clinical education in the OR, residency/career advice, and research. Visit www.asahq.org for more information.

3 Jessica Barnes, a graduate of the Texas A & M College of Medicine, describes the impact her mentor had on her ability to match into anesthesiology. "I had a fantastic mentor that led me to choose anesthesiology. When I had questions about my career choice and even concerns about the specialty I was choosing, he was able to give some advice regarding my concerns. They can often give you real life expectations and provide you contacts around the country which is important for interviewing for residency positions."[26]

4 Opportunities to participate in anesthesiology research during the summer between your first and second years are available at many medical schools.

5 The Foundation for Anesthesia Education and Research (FAER) offers the Medical Student Anesthesia Research Fellowship to students interested in a career in anesthesiology research and perioperative medicine. This is a two-month research experience with the opportunity to present findings at the ASA annual meeting.

6 Joining your school's Anesthesiology Interest Group is an excellent way to learn more about the specialty, and may offer the chance to meet faculty. In a survey of students applying to the Beth Israel Deaconess Medical Center in Boston, only 64% of respondents attended a school where there was an Anesthesiology Interest Group.[27] If your school doesn't have a group, a guide to help establish one is available at the website for the American Society of Anesthesiologists (www.asahq.org).

7 Opportunities to learn more about the specialty, present research findings, and network with those in the field are also available to students who attend the ASA Annual Conference held in October.

8 The ASA has a Medical School Component, and you can take a more active role in this organization by running for one of six positions available in the Medical Student Governing Council.

9 Shadow one of your school's anesthesiologists. Shadowing can be arranged by contacting your school's anesthesiology department or joining the Anesthesiology Interest Group. According to the Ohio State University Department of Anesthesiology, "Shadowing does help! If a student is interested in anesthesiology, many would recommend shadowing because one day actually may be enough to get a feel for what anesthesiologists do. By shadowing for a short amount of time, a student would be able to better assess whether he/she would want to select anesthesiology as a third year elective."[28]

10 Some medical schools have created a list of faculty members interested in mentoring students. For example, LSU medical students can find anesthesiology mentors through the LSUHSC Mentors program. If there's no such list at your school, you'll have to take the initiative to create your own. You may meet potential mentors through lectures, preceptorships, or interest groups. You may identify potential mentors by speaking with third or fourth year students. You can also schedule a meeting with the clerkship director or program director at your institution, and seek advice on potential advisors.

Dermatology: 10 Ways to Explore the Specialty as a Preclinical Student

"It's also one of the last corners of medicine where there is what I call 'real medicine', clinical medicine, where you look at the problem; analyze it with your eyes. You're not forever writing lab tests and sending people off to have fancy scans here, there and everywhere. You look with your eyes, listen with your ears, touch with your fingers and you figure out what is wrong with the patient, and that is fascinating and satisfying."[29]

Dermatology is a highly competitive specialty. In the 2011 NRMP Match, approximately 370 positions were available. However, 21% of U.S. senior medical students failed to match. In 2010, there were a total of 1,040 residents training in 114 allopathic dermatology residency programs.[23] Ninety-five percent were U.S. MDs, 3.7% were IMGs, 1.3% were osteopathic graduates, and 0.1% were Canadian graduates. There are also twenty osteopathic residency programs offering positions through the AOA Match.

At most schools, students won't be able to complete a dermatology rotation until the end of their third year. However, for students who take the initiative, there are multiple opportunities to explore the field now.

1 Almost all applicants to dermatology will have performed research, and therefore if you're considering dermatology as a career, you may wish to participate in research between the first and second years of medical school. In a 2002 survey of 36 departments of dermatology, 21 reported at least one first- or second-year student involved in a case report or series.[30] Research experience has significant educational benefits. Beyond those benefits, research allows a student the chance to develop a relationship with their research supervisor. Establishing a mentor-mentee relationship will prove useful during the residency application process when your mentor can provide a strong letter of recommendation, based on significant personal interaction, as well as advocate on your behalf at other programs.

2 There are several sources of funding, such as the Medical Student Grant Targeting Melanoma sponsored by the American Skin Association. Strive for publication in the field. If publication isn't possible, seek out other opportunities to present your research. Poster presentations or oral presentations at conferences are valuable experiences.

3 Since most dermatology applicants have outstanding USMLE Step 1 scores and grades, the depth of your involvement in extracurricular and community service activities can help you stand out from a sea of highly qualified applicants. The demands of the clinical years can make it difficult to participate in these activities. Your involvement now as a preclinical student can aid significantly when you're ready to apply.

4 Dermatologists are active in the community, and students have opportunities to take part. Students can participate in Camp Discovery, Camp Horizon, Camp Sundown, and Camp Wonder, all of which provide wonderful experiences for children with a variety of skin diseases. Through the Melanoma Awareness Project, medical students teach children about the sun's effects on the skin, sun protection, and skin cancer. Miles for Melanoma is a program to raise funds for the Melanoma Research Society. You can seek out local opportunities as well. A number of dermatologists are involved in local clinics that provide care for the uninsured.

5 Since dermatology is often considered the most competitive specialty, find and establish a relationship with a mentor early. Introduce yourself to the dermatology department at your school. Take advantage of any opportunities to meet with the program director and chairman. "Meeting a supportive mentor early in medical school gives one a significant advantage over other applicants who do not find a mentor until much later."[31]

6 The Women's Dermatologic Society sponsors the Medical Student Awareness Program. Participants learn about the specialty by working with a dermatologist in academics or private practice.[32] This program "targets medical students in schools that lack a division or department of dermatology." First- and second-year students are given preference for the program.

7 The American Academy of Dermatology (AAD) has a Diversity Medical Student Mentorship program. This program allows students from "ethnically and socioeconomically diverse backgrounds to gain exposure to the specialty of dermatology by providing a firsthand, one-on-one mentorship experience with the dermatologist of the student's choice."[33]

8 Shadow a dermatology faculty member at your own school, or in the local area, to learn more about the specialty. Arrange a shadowing experience by contacting your school's dermatology department or joining the Dermatology Interest Group.

9 Joining your school's Dermatology Interest Group is an excellent way to learn more about the specialty. According to the Dermatology Interest Group Association (DIGA), 63 medical schools have an interest group. If you'd like to establish a group at your own school, a guide is available at the DIGA website.

10 Attend a conference. The American Academy of Dermatology holds its annual meeting in February. A Summer Academy Meeting takes place in August. Students can present their research findings at these meetings, and network with physicians in the field. The American Osteopathic College of Dermatology holds its annual meeting in October.

Emergency Medicine: 10 Ways to Explore the Specialty as a Preclinical Student

Dr. Sorabh Khandelwal, Director of the Emergency Medicine Clerkship at Ohio State University, describes what draws many medical students to the specialty. "It is a field that is full of excitement. It truly is a constant adrenaline rush. Life and death decisions are made at the bedside literally in seconds in many patients and this truly is a powerful and humbling experience at the same time. Our field covers an amazing breadth of medicine. Almost every journal in any specialty will have some article that is useful to an emergency physician. Perhaps you have heard the phrase regarding an emergency physician, 'jack of all trades, master of none'. It is true to an extent, however we believe we are masters at resuscitation and acute care medicine. Aside from a challenging work arena, emergency medicine allows for an active social life outside of medicine. This is a big reason why many people choose Emergency Medicine."[34]

Emergency medicine is a moderately competitive specialty. In the 2011 NRMP Match, there were over 1,600 available residency positions. However, nearly 10% of U. S. seniors failed to match. In 2010, there were 5,119 residents training in a total of 155 allopathic emergency medicine residency programs.[23] Eighty-one percent were U.S. MDs, 7.4% were IMGs, 11.5% were osteopathic graduates, and 0.1% were Canadian graduates. There are also over 40 osteopathic residency programs offering positions through the AOA Match.

At most schools, exposure to emergency medicine is limited until the fourth year, when students have greater flexibility to participate in an EM clerkship. However, opportunities to explore the field are available earlier. Dr. Shahram Lotfipour, Associate Dean for Clinical Science Education and Clinical Professor of Emergency Medicine at the University of California – Irvine, offers the following advice for preclinical students.[35] "Students exploring EM should seek out clinical exposure, interact with EM faculty, participate in EM organizations, and increase their knowledge of EM literature."

1 Given the competitiveness of the specialty, establishing a relationship with a mentor early in the process will be helpful. According to Dr. Gus Garmel, Co-Program Director of the Stanford-Kaiser Emergency Medicine Residency Program, finding a mentor is not easy.[36] "How students find faculty mentors is challenging, because their exposure to a broad selection of emergency medicine faculty may

be limited early in their training." Dr. Garmel encourages students "to seek out mentors from faculty committed to their well-being, personal and professional growth, and success within the specialty."

2 The Society for Academic Emergency Medicine (SAEM) has a virtual advisor program. This program allows students who attend schools without an emergency medicine residency program to interact with faculty elsewhere. For DO students interested in the field, the American College of Osteopathic Emergency Physicians (ACOEP) has established a mentor program for students. There are over 2,000 osteopathic emergency medicine physicians.

3 Most medical schools have an Emergency Medicine Interest Group. Membership allows students opportunities to explore the specialty further by engaging in clinical observation, research, and community service. Leadership positions are also available.

4 While many students have an idea of what emergency medicine involves, there's no substitute for real-life experience. That's why shadowing EM physicians becomes so important. In a study done at the University of Toronto, preclinical students participated in an EM observorship experience.[37] Researchers found that this experience allowed students to make more informed decisions with respect to EM as a career.

5 Dr. Jamie Collings, former Program Director of the EM residency at Northwestern University, states that "I think that students should spend time shadowing, but also talking to practicing EM physicians about the good and the bad of the specialty. Also, if you are really interested in EM, make sure you shadow on a Friday or Saturday during the night (a room full of drunk patients may not be what you envision)."[38]

6 At schools with academic emergency medicine departments, there are often opportunities to participate in research during the summer between first and second year. If you're interested in performing EM research during this time, consider applying for the Medical Student Research Grant, which is jointly sponsored by SAEM and the Emergency Medicine Foundation. Medical students are also eligible to apply for a Research Grant from the Emergency Medicine Residents' Association (EMRA).

7 Research findings may be presented at the American College of Emergency Physicians (ACEP) Research Forum. The Best Medical Student Paper award is given at the meeting.

8 For students interested in community service, Local Action Grants are available through EMRA. Grants are awarded to students for projects that improve community health, such as through education, direct services, or preventive programs. Grants are also awarded for projects that support the specialty through community awareness, advocacy, or involvement with local and state government.[39]

9 To learn more about the specialty, consider attending the American College of Emergency Physicians Scientific Assembly meeting (October), SAEM Annual Meeting (June), and American Academy of Emergency Medicine (AAEM) Scientific Assembly (February). The American College of Osteopathic Emergency Physicians has two annual conferences – the Fall Scientific Assembly and the Spring Conference. Both conferences offer students opportunities to interact with residency programs and faculty.

10 For students interested in taking a more active role in the American Academy of Emergency Medicine, consider running for a position in the Medical Student Council.

Family Medicine: 10 Ways to Explore the Specialty as a Preclinical Student

Dr. Cynthia Romero is a family physician and Chief Medical Officer of the Chesapeake Regional Medical Center. After graduating from Eastern Virginia Medical School, she completed a residency in family medicine. As a family physician, she enjoys the continuity of care the specialty provides. "The best part of being a primary care physician is the continuity of care that I can have with my patients – being able to both prevent injury and illness through health maintenance and take care of people when they are sick. Caring for all of my patients' needs is very rewarding and satisfying. I get to know them as individuals."[40]

Family Medicine is not a competitive specialty. However, securing a position in highly coveted residency programs is difficult. In the 2011 NRMP Match, there were approximately 2,700 residency positions available. In 2010, there were 9,583 residents training in a total of 451 allopathic family medicine residency programs.[23] Forty-four percent were U.S. MDs, 39.1% were IMGs, 16.7% were osteopathic graduates, and 0.1% were Canadian graduates. There are also over 80 osteopathic residency programs offering positions through the AOA Match.

1 Family physicians are active in the community, and many welcome student participation. Through the American Association of Family Physicians (AAFP) Tar Wars program, health care professionals annually reach out to over 500,000 fourth and fifth-grade students to discourage children from smoking. Since most Family Medicine Interest Groups are involved in community service, joining your school's group is an excellent way to learn how family medicine physicians are able to impact their communities.

2 You can learn more about the specialty by joining your school's Family Medicine Interest Group. For information on how to establish or maintain an FMIG at your school, a useful resource is the FMIG Manual, available at http://fmignet.aafp.org. If your school has an established group, you'll have the opportunity to run for officer positions, such as president, community service coordinator, and student membership coordinator. According to the Virtual Family

Medicine Interest Group website, "many FMIG leaders go on to hold leadership positions at the state and national levels of the AAFP throughout their careers."[41]

3 As with any field of medicine, one of the best ways to learn about the field is to observe and speak with practicing physicians. Family medicine physicians are actively involved in preclinical education through Physical Diagnosis and Introduction to Clinical Medicine courses. You can approach these faculty and ask about shadowing opportunities. You can also identify opportunities through your school's Family Medicine Interest Group.

4 While preclinical interactions can help you identify potential mentors, you can also directly introduce yourself to the family medicine department. Osteopathic students can identify mentors through the Mentor Exchange program developed by the American Osteopathic Association. The American College of Osteopathic Family Physicians is another organization that can help students locate mentors. State organizations are also involved in mentoring. For example, the Osteopathic Surgeons and Physicians of California has a mentoring program for students who are members of the organization.

5 Most schools provide opportunities to perform family medicine research during the summer between the first and second years of medical school. Organizations such as the American Academy of Family Physicians (AAFP), Society of Teachers of Family Medicine (STFM), and the North American Primary Care Research Group (NAPCRG) also provide students with research opportunities.

6 Funding for your research project may be provided by your school. You can also apply for external grants or awards. The AAFP awards Student Externship Matching Grants to support students pursuing research opportunities in Family Medicine. State chapters are another source. For example, the Minnesota Academy of Family Physicians awards grants to students interested in family medicine research projects through their David Mersy, M.D. Student Externship Program.

7 Students who have performed family medicine research may be eligible for the NAPCRG Student Family Medicine/ Primary Care Research Award.

8 Research may be published in journals or presented at conferences. These include the AAFP Scientific Assembly (fall), National Conference of Family Medicine Residents & Students (early August), AMSA National Conference, NAPCRG Annual Meeting, and the American College of Osteopathic Family Physicians Annual Convention. Opportunities to present research may also be available at state meetings and conferences. For example, the Arizona Osteopathic Medical Association has an Annual Clinical Case and Poster Presentation.

9 Student chapters of the American College of Osteopathic Family Physicians (ACOFP) exist at many osteopathic schools. ACOFP encourages students to "build leadership skills by participating and running for office in the ACOFP student chapter on campus."

10 The AAFP holds its annual meeting in the fall. It also holds the National Conference for Medical Residents and Students in August. The AAFP Foundation provides scholarships for students to attend the National Conference. The AAFP writes that these funds enable students "the opportunity to explore Family Medicine through clinical sessions, procedural workshops and interaction with family physicians across the country." The American College of Osteopathic Family Physicians holds its Annual Convention in March. The convention's Residency Fair allows students to meet with program directors and residents representing many of the 150 AOA-approved programs.

Internal Medicine: 10 Ways to Explore the Specialty as a Preclinical Student

Dr. Robert Waterbor is an internist at the Eisenhower Medical Center in California. As a medical student at Duke University, he was attracted to internal medicine for several reasons. "I went into internal medicine because I believe a good internist is equipped to be a good detective. We see whatever comes through the door, and it can be anything from a surgical problem to an obscure medical diagnosis, and part of our job is to be able to recognize when something serious may be going on....Besides liking the detective aspect of the field, I do like the long-term commitment to patients that goes along with it. Getting to know patients is not only gratifying in its own right, but really enables me to assess their health a lot more easily."[42]

Internal Medicine is not a competitive specialty. However, top tier residency programs receive thousands of applications for a small number of positions, and matching with one of these programs is difficult. In the 2011 NRMP Match, there were approximately 5,100 available residency positions. In 2010, there were 22,415 residents training in a total of 380 allopathic internal medicine residency programs.[23] Forty-nine percent were U.S. MDs, 44.6% were IMGs, 6.4% were osteopathic graduates, and 0.1% were Canadian graduates. There are also over 100 osteopathic residency programs offering positions through the AOA Match.

Following an internal medicine residency, graduates may practice as internists (outpatient primary care, hospitalist) or pursue fellowship training in a subspecialty. Subspecialties of internal medicine include allergy, cardiology, endocrinology, gastroenterology, geriatric medicine, hematology/oncology, infectious disease, nephrology, pulmonary medicine, and rheumatology.

Polls of the general public have demonstrated a poor understanding of what internists do. New med students are often confused as well. Dr. Mahendr Kochar, Senior Associate Dean for Graduate Medical Education at the Medical College of Wisconsin, says that "if you ask members of the general public, they don't have a clue, unless they are already under the care of an internist. Even incoming medical students are at a loss when you ask them what internal medicine is."[43] In this section we provide suggestions on ways to learn about the specialty.

1 The American College of Physicians (ACP) has created a Mentoring Database. To access the database, which includes program directors, clerkship directors, chairs of medicine, practicing internists, and residents, you must be a member. Mentors are available to answer "specific questions about scheduling your summer preceptorships, getting through the match, and preparing for clerkships and residency interviews..."[44] The database allows you to narrow the list of potential mentors based on specialty, geographic location, type of practice, gender, ethnicity, and other factors. If you're not sure how to select a mentor from the database, ACP can pair you with an appropriate individual depending on your interests or specific questions.

2 Participation in research is an excellent way to explore internal medicine or one of its subspecialties. Medical schools often provide summer research experiences in internal medicine. The Ohio State University Department of Internal Medicine has funded positions for entering second year students. Students may conduct a basic science or clinical research project. "The student will play a participatory role and take an active part in reviewing literature, executing experiments, collecting data, analyzing, interpreting results and writing manuscripts. Dissemination of results through publication and presentations is expected and advantageous to a student's career."[45]

3 Medical student members of the ACP may enter abstract competitions at both the local and national level. Abstracts can be submitted in one of four categories – clinical vignette, basic research, clinical research, and quality improvement/patient safety. Winners of the National Clinical Vignette and National Research Paper competitions are showcased at the ACP annual scientific meeting.

4 ACP IMpact is an internal medicine newsletter published monthly by the American College of Physicians. The newsletter does accept submissions from medical student members. Through past articles, students have shared study tips, informed colleagues of helpful resources, and offered tips to survive medical school.

5 Networking opportunities are available to students who attend national conferences. At the annual scientific meeting of the ACP, students can interact with physicians in the field, meet residency program personnel at the Internal Medicine Residency Fair, and attend a Medical Student Mentoring Breakfast.

6 Shadowing is an excellent way to explore the specialty. Nearly all medical schools have an Internal Medicine Interest Group, and opportunities to shadow are often available through the group. At the Uniformed Services University of the Health Sciences, students can arrange such experiences by contacting the leadership of their Club Med organization. "Our faculty are eager to have students visit their clinics and procedure suites to see first-hand what internists do!" USUHS students have seen patients on the general medicine wards and subspecialty clinics. They have also observed a variety of procedures, including cardiac catheterization, video bronchoscopy, and gastrointestinal endoscopy.[46]

7 Your Student Affairs Office may have a list of internal medicine physicians who are interested in having students shadow them. Dr. Isaac Wood, Associate Dean of Student Affairs at Virginia Commonwealth University School of Medicine, has created the guide *Exploring Career Options in Medicine*.[47] In the guide, he lists "contact information for faculty who would be happy to meet with you, talk about their work and arrange a shadowing experience so you may become better informed."

8 If your school has an established mentoring program, you may be able to identify a mentor in the field through the program. Another option is to approach your advising or student affairs dean for his or her advice. Since physicians practicing internal medicine or a subspecialty are often heavily involved in the preclinical curriculum, you may encounter potential mentors through your courses, small group discussions, and preceptorships. Mentors may also be identified through internal medicine interest groups, school alumni offices, and referrals from junior and senior medical students.

9 Internal Medicine Interest Groups (IMIGs) are well-established at U.S. medical schools. If your school doesn't have a group, turn to the IMIG Resource Guide available at the ACP website for information on bringing a new group to life. ACP's IMIG Sponsorship Program provides funding for groups, and additional funds are made available to groups who reach certain recruitment levels. Participation in your school's IMIG will provide exposure to the specialty, provide opportunities to network with residents and faculty, facilitate shadowing, and allow you to run for leadership positions.

10 Osteopathic medical students interested in internal medicine can become members of the American College of Osteopathic Internists (ACOI). Through the organization's mentoring program, you can be paired with a physician in the field. Chapters of the student branch, known as the Student Osteopathic Internal Medicine Association (SOIMA), are active at osteopathic schools.

Neurology: 10 Ways to Explore the Specialty as a Preclinical Student

Dr. George Richerson is Professor and Chair of the Department of Neurology at the University of Iowa. He was drawn to the specialty of neurology because he found that the brain was more interesting than any other organ in the body. "I was attracted to the challenge of understanding how it works and curing diseases that affect it," says Dr. Richerson. "Patients with disorders of the nervous system often present with unusual symptoms and signs and can be challenging and fun to diagnose. There are already treatments for many of these patients. Recent progress in developing treatments for others has been astounding, and is continuing at a pace much faster than most fields in medicine. It is exciting to be part of that progress and to try to contribute to it. It is also gratifying to be able to treat patients with neurological diseases that other physicians either do not recognize or don't understand well enough to know how to manage."[48]

Neurology is not a competitive field. In the 2011 NRMP Match, approximately 600 positions were available. Ninety-eight percent of U.S. seniors successfully matched. However, highly coveted neurology residency programs remain quite competitive, and it is challenging to secure a position in these programs. In 2010, there were 1,928 residents training in a total of 126 allopathic neurology residency programs.[23] Fifty-five percent were U.S. MDs, 36.6% were IMGs, 7.9% were osteopathic graduates, and 0.1% were Canadian graduates. There are also 7 osteopathic residency programs offering positions through the AOA Match.

Neurology is heavily covered in U.S. medical schools during the preclinical portion of the curriculum. Neuroanatomy and neurophysiology may be a component of anatomy and physiology courses, or may be covered in a separate neuroscience course. If you have an early interest, there are considerable opportunities to explore the field as a preclinical student.

1 Research in the field can provide significant exposure and the opportunity to work closely with faculty members. In many schools, students can perform research in the summer following first year. Funding to support research may be available through schools or through external sources such as the American Academy of Neurology (AAN). Students who are members of their school's Student Interest

Group in Neurology are eligible to apply for the Medical Student Summer Scholarship sponsored by the AAN.

2 Preclinical students are eligible to apply for the Summer Program in the Neurological Sciences sponsored by the National Institute of Neurological Disorders and Stroke.

3 The Child Neurology Foundation offers the Swaiman Medical Scholarship. This is a summer clinical research experience open to first and second year medical students.

4 The Parkinson's Disease Foundation has a Summer Fellowship Program for students interested in performing Parkinson's-related summer research.

5 For students interested in researching myasthenia gravis or a related neuromuscular disorder, consider the Myasthenia Gravis Foundation of America's Henry R. Viets Medical/Graduate Student Research Fellowship.

6 The American Brain Tumor Association (ABTA) offers the Medical Student Summer Fellowship program for students interested in performing neuro-oncology research. At the end of the fellowship, students are required to submit a report. Following review of these reports, an outstanding medical student is chosen to receive the ABTA Lucien Rubenstein Award.

7 With over 150 chapters in the United States and Canada, it's likely that your school has a Student Interest Group in Neurology (SIGN). Membership allows opportunities to shadow neurologists, learn more about the field through lectures and presentations, and apply for SIGN scholarships. For information on starting or running a chapter, the American Academy of Neurology (AAN) has developed the SIGN Reference Manual, available at their website.[49]

8 First-hand observation of a neurologist in clinical practice is invaluable. You can often arrange shadowing experiences with faculty members at your institution. According to the American Academy of Neurology, shadowing will allow you to "get a glimpse of a-day-in-the-life of your potential future profession."[50]

9 Since members of the neurology faculty are often involved in preclinical education, you may be able to meet and establish mentor-mentee relationships through these interactions. The American Academy of Neurology recommends that you "choose a mentor who makes you comfortable, shares your interests, and has an interest in you. Get to know the neurology faculty at your medical school by attending Grand Rounds, resident teaching conferences, or SIGN events."[50]

10 The AAN holds its Annual Meeting in April. The AAN and the Association of University Professors of Neurology have combined their efforts and make scholarships available to fund students interested in attending the meeting.

Neurological Surgery: 10 Ways to Explore the Specialty as a Preclinical Student

According to the Women in Neurosurgery organization, "neurosurgery appeals to those individuals who find the human brain fascinating and who enjoy the physical act of correcting abnormalities of the nervous system. Although the intellectual challenge of constant learning and change may draw an individual to neurosurgery, it must be coupled with a strong desire to be an interventionist, willing to make decisions and take responsibility for those decisions. No two operations are exactly the same, and much time is spent considering the various options before choosing an approach to a problem. Stress and the challenges of dealing with critically ill patients are everyday occurrences for neurosurgeons. They must be able to cope not only with death but also with the very real and difficult decisions regarding the most vital functions of the brain and spinal cord such as the ability to think, speak, see, move, and feel. Neurosurgeons are asked to communicate complex concepts to patients and family members about quality of life and risks versus benefits of surgical procedures on the most delicate organ in the body."[51]

Neurosurgery is a highly competitive specialty. In the 2011 NRMP Match, 195 positions were available. However, 14% of U.S. seniors did not match. In 2010, there were 1,140 residents training in a total of 101 allopathic neurological surgery residency programs.[23] Eighty-nine percent were U.S. MDs, 10.5% were IMGs, 0.4% were osteopathic graduates, and 0.1% were Canadian graduates. There are also 11 osteopathic residency programs offering positions through the AOA Match.

In a survey of U.S. medical schools, only 33% of schools offered neurosurgery rotations to third year students.[52] Therefore, most students won't have the opportunity to perform a neurosurgical rotation until their fourth year. If you've developed an early interest in the field, however, there are a number of ways to explore the field prior to your clinical rotation.

1 In the document *So, You Want to be a Neurosurgeon,* the Women in Neurosurgery organization encourages students to "get to know neurosurgeons in active practice and spend time with them and residents training in neurosurgery. There are many different styles of practice and a wide variety of personalities can be found in neurosurgery...Shadow a neurosurgeon to see what his or her life is like."[51]

2 Not every medical school has a neurological surgery residency program. If you don't have access through your school, organizations that can put you into contact with neurosurgeons include the American Association of Neurological Surgeons, Congress of Neurological Surgeons (CNS), Women in Neurosurgery, and Council of State Neurosurgical Societies (CSNS).

3 The NYU Department of Neurosurgery offers a Summer Intensive in Neurosurgery. During this 8-week rotation at Tisch Hospital, students are active members of the neurosurgical team, working closely with both residents and attending physicians. The goal of the intensive is for students "to fully understand what neurosurgery is all about so they can make an educated decision about whether it is for them or not." Although priority is given to NYU students, the program is open to other U.S. medical students.[53]

4 Dr. Ellen Shaver, Associate Professor of Neurosurgery at the Medical College of Georgia, writes that "in the preclinical years, it is helpful to identify a mentor or faculty advisor to recommend possible electives, research opportunities and residency programs of interest to you."[54] Because you may have limited interaction with neurosurgical faculty until third or fourth year, your initiative will be key to establishing a relationship with a mentor early in your education. Introduce yourself to the neurosurgery department at your school. In particular, take advantage of any opportunities to meet with the program director and chairman.

5 The Women in Neurosurgery organization has developed a mentoring program that pairs the medical student with an experienced neurosurgeon.

6 Schools with neurosurgery departments often provide opportunities to perform research during the summer following first year. Preclinical students are eligible to apply for the Campagna Scholarship, which supports a 10-week summer neurosurgical research experience with a mentor at the Oregon Health & Science University.

7 The Department of Neurosurgery at Cedars-Sinai Medical Center offers the Pauletta and Denzel Washington Family Gifted Scholars in Neuroscience Award. During this summer fellowship, awardees work in a research laboratory at Cedars-Sinai under the supervision of Dr. Keith Black. "Awardees are expected to submit an abstract or scientific paper on their research to a national neuroscience, cancer, or neurosurgery meeting."[55]

8 The American Association of Neurological Surgeons offers summer fellowships for medical students who want to perform neurosurgical research (Medical Student Summer Research Fellowship Program). CNS and CSNS offer the Medical Student Summer Fellowship in Socioeconomic Research, an award given to students conducting research on a socioeconomic issue affecting neurosurgical practice.

9 Joining your school's Neurosurgery Interest Group will help you learn more about the specialty. However, many schools lack a group or have groups that have become inactive. Explore ways to start a group at your school.

10 The Congress of Neurological Surgeons holds its annual meeting in October. The Annual Meeting of the American Association of Neurological Surgeons takes place in April. Students may be able to present their research findings at these meetings and network with physicians in the field.

Obstetrics and Gynecology: 10 Ways to Explore the Specialty as a Preclinical Student

In reflecting on his career in obstetrics and gynecology, Dr. Mark Rowe, a faculty member at the Texas A & M Health Science Center College of Medicine, could not imagine choosing a specialty more exciting. "What could be more exciting than looking back over a generation of deliveries?" says Dr. Rowe. "I have had the opportunity to bring many new lives into the world and have on occasion seen some back as grown-up patients." For Dr. Rowe, the specialty "was the right combination of basic science of reproductive medicine and the clinical practice of medicine. The science that forms the basis for the specialty is intellectually stimulating and the patient relationships are personally satisfying."[56]

Obstetrics and gynecology is a moderately competitive specialty. In the 2011 NRMP Match, there were approximately 1,200 available residency positions. Six percent of U.S. senior medical students failed to match. In 2010, there were 4,884 residents training in a total of 243 allopathic obstetrics and gynecology residency programs.[23] Seventy-four percent were U.S. MDs, 16% were IMGs, 9.5% were osteopathic graduates, and 0.1% were Canadian graduates. There are also 29 osteopathic residency programs offering positions through the AOA Match.

Obstetrics and gynecology is a core clerkship, and all medical students are required to rotate through the field during the clinical years. For most students, this is often their first exposure to the specialty.[57] However, opportunities to explore obstetrics and gynecology are available to preclinical students, and are described below. "Exposing medical students to women's health care earlier in their career can help encourage greater awareness, interest, and motivation, while helping to avoid misperceptions," writes Dr. Peter Schnatz.[58]

1 The American Congress of Obstetricians and Gynecologists (ACOG) has produced a video for medical students. Titled "Choose Ob-Gyn for Women's Health," the video is available at www.acog.org.

2 The Association of Professors of Gynecology and Obstetrics (APGO) has developed several documents of interest for students – *Basic Science Prerequisites to a Clerkship in Obstetrics and Gynecology* and *Comprehensive Women's Health Care: A Career in Obstetrics and Gynecology.* These documents are available at www.apgo.org.

3 Preclinical students often take lectures or courses on Women's Health, and you'll have opportunities to meet OB/GYN faculty through these interactions. Other opportunities include welcome lunches, career panel discussions, and meetings of the medical student OB/GYN interest group. "Shadowing a physician in private practice, doing some research for a summer, and talking to a student-friendly faculty member in giving advice are good ways to gain exposure," says Dr. Eugene Toy, Residency Program Director of OB/GYN at The Methodist Hospital in Houston.[59]

4 Schools often provide opportunities to perform research during the summer between the first and second years of med school. In the Obstetrics and Gynecology Summer Research Program at Jefferson Medical College, students work with a research-oriented faculty member and have opportunities to "shadow, observe, and become involved in the clinical offices, operating room, labor and delivery, grand rounds, journal club and clinical meetings."[60]

5 At ACOG's Annual Clinical Meeting, students can attend the medical student course and luncheon, residency fair, and student workshops. Registration and membership are free for students. ACOG divides its members into regions or districts based on geography. Medical student members can also attend their Annual District Meeting.

6 ACOG has developed a list of obstetricians and gynecologists interested in mentoring students. To access the list, you must become an ACOG member. Dr. Eugene Toy offers advice for students seeking a mentor. "The two most important factors are availability/interest of the faculty member, and experience/expertise of the faculty member to give good advice. Other factors include honesty and integrity, confidentiality, and the mentor's placing the students' interests as higher than one's own or the institution's."[59]

7 Learn more about the specialty by joining your school's interest group. There are over 120 active medical student OB/GYN interest groups. A guide to starting a new group is available at the ACOG website.

8 Obstetricians and gynecologists are active in the community, and in many cases students may join them. At UCSF, students can volunteer in the Women's Clinic of the Homeless Clinic. At the University of Kansas, students provide Women's Health education at a local women's shelter and participate in the Susan G. Komen Race for the Cure.

9 Osteopathic students may learn more about the specialty by becoming members of the American College of Osteopathic Obstetricians & Gynecologists.

10 Students can explore residency programs through an online residency directory available at the APGO website.

Ophthalmology: 10 Ways to Explore the Specialty as a Preclinical Student

Dr. Adam Abroms is an ophthalmologist in private practice in California who completed his residency training in the Department of Ophthalmology at the University of California Irvine. "I have always had a passion for fixing things," says Dr. Abroms. "As an ophthalmologist, I am challenged by fixing complicated medical problems. Today, with so many exciting technologies available, the solution to vision problems has never been more within reach."[61]

Ophthalmology is a highly competitive field. In the 2011 NRMP Match, there were approximately 460 available residency positions. However, 12% of U.S. senior medical students did not match. In 2010, there were 1,268 residents training in a total of 117 allopathic ophthalmology residency programs.[23] Ninety-three percent were U.S. MDs, 6.5% were IMGs, 0.9% were osteopathic graduates, and 0.1% were Canadian graduates. There are also 13 osteopathic residency programs offering positions through the AOA Match.

In 2000, 68% of medical schools required an ophthalmology rotation. By 2004, the percentage had decreased to 30%.[62]

1 At the American Academy of Ophthalmology (AAO) website, information is available for students interested in the specialty. Students can learn about the practice of ophthalmology, subspecialties, and the basics and structure of residency programs.

2 Ophthalmologists are involved in service work in the United States and abroad through such organizations as Unite for Sight, Operation Access, ORBIS, Volunteer Eye Surgeons International, Eye Care America, and Prevent Blindness America. Medical students can also participate. Participation in community service can enhance your ophthalmologic knowledge and eye examination skills while providing a much needed service.

3 Shadow an ophthalmologist. According to Dr. Andrew Lee, Chairman of the Department of Ophthalmology at The Methodist Hospital, "shadowing both a private practice eye MD or an academic faculty member might allow the student an insider glimpse into the practice of ophthalmology, and can create a mentoring opportunity that could lead to an important and convincing letter of recommendation downstream."[63]

4 Many schools have an Ophthalmology Student Interest Group (OSIG). Through your involvement in this group, you can learn more about the specialty and gain access to busy clinical faculty. Exposure to the specialty will allow you to assess whether your "personality matches the 'ophthalmology personality type'" says Dr. Lee.[63]

5 Schools often provide opportunities to perform research during the summer between the first and second years of medical school.

6 Summer Student Fellowships are available to med students interested in eye research through Fight for Sight. The organization has also partnered with WomensEyeHealth.org to offer a summer fellowship entitled "Understanding Gender Disparities in Eye Health." Fellowships are also available in ocular immunology and cornea study.

7 The Bascom Palmer Eye Institute, affiliated with the University of Miami Miller School of Medicine, offers short or long-term research training opportunities for medical students.

8 Research grants for medical students are also available through the Sjogren's Syndrome Foundation.

9 For students interested in a longer period of research, Research to Prevent Blindness offers a one-year fellowship with $ 30,000 grant support.

10 Medical students can present their research at local, regional, and national conferences such as the Association for Research in Vision and Ophthalmology.

Orthopedic Surgery: 10 Ways to Explore the Specialty as a Preclinical Student

Dr. Stephen Ritter is an orthopedic surgeon with Methodist Sports Medicine in Indiana. As a medical student at the University of Iowa, he recalls being attracted to the field of orthopedics because "it combines both the science and the art of medicine. The ability to alter form to improve function requires skill, attention to detail and an appreciation of what an elegant and intricate structure the human body is. When you are responsible for trying to help a patient return to their normal lifestyle, it is very important that they receive nothing less than complete honesty."[64]

Orthopedic Surgery is a highly competitive specialty. In the 2011 NRMP Match, approximately 670 residency positions were available. However, 23% of U.S. senior medical students failed to match. In 2010, there were 3,412 total residents training in 152 allopathic orthopedic surgery residency programs.[23] Ninety-six percent were U.S. MDs, 2.9% were IMGs, and 1.0% were osteopathic graduates. There are also 33 osteopathic residency programs offering positions through the AOA Match.

In a survey of U.S. medical schools, only 55% had mandatory instruction in musculoskeletal medicine, defined as "a preclinical module or clinical clerkship in orthopedic surgery" or related field.[65] According to Dr. Peter Stern, Chairman of Orthopedic Surgery at the University of Cincinnati, "orthopedic surgeons are underrepresented on curriculum committees, resulting in underexposure of students to orthopedic practice during the preclinical years."[66] Therefore, many students won't gain exposure to the specialty unless they actively seek out experience. Dr. Chris Reilly, a faculty member in the Department of Orthopedics at the University of British Columbia, writes that "students may be exposed to a specialty late in their education," and this may result in less competitive applications.[67] For students who may be considering this field, it's therefore important to begin exploring opportunities now.

1 Because you may have limited interaction with orthopedic surgery faculty until third or fourth year, your assertiveness will be key to establishing a relationship with a mentor early in your medical education. According to the Department of Orthopedic Surgery at Wake Forest University School of Medicine, "make yourself known to the orthopedic faculty at your own institution. Contact one or more of the attendings and introduce yourself as a prospective orthopedic residency candidate. Just get to know them and allow them an opportunity to know you."[68] In particular, take advantage of any opportunities to meet with the program director and chairman. Some students are able to establish a mentor-mentee relationship with the help of their school's orthopedic surgery interest group.

2 The American Academy of Orthopedic Surgeons (AAOS) has created a Mentoring Program. Information about the program, which was developed primarily for minorities and women, is available at their website.

3 The J. Robert Gladden Orthopedic Society is an organization that seeks to increase diversity in the specialty, and offers mentoring and networking programs for medical students.

4 There's no better way to begin learning about the field than by watching an orthopedic surgeon in action. Many faculty members welcome student observers. To arrange a shadowing experience, begin by checking with your dean's office. Some will maintain a list of faculty members with an interest in having student observers. If there's no such list, you can directly contact the orthopedic surgery department.

5 According to Dr. Nitin Bhatia, Program Director of the University of California Irvine residency program, performing research in the field will definitely improve your chances for obtaining a residency position.[69] Schools with orthopedic surgery departments often provide students with opportunities to perform research during the summer between the first and second years of medical school.

6 The Hospital for Special Surgery sponsors the Medical Student Summer Research Fellowship, a two-month program for students who have completed their first year of medical school. Students have opportunities to perform basic science, translational science, or clinical research under the supervision of a faculty mentor. Observation of orthopedic surgical procedures is also available. Although Weill Cornell Medical College students are given preference, the program is open to students at other schools.

7 The Children's Hospital of Philadelphia (CHOP) has an orthopedic surgery research program open to students attending accredited medical schools.[70] According to the program, "the ideal time commitment is at least three months with a minimum goal of having a published article or public presentation on the obtained results." For students interested in a longer period of research, CHOP also offers the Orthopedics Medical Student Clinical Research Award. This is a one-year experience dedicated to performing clinical research before either the third or fourth year.

8 The AAOS holds its Annual Meeting in February. To offset the costs of attending the conference, the Ruth Jackson Orthopedic Society provides up to $ 1500 each to two students.

9 The American Osteopathic Academy of Orthopedics holds its annual meeting in conjunction with the American Osteopathic Association in October. Students may have opportunities to present their research findings at these meetings, and network with physicians in the field.

10 Joining your school's Orthopedic Surgery Interest Group is an excellent way to learn more about the specialty. However, many schools lack a group or have groups that have become inactive. If your school does not have a group, consider starting one. Doing so may fulfill a need at your school, much like the Vanderbilt Orthopedic Interest Group has done. Through the efforts of the group, Vanderbilt medical students gain early exposure to the field by linking students with mentors and introducing students to orthopedic research.

Otolaryngology: 10 Ways to Explore the Specialty as a Preclinical Student

Dr. David Oliver is an otolaryngologist in private practice in Savannah, Georgia. He is a graduate of the Medical University of South Carolina otolaryngology residency program. In medical school, he was intrigued by the specialty, and remains attracted to otolaryngology for the same reasons. "I went to medical school and became intrigued by the diversity of the ENT specialty. I treat every age group from newborns to the elderly, men and women, have a significant office practice, and perform a variety of surgeries. I was also attracted to the complexity of the ENT specialty. The anatomy and physiology of ear, nose, and throat are poorly understood by patients and other doctors and the management is intricate. There are many special sense (smell, taste, hearing, special, singing, etc.) and cosmetic concerns in the ear, nose, and throat."[71]

Otolaryngology, commonly referred to as ENT [ear, nose, and throat] is considered a highly competitive specialty. In the 2011 NRMP Match, approximately 280 positions were available. Fourteen percent of U.S. senior applicants failed to match. In 2010, there were a total of 1,424 residents training in 103 allopathic otolaryngology residency programs.[23] Ninety-seven percent were U.S. MDs, 2.6% were IMGs, 0.2% were osteopathic graduates, and 0.2% were Canadian graduates. There are also 15 osteopathic residency programs offering positions through the AOA Match.

In all of the highly competitive specialties, an early start can provide a strong advantage in the residency match. Early involvement in the field can lead to important connections, mentoring, research opportunities, and opportunities for leadership, publication, presentations, or awards. An early start can be difficult in ENT, though. In a survey of U.S. medical schools, otolaryngology was a required third-year rotation at only 33.6% of schools.[72] Therefore, most students won't be able to rotate through the ENT department until their fourth year of medical school. We've outlined ways in which preclinical students can develop their own opportunities to explore the field and excel in the field.

1 In order to learn more about the field, it's best to speak with and observe ENT physicians. Shadowing experiences can be ideal, and most students can find opportunities to shadow faculty at their own institution. However, not every medical school has an otolaryngology surgery residency program or department. If you don't have access through your school, the American Academy of Otolaryngology – Head and Neck Surgeons may be able to help you.

2 Students can also work with otolaryngology residents. Some schools provide formal opportunities to do so, while at other institutions you'll have to arrange your own experiences. At the University of Pittsburgh, preclinical students can observe and assist ENT residents in their on call duties on weeknights and weekend days through the ENT Buddy Call program.

3 Most students will have limited interaction with ENT faculty until the third or fourth year of med school. Therefore, you'll need to take the initiative to identify potential advisors and mentors, and establish those relationships. Most students begin by scheduling a meeting with the designated student contact in the ENT department. This may be a faculty member, chairman, program director, or clerkship director. During your preclinical years, you should also take advantage of any opportunities to meet with these individuals. Since otolaryngologists are sometimes involved in preclinical education through anatomy lectures and physical diagnosis instruction, you may be able to meet and establish relationships through these venues.

4 Almost all students who apply to otolaryngology will have performed research. Starting early can provide students with more significant opportunities to participate. Many schools with ENT departments provide opportunities to perform research during the summer after first year. Dr. Venu Divi, Program Director of the otolaryngology residency program at Drexel University, encourages students to be productive in research. "Ideally the research should be completed and published by the time the application is due. Research specific to otolaryngology is best, but experience which can be utilized for future projects, such as basic science research, is also useful."[73]

5 Preclinical students who are members of underrepresented minority groups are eligible to apply for the Johns Hopkins Department of Otolaryngology Medical Student Mentoring Clerkship Program.

Through this program, students may perform a three-month clinical and/or research rotation at Hopkins. Students must have completed at least one year of medical education to be considered.

6 Funding for medical student research is available through several organizations, including the American Academy of Otolaryngology - Head and Neck Surgery, American Head and Neck Society, and American Academy of Otolaryngic Allergy. Students seeking funding for one year of research can apply for the American Head and Neck Society – Pilot Grant.

7 Interest groups provide valuable opportunities, starting with the chance to learn more about the specialty. Some schools lack ENT interest groups, or have inactive groups. If that's the case, you can start one and thereby fulfill a need at your school. The purpose of the ENT interest group at the University of Virginia School of Medicine is to "expose students to this exciting field" and "foster shadowing, mentoring, and research opportunities between faculty and students."[74]

8 The American Academy of Otolaryngology – Head and Neck Surgeons holds its Annual Meeting in September. Students may be able to present their research findings at these meetings, and network with physicians in the field.

9 The American Academy of Otolaryngology – Head and Neck Foundation offers a Medical Student Research Paper Prize.

10 The Association for Research in Otolaryngology has offered awards to students in recognition of research contributions. Glenn Schneider, a medical student at the University of Rochester, received a fellowship award to cover travel expenses so that he could attend the organization's annual meeting. There, he was able to present the results of his research project on deafness.[6]

Pathology: 10 Ways to Explore the Specialty as a Preclinical Student

Dr. Justin Bishop is a chief resident in the Johns Hopkins pathology residency program. He discovered a passion for pathology during his pathology elective. "During my pathology elective it became clear that it was the field for me. The importance of the pathologist's diagnosis was astonishing; the course of treatment, along with the patient's prognosis, was entirely dependent on the impression of the pathologist, the ultimate consultant. The field struck me as very cerebral; pathologists are required to have knowledge of virtually every disease process that can affect every organ in order to diagnose them. Finally, I was struck by how vast the field was. Even though at that time I did not know what subspecialty of the field I would go into, I discovered that Pathology encompassed areas ranging from molecular diagnostics to clinical chemistry to forensic pathology. I knew that I would find my niche."[76]

Although pathology is a course taken by students during the preclinical years, study of the subject matter, in and of itself, won't allow students to properly explore the specialty as a possible career choice. In a survey of second-year students from 5 medical schools, Dr. Lorne Holland, Assistant Professor in the Department of Pathology at the University of Colorado, found that students often had misconceptions of the field.[77] He concluded that "better education about the practice of pathology in the second year" is needed. Similar findings were found when researchers met with focus groups of senior medical students.[78] "This study indicates that despite relatively abundant preclinical exposure to pathology, students 'don't even get what pathologists do.'"

Pathology is not a competitive specialty. However, securing a position in one of the top tier programs remains challenging. In the 2011 NRMP Match, approximately 520 positions were available. In 2010, there were 2,355 residents training in a total of 147 allopathic pathology residency programs.[23] Sixty-two percent were U.S. MDs, 31.3% were IMGs, and 6.5% were osteopathic graduates.

1 Explore the specialty by reading *Pathology as a Career in Medicine* published by the Intersociety Council for Pathology (ICPI). Other publications worth reading include *A Career as a Pathologist* and *Top 10 Myths about Pathology*. Both are available at www.asip.org.

Budding clinician scientists will be particularly interested in *The Road to Becoming a Clinician Scientist in Pathology and Laboratory Medicine* published by the American Society for Investigative Pathology (www.asip.org). Among the questions addressed in the publication are "Why choose academic pathology and laboratory medicine?" and "Is a physician scientist career for me?"

2 Membership in the American Society for Clinical Pathology is complimentary for medical students, and is an excellent way to learn more about the field (www.ascp.org). For students who have a specific question about pathology, the College of American Pathologists has an "Ask a Pathologist Your Question" service.

3 To observe the responsibilities of a practicing pathologist, start by checking with your school for a list of pathologists able to provide shadowing experiences. You may also be able to identify a pathologist open to observers through the interest group at your school. Some pathology departments, such as that at the University of Massachusetts, have developed formal observership programs for preclinical students. The Department of Pathology writes that "most students go through medical school, especially the first 2 years, having little exposure to pathology as a medical specialty. The observership will provide an opportunity to see what pathologists really do in their day-to-day life – the important role they play in patient care, what type of 'lifestyle' they have, etc."[79]

4 Establishing a relationship with a mentor is an excellent way to learn more about the field. Since pathologists are often actively involved in preclinical education, you may be able to identify a mentor through your coursework. Students are also encouraged to visit their school's department of pathology, and initiate relationships with key faculty, such as the program director or chairman. According to the University of Chicago, "specialty advisors should be experienced in the appropriate clinical arena, have time and 'chemistry' with the student, and have a broad view of the field."[80]

5 Join your school's pathology interest group. If no chapter exists at your school, consider starting one. ICPI provides Medical Student Interest Group (MSIGs) Grants to schools to start new groups or enhance existing groups.

6 In schools with academic pathology departments, students will often find opportunities to participate in pathology research during the summer following their first year. The American Society for Investigative Pathology (ASIP) sponsors the Summer Research Opportunity Program in Pathology. This program, which targets underrepresented minority students, allows students to participate in research at prominent institutions. For students interested in a longer period of research, some schools offer a one year experience.

7 Medical students may be honored with the Award for Academic Excellence and Achievement by the ASCP. Each medical school's pathology department can nominate a single second-year student. To be eligible, students must attend school in the US, Canada, or Puerto Rico. Recently, 47 second-year students were honored.

8 Wondering about work-life balance as a leader in the field? In the February 2011 ASIP Trainee Newsletter, Dr. Dani Zander, Chair of the Department of Pathology at Pennsylvania State College of Medicine, offers her perspective.[81]

9 The ASCP Resident Council annually surveys residents and fellows about the fellowship application process and job market for pathologists. Survey results are available at www.ascp.org.

10 Concerned about the cost associated with attending a pathology conference? ICPI offers the ICPI Trainee Travel Award to support trainees who wish to participate in scientific meetings of one of the member societies.

Pediatrics: 10 Ways to Explore the Specialty as a Preclinical Student

Dr. Steven Czinn is Chair of Pediatrics at the University of Maryland. Soon after starting medical school, he discovered his love for pediatrics. "When I was in school, I saw that there is nothing more rewarding than taking a child who is ill or suffering, and making him feel better. To see the look on the child's face, and the look on the parents' face, is such an extremely satisfying feeling. I decided then that this was what I wanted to do."[82]

In a survey of over 900 students attending 15 U.S. medical schools, pediatrics was the most commonly chosen specialty choice among freshman medical students.[1]

Pediatrics is not a competitive specialty. However, securing a position in a highly coveted residency program is difficult. In the 2011 NRMP Match, nearly 2,500 positions were available. In 2010, there were 8,140 residents training in a total of 198 allopathic pediatrics residency programs.[23] Sixty-seven percent were U.S. MDs, 23.9% were IMGs, 9.3% were osteopathic graduates, and 0.2% were Canadian graduates. There are also 17 osteopathic residency programs offering positions through the AOA Match.

1 Since many schools have incorporated primary care preceptorships into the preclinical curriculum, you may be able to request a pediatrics preceptor. You may also locate preceptorships separate from your medical school. The Texas Pediatric Society has implemented a General Pediatric Preceptorship Program (www.txpeds.org). Through this program, students "are placed with pediatricians in private practice for a four-week period to learn at a practical level about general pediatric practice."[83]

2 To arrange a shadowing experience, check with the dean's office for a list of interested faculty members. If there's a Pediatrics Interest Group at your school, you may locate a physician to shadow through the group. You can also arrange to shadow by directly contacting your school's pediatrics department.

3 Since pediatricians are actively involved in preclinical education, you may locate a mentor through your coursework. In a survey of pediatric clerkship directors, it was learned that 63% taught in the preclinical years, with 23.5% having administrative responsibility for a preclinical course.[84] Some schools have created a list of faculty members interested in mentoring students. If no such list exists, you may directly introduce yourself to your pediatrics department. Take advantage of any opportunities to meet with the program director, chairman, or clerkship director. Mentors may also be located through your school's Pediatric Interest Group.

4 Pediatricians are active in the community, and students have opportunities to take part. You can directly contact the involved pediatricians, or you may be introduced to these activities through your involvement in a pediatrics interest group. According to the American Academy of Pediatrics, these groups offer "numerous opportunities to serve the public and children through community-oriented projects. Some of these projects give you practical training interacting with pediatric populations."[85]

5 In her second year, Georgetown student Allison Heinly was actively involved in community service through her school's interest group. "This past year she has headed the pediatric interest group, which hosts holiday activities, coordinates a book drive, and donates proceeds to the pediatric inpatient unit at Georgetown University Hospital. She also volunteers with the Georgetown Medical Student – Patient Partners Program, in which medical students are paired with pediatric patients suffering from chronic illness. The students offer their time and support to the children, helping to ease their time while in the hospital."[86]

6 Joining your school's Pediatric Interest Group is an excellent way to learn more about the specialty. For information on how to establish or maintain a group at your school, a useful resource is the Pediatric Interest Group Resource.[87]

7 Many osteopathic schools have pediatric student clubs. If your school doesn't, the American College of Osteopathic Pediatricians has created a Student Chapter Manual with information on how to organize and run a club.[88]

8 Although research in pediatrics isn't required to secure a residency position, there are many benefits to research participation. The Department of Pediatrics at the Medical College of Georgia writes that summer research projects "add science to the art of medicine, build rapport with advisors and potential mentors, and enhance one's competitiveness for matching in first choice residency programs after medical school. We believe that getting involved in research during the summer will enhance the quality of your work as a future pediatrician or other clinical practitioner."[89] Most schools provide students with opportunities to perform pediatrics research during the summer between the first and second years.

9 The American Pediatric Society and the Society for Pediatric Research jointly sponsor the Student Research Program. There are currently research opportunities at over 300 institutions in the United State. A strong effort is made to link the student with the research group of his or her choice. Accepted students receive a stipend to support a two to three month experience. Of note, the experience takes place at an institution other than the student's own medical school. For more information, visit https://www.aps-spr.org.

10 The American Academy of Pediatrics holds its National Conference in October. Several years ago, the Academy developed the Medical Student Subcommittee, which has worked on developing resources for medical students. Students interested in applying for a position should visit www.aap.org. The American College of Osteopathic Pediatricians holds its Spring Conference in April. Students may be able to present their research findings at these meetings, and network with physicians in the field.

Physical medicine and Rehabilitation: 10 Ways to Explore the Specialty as a Preclinical Student

Dr. Sarah Knievel is a fourth-year resident in the Department of Physical Medicine and Rehabilitation at the Mayo Clinic. For Sarah, "the decision to enter physical medicine and rehabilitation (PMR) was an easy one. PMR is a specialty that focuses primarily on the restoration of function. It is fascinating to work with complex patients with the intent to restore mobility, independence, and their ability to reach personal goals. Patient success ranges from resuming the activities of daily living to obtaining a personal record in a 10K race. I enjoy both the diagnostic and therapeutic aspects of my job that ultimately provide patients with tools to help themselves."[90]

Physical medicine and rehabilitation is a moderately competitive specialty. In the 2011 NRMP Match, approximately 370 positions were available. In 2010, there were a total of 1,228 residents training in 77 allopathic physical medicine and rehabilitation residency programs.[23] Fifty-five percent were U.S. MDs, 19.2% were IMGs, 25.7% were osteopathic graduates, and 0.1% were Canadian graduates. There are also three osteopathic residency programs offering positions through the AOA Match.

Exposure to physical medicine and rehabilitation during the preclinical years is often limited. To learn more about the specialty, the American Academy of Physical Medicine and Rehabilitation offers the following advice.[91] "As a first or second year medical student, exploring PM&R as an option can be done through shadowing, contacting local residents and faculty, and through pursuing research on a relevant topic. There are some 'externships' in PM&R available to first year medical students during the summer between first and second year."

1 Most students begin their exploration of the specialty by shadowing practicing physicians. Your dean's office may provide a list of faculty members who provide such experiences, or you may locate a physician through your school's interest group. You can also contact the PM&R department directly. In some cases, formal programs may be available. For example, the Department of Physical Medicine and Rehabilitation at the Indiana University School of Medicine offers a Summer Scholarship Program. This is a one-month experience in which students observe a faculty member in day-to-day activity.

2 The Department of Physical Medicine and Rehabilitation at Northwestern University sponsors the Rehabilitation Institute of Chicago Summer Externship Program. This program offers preclinical students the opportunity to assist in the clinical management of patients. Students are also able to participate in a research project.

3 Mentors are valuable resources, and can provide advice, guidance, and application support. In a survey of PM&R residents, only 35.4% of respondents reported having had a mentor before beginning residency training.[92] However, among those who had a mentor, 75.9% indicated that their relationship with a mentor had a positive effect on their career decision. Some medical schools have created a list of faculty members who are interested in mentoring. If no such list exists, you can express your interest in the field and schedule a meeting with a faculty member in the department.

4 The American Academy of Physical Medicine and Rehabilitation has created a mentor program. Mentors are grouped according to their areas of interest in the field, and are available to answer questions about the specialty, residency programs, and the application process. Osteopathic students can also find a mentor through the American Osteopathic College of Physical Medicine and Rehabilitation's mentor program.

5 Opportunities to participate in PM&R research are available at many med schools, and students often take advantage of the summer following first year to participate in a focused research experience.

6 The Association of Academic Physiatrists (AAP) and the Foundation for PM&R offers students a summer externship (Rehabilitation Research Experience for Medical Students) following the first year of medical school at participating host institutions. During this externship, students are expected to complete a scholarly project. After completion of the project, students are expected to submit a research paper to the AAP Best Medical Student Paper Competition. Students are able to present their findings at the organization's Annual Assembly.

7 Students interested in research should also investigate the Medical Student Research Grant sponsored by the Education and Research Fund of the Foundation for Physical Medicine and Rehabilitation.

8 Interest groups provide a number of opportunities to explore the field in more depth. If your school does not have an active chapter, a guide to help you establish one is available at the website for the Association of Academic Physiatrists.[93]

9 Osteopathic students may also learn more about the field through student chapters of the American Osteopathic College of Physical Medicine and Rehabilitation (AOCPMR), which have been established at many schools.

10 At the Annual Meeting of the Association of Academic Physiatrists, students may have opportunities to present their research, network with physicians in the field, and meet additional mentors. Opportunities to learn more about the specialty and network with those in the field are also available to students who attend the AOCPMR conference held in April. At the 2010 conference, students were given an overview of the field, tips to ace their PM&R clerkship, and insight into the application process from the perspective of program directors.

Plastic Surgery: 10 Ways to Explore the Specialty as a Preclinical Student

Dr. Trung Le is a plastic surgeon in private practice in Massachusetts. He was initially drawn to the specialty after being involved in the care of a woman who had breast cancer. "After the plastic surgeon performed breast reconstruction on her, you could see a big difference of how she viewed herself and her relationship with her husband. It was very inspiring," recalls Dr. Le.[94]

Plastic surgery is a highly competitive specialty. In the 2011 NRMP Match, approximately 100 positions were available for new graduates. In 2010, there were a total of 345 residents training in 71 allopathic plastic surgery residency programs.[23] Eighty-six percent were U.S. MDs, 11.9% were IMGs, 1.7% were osteopathic graduates, and 0.3% were Canadian graduates. There are also three osteopathic residency programs offering positions through the AOA Match.

At most schools, plastic surgery is not a required or core rotation. However, some third-year students are able to rotate through the field during their surgery core clerkship. If not, you'll have to wait until the beginning of your fourth year. However, there are considerable opportunities to explore the field as a preclinical student. In a survey of medical students, Dr. Greene, a faculty member in the Division of Plastic Surgery at the Harvard Medical School, found that "medical student exposure to plastic surgery is the most influential factor in a student's decision to pursue a career in plastic surgery."[95]

1 Plastic surgeons are often active in the community. Students can witness the benefits they provide, and may be able to participate. Operation Smile offers medical mission opportunities to medical students. The organization is well-known for providing free cleft lip and palate repair surgery to children all over the world.

2 At the Annual Meeting of the American Society of Plastic Surgeons, which takes place in September, the Young Plastic Surgeons Forum holds its popular Medical Students Day. On this day, students can meet recognized leaders in the field, receive an overview of the residency training programs, learn about research opportunities, and attend a Q & A session with residents.

3 The American Society for Aesthetic Plastic Surgery invites medical students interested in plastic surgery as a career to attend The Aesthetic Meeting free of charge. At the scientific meeting, students are allowed to attend the Welcome Reception, visit exhibits, and interact with residents, fellows, and plastic surgeons. The meeting takes place in April or May.

4 Students interested in the field should explore the specialty further through shadowing. You can contact your dean's office or the plastic surgery department, and explain your interest in the field. Many faculty members are open to such requests, and some will have listed their interest with the dean's office.

5 Given the competitiveness of plastic surgery, locating a mentor and developing a relationship is important. By cultivating the relationship over time, your mentor will be able to write you a strong letter of recommendation when it comes time to apply for a residency position. In a survey of plastic surgery program directors, Dr. Jeffrey Janis, Program Director of the Plastic Surgery Residency at the University of Texas Southwestern Medical Center, found that high-quality letters of recommendation, performance on subinternship rotations, and interview score were the three most important resident selection criteria.[96]

6 "If a student is interested in plastic surgery, she or he should try and identify a mentor early," write Dr. Jennifer Walden, Program Director of the Aesthetic Surgery Fellowship at the Manhattan Eye, Ear, and Throat Hospital, and Dr. Linda Phillips, Chief of the Division of Plastic Surgery and Senior Associate Dean for Faculty Affairs at UTMB.[97]

7 At the "Becoming a Plastic Surgeon" blog, Dr. Charles Lee describes the benefits of a mentor relationship. "In medical school, you will be studying twice as hard, but should still find the time to identify a mentor, preferably at this time a plastic surgeon, with whom you can identify and begin some research projects. This will prepare you in multiple ways. It will allow you to see the process of residency training in plastic surgery, spend time with your role model to see what their professional career is like, and begin delving deeper into the science of plastic surgery. The mentor in this position will be critical in helping you obtain a spot in the most competitive residency in medicine."[98]

8 Opportunities to participate in plastic surgery research during the summer between your first and second years are available at some schools. Research leading to publication is highly valued in the plastic surgery residency selection process. In a survey of program directors, among the objective criteria used to evaluate applicants, publications in peer-reviewed journals ranked second in importance behind only membership in the Alpha Omega Alpha Honor Society.[99]

9 Many students interested in the field will join their school's Plastic Surgery Interest Group. Through lectures, community service projects, other experiences, and the opportunity to speak directly with plastic surgeons, students can gain a more extensive overview of the field. Unfortunately, many schools lack such a group. If so, you may consider starting your own chapter. A list of active and inactive groups is available at The American Society for Aesthetic Plastic Surgery website (www.surgery.org).

10 Note that leadership capabilities were considered the most important subjective criterion used by program directors to evaluate applicants during the residency interview.[99] The preclinical years are an excellent time to actively participate in student organizations and run for leadership positions.

Psychiatry: 10 Ways to Explore the Specialty as a Preclinical Student

Dr. Sarah Whitman, a psychiatrist in private practice in Pennsylvania, recalls how her initial interest in the specialty developed. "When I entered medical school, I really knew nothing about psychiatry. I had taken psychology courses in college, but didn't know about psychiatry as a field. In the 3rd year of medical school, my psychiatry rotation was seeing patients who were on the medical units of the hospital about whom the staff had some psychiatric concerns or questions. For example, if someone had just been diagnosed with cancer and didn't seem to handle that well. Or a patient was in the ICU and seemed to be out of it – what was going on. So these were people just like you and me who were having psychological problems while in the hospital. That intersection of psychiatry and medicine seemed really interesting to me. It also allowed me to continue to use my medical knowledge."[100]

Although psychiatry is not a competitive specialty, securing a position in a top tier residency program is difficult. In the 2011 NRMP Match, approximately 1,100 positions were available. In 2010, there were 4,865 residents training in a total of 182 allopathic psychiatry residency programs.[23] Fifty-seven percent were U.S. MDs, 33.2% were IMGs, 9.5% were osteopathic graduates, and 0.1% were Canadian graduates. There are also 12 osteopathic residency programs offering positions through the AOA match.

1 The most helpful way to begin learning about the specialty is to observe psychiatrists in practice. Psychiatrists are actively involved in the preclinical education of medical students through behavioral science and neuroscience courses, and you can ask these faculty members about shadowing opportunities. Opportunities may also be available through participation in your school's Psychiatry Interest Group.

2 The Summer Medical Student Fellowship sponsored by the American Academy of Child and Adolescent Psychiatry allows students to explore the field, gain clinical or research experience, and meet leaders in the field by attending the AACAP Annual Meeting.

3 The American Psychiatric Association has a Minority Medical Student Summer Mentoring Program for minority students. In the program, students work closely with a psychiatry mentor in a research, academic, or clinical setting.

4 The American Psychiatric Association has a Minority Medical Student Summer Externship in Addiction Psychiatry. Through this one-month program, minority medical students are able to participate in a clinical shadowing experience in services related to substance abuse treatment. The AACAP also sponsors the Jeanne Spurlock Minority Medical Student Research Fellowship in Substance Abuse and Addiction. This is a summer opportunity for minority medical students to perform research in substance abuse as it relates to child and adolescent psychiatry. Participants are expected to present their research at the Annual Meeting.

5 The Department of Psychiatry at Indiana University sponsors the Psychiatry Summer Internship Program. This program provides students with an opportunity to learn about research and clinical care in the field. The time is split evenly between clinical care and research. According to the department, "the expectation is that all participants will complete a paper ready for submission to a psychiatric journal during the 6-week program."[101]

6 Students benefit greatly when they receive advice and guidance from experienced psychiatry faculty. Mentors can also provide clinical and research opportunities, as well as advocate for students during the residency application process. Because psychiatrists at most schools are significantly involved in preclinical education, you may have opportunities to meet these physicians in small group sessions and lectures. Mentor relationships may be established through your school's psychiatry interest group. You can also introduce yourself to the psychiatry department, express your interest in the field, and ask for suggestions on possible advisors.

7 Dr. Angela Harper, a psychiatrist in private practice, was fortunate to have several wonderful mentors.[102] "I worked with a female psychiatrist in private practice as a medical student who first made me think, 'I want to be like her when I grow up." However, the mentor that has most impacted her personally and professionally was her third-year psychiatry clerkship director. "He has seen me through it all – the 'match,' my first night of call in the emergency room (when I was scared to death), professional successes and failures, deciding on a fellowship, moonlighting anxiety, career decisions, and personal anxieties and triumphs."

8 Several national organizations have established mentor programs. The American Academy of Child and Adolescent Psychiatry (AACAP) has started a program for medical students interested in child and adolescent psychiatry. The American Association for Geriatric Psychiatry also makes geriatric psychiatrists available to students for mentoring.

9 In order to learn more about the field, you should join your school's Psychiatry Interest Group. Membership will allow you to interact with others who share your interest in the field, shadow psychiatrists, and identify mentors. Most U.S. medical schools have active groups. Resources to help you start or grow a group are available at the Psychiatry Student Interest Group Network.[103]

10 The American Academy of Child and Adolescent Psychiatry has prepared materials to help students establish medical school groups to explore the field of child and adolescent psychiatry. The program is called the Special Interest Group Network (SIGN), and ideas for SIGN activities are available at www.aacap.org. The organization makes monetary grants (Medical Student – Psychiatry Special Interest Grant) available to those who wish to plan activities that would allow students to explore some aspect of the field.

Radiation Oncology: 10 Ways to Explore the Specialty as a Preclinical Student

Dr. Arpi Thukral is a radiation oncologist in Chicago. Recently she was asked why she chose to pursue a career in radiation oncology. "I am attracted to this specialty because it is an intellectual and technically-driven discipline with the physician-patient relationship at its core. As a radiation oncologist, I have the privilege and opportunity to help and support cancer patients and their families through the challenging treatment journey they endure."[104]

Radiation oncology is a highly competitive specialty. In the 2011 NRMP Match, approximately 170 positions were available. Fifteen percent of U.S. senior applicants failed to match. In 2010, there were 603 residents training in a total of 85 allopathic radiation oncology residency programs.[23] Ninety-six percent were U.S. MDs, 3.0% were IMGs, and 1.0% were osteopathic graduates.

Exposure to the specialty of radiation oncology is limited at many schools. Dr. Ariel Hirsch, Director of Education in the Department of Radiation Oncology at the Boston University Medical Center, wrote that "radiation oncology is a subject that is not widely taught in the mainstream undergraduate medical curriculum, nor is it well understood by medical students and physicians outside of the field. Although interest in radiation oncology has been increasing steadily over the past few years, it is generally only those medical students applying for radiation oncology residencies who rotate through specific radiation oncology electives. For the remainder of the medical student body, exposure to radiation oncology will be limited to none."[105]

1 Radiation oncology is a very competitive residency, and many students first hear about it because it is one of the fields associated with a controllable lifestyle and one in which physicians have significant impact on seriously ill patients. Since preclinical exposure to the field is typically non-existent, students with an interest in learning more about the field should begin by shadowing a practicing radiation oncologist. You can begin by asking your dean's office, or by approaching one of the faculty members at your school.

2 Because you may have limited interaction with radiation oncology faculty until fourth year, your initiative will be key to establishing a relationship with a mentor early in your medical education. Introduce yourself to the radiation oncology department at your school. Take advantage of any opportunities to meet with the program director or chairman. Dr. Dennis Hallahan, Chairman of Radiation Oncology at Washington University in St. Louis, credits his mentors for stimulating his interest in the field. "While I was training at the University of Chicago, I met some brilliant mentors in radiation oncology and decided to train with them as opposed to going into medical oncology."[106]

3 Some schools arrange career fairs or forums, and you may have an opportunity to meet faculty through these means. Performing research is yet another way to establish a relationship with a mentor.

4 Because radiation oncology is one of the most competitive specialties, students with an early interest in the field should seriously consider participation in research. Schools with academic radiation oncology departments often provide research opportunities for students following their first year.

5 Preclinical students are eligible to apply for the Simon Kramer Externship in Radiation Oncology. Through this program, students spend six weeks at an academic radiation oncology department working on a clinical research project and shadowing radiation oncologists.

6 Another program that provides early exposure to the specialty is the Ivan H. Smith Memorial Studentship (ISMS) program. In this program, students spend six to eight weeks shadowing oncologists and radiation oncologists in Canada. Although the emphasis of this experience is clinical, students are also encouraged to pursue a research project.

7 The American Society for Radiation Oncology offers the Minority Summer Fellowship Award to support medical students from underrepresented minority groups. Through this program, students are introduced to the discipline of radiation oncology early in their medical training. The experience allows students to receive "a unique training opportunity that focuses on mentoring and hands-on experience" in the field.[107]

8 The Radiological Society of North America encourages students interested in radiological sciences to apply for their Research Medical Student Grant. At least ten weeks must be spent on a full time basis performing research in a department of radiology, radiation oncology, or nuclear medicine.

9 Joining your school's Radiation Oncology Interest Group will provide opportunities to learn more about the specialty and meet faculty. However, many schools lack a group or have groups that have become inactive. If so, you can restart a group, or become the founder of a new group.

10 The Pediatric Oncology Education Program at St. Jude Children's Research Hospital offers short-term training experience in clinical or laboratory research in a variety of disciplines, including radiation oncology.

Radiology: 10 Ways to Explore the Specialty as a Preclinical Student

Dr. Alan Zuckerman is an interventional radiologist in Atlanta. He was drawn to the specialty because of the integral role radiology plays in patient care. "As a medical student, I was attracted to radiology because it seemed to me that many diagnoses and decisions were being made on the basis of patients' radiology exams. Treatment options became clear once the radiology results were in, so the radiology department was an important, almost powerful, place. I have not been disappointed by radiology as a career. The technology revolution that has brought us the Internet and e-mail also propels diagnostic imaging forward. Of course, this improves healthcare for the public, but it also makes radiology a consistently stimulating profession."[108]

Diagnostic radiology is a moderately competitive specialty. In the 2011 NRMP Match, over 1,100 positions were available. In 2010, there were 4,531 residents training in a total of 187 allopathic diagnostic radiology residency programs.[23] Eighty-eight percent were U.S. MDs, 8.0% were IMGs, 3.9% were osteopathic graduates, and 0.2% were Canadian graduates. There are also fifteen osteopathic residency programs offering positions through the AOA Match.

According to Dr. Barton Branstetter, Associate Professor of Radiology at the University of Pittsburgh, "in most traditional medical school curricula, radiology is not formally introduced to students until their clinical rotations."[109] Although exposure to the specialty may be limited through your preclinical coursework, for students with an interest in the field, opportunities to explore the specialty are available during the basic science years.

1 Most students begin to learn more about the actual practice of radiology through observation. If your school has an Office of Career Development, you may be able to arrange a shadowing experience through this office, such as at Oklahoma State University College of Osteopathic Medicine. At some schools, students are asked to contact the department of radiology directly to arrange the experience. Another option is to join your medical school's radiology interest group. Many of these groups have established shadowing programs. For example, the Radiology Society at Northwestern University Feinberg School of Medicine has a shadowing program that links preclinical students with radiologists.

2 Mentoring relationships are valuable for a number of reasons, but will require initiative to establish, especially since you may have limited interaction with radiology faculty until the third or fourth year of medical school. Introduce yourself to the Radiology department at your school. In particular, take advantage of any opportunities to meet with the program director or chairman. You may also identify mentors through participation in your school's radiology interest group. Once established, the mentoring relationship may have significant impact, as the following student describes:[110]

My mentor permitted me to see every aspect of her job, including her clinical work, teaching, didactic lecturing, and research. I saw that there are differences in how clinical work is done. I also found her to be very generous of her time, as she never said no to anyone asking for her expertise or any opportunity to teach... Being with someone who is so diligent can be very inspirational and makes you want to work hard. It incites you to want to teach, be involved in research, and give something back as a mentor to someone else.

3 Although students can match into the specialty without research, such experience, particularly if it leads to publication, can significantly strengthen your chances. Note that some academic programs may be very research-oriented. At these programs, lack of research may eliminate you from further consideration.

4 Students with an early interest in the field should consider involvement in research. Dr. Judith Amorosa, a faculty member in the Department of Radiology at UMDNJ/Robert Wood Johnson, offers a strong argument for performing research early in medical school. She writes that "starting a research elective near the end of the third year of medical school can be challenging. If there is adequate infrastructure and close mentoring, it is possible to accomplish a project that may even be submitted to a national meeting and eventually be published."[111] Schools with academic radiology departments often provide students with opportunities to perform research during the summer following first year.

5 The Radiologic Society of North America sponsors the Research Medical Student Grant, which provides support for a research project.

Applicants must be students at an accredited North American medical school, and perform research for a minimum of 10 weeks.

6 The Mallinckrodt Institute of Radiology at Washington University in St. Louis offers the Radiology Summer Research Program to medical students.

7 The Department of Radiology at the University of Cincinnati College of Medicine has set aside funds for medical students interested in performing clinical and/or translational research in the radiologic sciences.

8 The Society for Interventional Radiology has created the Student Research Grant to provide funding for a summer research project in an area important to the advancement of interventional radiology.

9 The Penn Interventional Radiology Department offers the Summer Scholars Program for students between their first and second years of med school. Through this experience, students carry out a clinical research project. An abstract is prepared and submitted to the Society of Interventional Radiology meeting. If accepted, students may have an opportunity to present their research at the meeting. The work of many students has culminated in the publication of a manuscript.

10 Many schools have established radiology student interest groups, and you can learn more about the specialty through involvement. If your school doesn't have a group, you may choose to start one. An excellent resource to help you create a new group or enhance an existing one was recently published in the journal *Academic Radiology*.[112]

General Surgery: 10 Ways to Explore the Specialty as a Preclinical Student

Dr. Michael Awad is a faculty member in the Department of Surgery at Washington University in St. Louis. As a medical student, he was unsure of his specialty choice entering clerkships. "I was undecided going into my third year of medical school at Brown University, so I kept my options open. I enjoyed both my pediatrics rotation and internal medicine rotation --but after my surgical rotation, I knew I had found my specialty. I appreciated the ability to have a direct and immediate impact on the course of someone's condition or disease. I had great mentors in surgery that showed me the art of the field. They loved their work and at the same time were caring and communicative people. This is what sent me down the path of general surgery."[113]

General surgery is a highly competitive specialty. In the 2011 NRMP Match, over 1,100 positions were available. However, 20% of U.S. senior medical school applicants failed to match. In 2010, there were 7,671 residents training in a total of 247 allopathic general surgery residency programs.[23] Seventy-nine percent were U.S. MDs, 17.8% were IMGs, 2.7% were osteopathic graduates, and 0.1% were Canadian graduates. There are also over 40 osteopathic residency programs offering positions through the AOA Match.

In a survey of over 900 students at 15 U.S. medical schools, surgery was the second most common specialty choice among first year students.[1] According to Dr. Riboh, a faculty member in the Department of Surgery at Stanford University, there is "no shortage of highly motivated preclinical medical students searching for opportunities in surgery."[114]

1 Despite significant early interest in the field, preclinical students often report difficulty exploring the specialty because of limited exposure to surgeons. However, "many hospitals and departments of surgery have allowed MS-1 and MS-2 students who are on summer rotations the opportunity of working in operating rooms, research laboratories, and other employment in the surgical work environment" writes Dr. Kirby Bland, Chairman of the Department of Surgery at the University of Alabama – Birmingham School of Medicine.[115]

2 If you're interested in surgery, you should take the initiative and arrange to shadow a surgeon. Shadowing opportunities aren't typically publicized, and it's up to each individual student to contact faculty members directly. You can start with your dean's office, as many maintain lists of faculty members open to medical student observers. You may also contact the department of surgery, and ask which faculty members you should approach about shadowing.

3 Because you may have limited interaction with surgery faculty until third or fourth year, you'll have to be pro-active if you wish to identify and work with a mentor early in your medical education. You can begin by introducing yourself to the surgery department at your school. In particular, take advantage of any opportunities to meet with the program director and chairman, as these individuals are fully involved in the residency selection process and can provide valuable guidance.

4 You may also identify mentors by joining your school's surgery interest group. The University of Texas Medical School at San Antonio has established its Longitudinal Surgical Mentorship Program to link new students with surgical mentors from Day 1 of medical school. Once established, the mentoring relationship may have a profound effect, as Dr. Elizabeth Stephens writes in a tribute to her mentor, Dr. Charles Fraser, Chief of the Texas Children's Hospital Cardiac Surgery Department:[116]

It was a clear, cool fall morning of my first year in medical school. I had remembered that we were scheduled to have a special guest for our 8 AM lecture that morning, but little did I know how much that lecture would change my life...As I approached Dr. Fraser at the conclusion of his lecture, I did not even know what to ask. All I knew was that I had been fascinated by what I saw and wanted to know more. Dr. Fraser, in his gentle, encouraging way, offered to meet with me to answer my questions...What struck me most about meeting with him was how generous he was with his time and his genuine interest in me and my career aspirations...He was also genuinely interested in me and my goals and was interested in supporting me regardless of my ultimate decision.

5 Your school's Surgery Interest Group can provide a number of opportunities to learn more about the field. The Surgical Society at the University of Colorado School of Medicine offers this advice. "You should take advantage of every opportunity to expose yourself to that field. For surgery, you should take advantage of the Surgical Society's Preceptor for a Day and Night On-Call with a Resident Programs, monthly lectures, suture clinics, laparoscopic workshops, surgical instruments workshops, and faculty-student receptions."[117]

6 Opportunities to perform research following first year are available at U.S. medical schools. Research may also be arranged through national organizations. The American Society of Colon and Rectal Surgeons offers the Medical Student Research Initiation Grant to medical students interested in performing clinical or laboratory-based research on diseases affecting the colon, rectum, and anus. Preclinical students may participate in the Summer Intern Scholarship Program established by the American Association for Thoracic Surgery. This program introduces students to cardiothoracic surgery. Medical students interested in vascular surgery may apply for the William J. von Liebig Summer Research Fellowship at Harvard Medical School.

7 Pablo Guzman, a medical student at the University of California San Francisco, arranged a four-week surgical rotation in Colombia following his first year of medical school. His goal was to combine his interest in surgery with his desire "to participate in international volunteer activities."[118] To arrange the experience, Pablo first visited the Office of International Programs where he was referred to a Colombia-trained pediatrician currently training as a pediatric critical care fellow at UCSF. The fellow was able to put him into contact with a colleague in Colombia, and, through her assistance, Pablo was able to organize a summer surgery internship abroad.

8 The Division of Thoracic Surgery at Massachusetts General Hospital has a Thoracic Surgery Summer Scholars Program in which preclinical students are able to spend the summer with thoracic surgeons rounding, taking care of patients, and observing in the operating room. Opportunities to perform a clinical research project are also available.

9 The Association of Women Surgeons encourages female medical students to participate in the Medical Student and Resident Poster Competition. This event is held annually, and selected students are able to present their research at the AWS meeting.

10 Medical students interested in a surgical volunteer experience can search through a database of opportunities at the Operation Giving Back website.[119] Operation Giving Back is a program of the American College of Surgeons. The database can be searched based on geographic location and specialty. Through Operation Smile, medical students interested in reconstructive surgery can observe operations in 25 different countries. The Cinterandes Foundation, based in Ecuador, provides free surgical services to patients in rural areas. Through their "Mobile Surgery" program, patients living in rural areas without access to surgery can undergo operations in a mobile operating room housed in a van. The Foundation has teaching programs for medical students which are typically 8 weeks in length.

Urology: 10 Ways to Explore the Specialty as a Preclinical Student

Dr. Karen Boyle is a urologist specializing in male infertility. Entering medical school at Albany Medical College, she anticipated pursuing a career in pediatric oncology. "But a urology rotation in my third year made me change course. I had an amazing mentor who later became their dean. He helped me appreciate the diversity of the surgeries one performs as a urologist. In urology you can develop a long-term bond with patients because you treat them both medically and surgically. I also enjoyed the technology, like minimally invasive surgery, and the diverse patient population."[120]

Urology is a highly competitive specialty. In the 2012 Match, there were 278 available positions. Twenty-three percent of U.S. senior medical students failed to match. In 2010, there were 1,069 residents training in a total of 122 allopathic urology residency programs.[23] Ninety-five percent were U.S. MDs, 3.9% were IMGs, 0.7% were osteopathic graduates, and 0.1% were Canadian graduates. There are also nine osteopathic residency programs offering positions through the AOA Match.

At most schools, urology is not a required or core rotation. However, some third year students are able to rotate through the field during the surgery core clerkship. According to Dr. Anurag Das, Assistant Professor of Urology at Harvard Medical School, "for many students, their initial exposure to urology is on their third-year rotations in surgery. Unfortunately, at many institutions, most students are never exposed to urology and never get a chance to consider it as a career choice."[121]

1 Given the competitiveness of urology, finding a mentor early in medical school is important. Dr. Martha Terris, a faculty member in the Department of Urology at the Medical College of Georgia, writes that preclinical students "should identify members of the urology faculty at their medical school who are willing to review their curriculum vitae and offer specific advice regarding enhancing their application."[122]

2 Establishing a relationship with a mentor may require significant initiative on your part, since contact with urology faculty may be limited during the preclinical years. In a survey of medical school urology departments, Dr. Loughlin, a faculty member in the Division of Urology at the Harvard Medical School, found that students at many schools did not have exposure to urologists during the preclinical years.[123] Thirty-two percent of schools had no urology faculty lectures and 50% had no urology lecture in the physical diagnosis course. Sixty-five percent of respondents reported that it was possible to complete medical school without any clinical exposure to the field.

3 If you're interested in the field, you have to learn what the daily practice of urology entails. Check with your school for a list of urology faculty members who are able to provide shadowing experiences. Shadowing can also be arranged by contacting your school's urology department. If there's a urology interest group at your school, you may be able to identify a faculty member to shadow through the group.

4 You may be able to identify mentors through national organizations. For example, the Society of Women in Urology has a Mentor Program. To be eligible for the program, you must become a member of the society. For more information, visit www.swiu.org.

5 Role models were one of the most important factors that led Dr. Cathy Naughton, Assistant Professor in the Department of Urology at the Washington University School of Medicine, to pursue urology as a career. "It takes one person to spark your interest in something. Mentorship is key."[124] According to Dr. Peter Schlegel, Chairman of the Department of Urology at the Weill Medical College of Cornell University, students should "learn as much about the field from residents, other students who have applied for residency positions, and local faculty members."[124]

6 Urologists are active in the community, and students may have opportunities to take part. For example, students in the Urologic Society at the Jefferson Medical College participate in the Prostate Cancer Run to raise money and awareness for prostate cancer. Recently, the group began the Testicular Disease Awareness Initiative. Through this program, students will visit Philadelphia high schools to educate students on testicular health, including the importance of self-examinations.

7 According to Dr. Roger Low, Program Director of the University of California Medical School at Davis, "research is highly desirable; most invited for interview are involved in research or have involvement in past publications."[125] Therefore, if you have an interest in urology, an ideal time to perform research in the field is the summer between the first and second years of med school.

8 Opportunities to participate in urology research during the summer following first year are often available at schools with academic urology departments. The American Urological Association Foundation offers the Herbert Brendler, MD Summer Medical Student Fellowship Program to students interested in performing urologic research. The Sexual Medicine Society of North America also offers funding through the Sexuality Research Grants Program.

9 Students attending medical school in the greater New York area (including New Jersey) may be eligible to receive funding through the Ferdinand C. Valentine Medical Student Research Grant in Urology. Participants are expected to present their research at the New York Academy of Medicine's annual Medical Student Forum.

10 You must develop relationships with faculty members to match into the field. Early development of these connections can help. By cultivating the relationship over time, your mentor will be able to write you a strong letter of recommendation when it comes time to apply for a residency position. At least two letters written by urology faculty are recommended by most residency programs.

References

[1] Compton M, Frank E, Elon L, Carrera J. Changes in U.S. medical students' specialty interests over the course of medical school. *J Gen Intern Med* 2008; 23(7): 1095-1100.

[2] Manuel R, Borges N, Jones B. Person-oriented versus technique-oriented specialties: early preferences and eventual choice. *Med Educ Online* 2009; 14: 4.

[3] Medical College of Wisconsin Alumni News: Alumni reflect on medical school courses that influenced them most. http://www.mcw/edu/display/docid23758.htm. Accessed January 24, 2012.

[4] Society for Education in Anesthesia Medical Student Guide to Anesthesiology. http://www.studentorg.vcu.edu/soaig/SEAMedicalStudentGuide2009.pdf. Accessed January 24, 2012.

[5] Hearst N, Shore W, Hudes E, French L. Family practice bashing as perceived by students at a university medical center. *Fam Med* 1995; 27(6): 366-70.

[6] Hunt D, Scott C, Zhong S, Goldstein E. Frequency and effect of negative comments ("badmouthing") on medical students' career choices. *Acad Med* 1996; 71(6): 665-9.

[7] Campos-Outclat D, Senf J, Kutob R. Comments heard by US medical students about family practice. *Fam Med* 2003; 35(8): 573-8.

[8] Katz L, Sarnacki R, Schimpfhauser F. The role of negative factors in changes in career selection by medical students. *J Med Educ* 1984; 59(4): 285-90.

[9] Holmes D, Turniel-Berhalter L, Zayas L, Watkins R. "Bashing" of medical specialties: students' experiences and recommendations. *Fam Med* 2008; 40(6): 400-6.

[10] 2010 AAMC Medical School Graduation Questionnaire. Available at: www.aamc.org. Accessed August 13, 2011.

[11] Kassebaum D, Szenas P. Medical students' career indecision and specialty rejection: roads not taken. *Acad Med* 1995; 70(10): 937-43.

[12] Medscape "How should I choose a medical specialty. Available at: http://www.medscape.com/viewarticle/544574. Accessed January 24, 2012.

[13] Association of American Medical Colleges (AAMC) Website. http://www.aamc.org/students/cim/about.htm. Accessed September 23, 2011.

[14] University of Virginia School of Medicine Medical Specialty Aptitude Test. Available at: http://www.med-ed.virginia.edu/specialties. Accessed January 24, 2012.

[15] Aagaard E, Hauer K. A cross-sectional descriptive study of mentoring relationships formed by medical students. *J Gen Intern Med* 2003; 18(4): 298-302.

[16] From Revolutionhealth. Interview with "Hopkins" ABC TV Real Life Doctor – Dr. Q. Available at: http://www.revolutionhealth.com/blogs/bradlyjacobsmdmph/interview-with-hopki-14503. Accessed January 24, 2012.

[17] Weinstein P, Gipple C. Some determinants of career choice in the second year of medical school. *J Med Educ* 1975; 50(2): 194-8.

[18]AAMC Choices Newsletter August 2010. Available at:
https://www.aamc.org/students/medstudents/cim/choicesnewsletter/august10/2
63054/ask_the_advisor_switching_specialties.html. Accessed January 24,
2012.

[19]Cardiothoracic Surgery Network "Why become a chest surgeon?" Available
at: http://www.ctsnet.org/sections/residents/newhorizons/article-3.html.
Accessed January 24, 2012.

[20]Schwartz R, Jarecky R, Strodel W, et al. Controllable lifestyle: a new factor
in career choice by medical students. *Acad Med* 1989; 64: 606-609.

[21]Dorsay E, Jarjoura D, Rutecki G. Influence of controllable lifestyle on recent
trends in specialty choice by US medical students. *JAMA* 2003; 290(9): 1173-8.

[22]New York Times. Call it a reversible coma, not sleep. Available at
http://www.nytimes.com/2011/03/01/science/01conv.html. Accessed January
24, 2012.

[23]Brotherton S, Etzel S. Graduate medical education, 2010-2011. *JAMA* 2011;
306(9): 1015-30.

[24]Lin S, Strom S, Canales C, Rodriguez A, Kain Z. The impact of the
anesthesiology clerkship structure on medical students matched to
anesthesiology. Abstract presented at the 2010 Annual Meeting of the
American Society Anesthesiologists. A1106.

[25]AMA Residency programs: an inside look. Available at: http://www.ama-
assn.org/ama/pub/about-ama/our-people/member-groups-sections/minority-
affairs-consortium/transitioning-residency/residency-programs-an-inside-
look.page. Accessed January 24, 2012.

[26]Premed Network Q & A with Dr. Jessica Barnes. Available at:
http://www.premednetwork.com/forum/topics/q-and-a-with-dr-jessica-barnes.
Accessed January 24, 2012.

[27]Barnett S, Mitchell J, Jones S. Is it time to unmask anesthesia in the medical
school curriculum? Abstract presented at the 2009 Annual Meeting of the
American Society Anesthesiologists. A1523.

[28]Ohio State University Department of Anesthesiology. Available at:
http://anesthesiology.osu.edu/11430.cfm. Accessed January 24, 2012.

[29]DrSkinLaser website. Available at:
http://www.doctorskinlaser.com/about/biography. Accessed January 24, 2012.

[30]Wagner R, Ioffe B. Medical student dermatology research in the United
States. *Dermatol Online J* 2005; 11(1): 8.

[31]Alikhan A, Sivamani R, Mutizwa M, Aldabagh B. Advice for medical
students interested in dermatology: perspectives from fourth year students who
matched. *Dermatol Online J* 2009; 15(7): 4.

[32]Women's Dermatologic Society. Available at: http://www.womensderm.org/.
Accessed February 9, 2012.

[33]American Academy of Dermatology. Available at:
http://www.aad.org/member-tools-and-benefits/residents-and-fellows/diversity-
mentorship-program-information-for-medical-students. Accessed January 24,
2012.

[34]Ohio State University College of Medicine Emergency Medicine Interest
Group. Available at: http://emig.org.ohio-state.edu/faq. Accessed January 25,
2012.

[35]Lotfipour S, Luu R, Hayden S, Vaca F, Hoonpongsimanont W, Langdorf M. Becoming an emergency medicine resident: a practical guide for medical students. *J Emerg Med* 2008; 35(3): 339-44.

[36]Garmel G. Mentoring medical students in academic emergency medicine. *Acad Emerg Med* 2004; 11(12): 1351-7.

[37]Penciner R. Emergency medicine preclerkship observerships: evaluation of a structured experience. *CJEM* 2009; 11(3): 235-9.

[38]The Successful Match: Getting into Emergency Medicine. Available at: http://studentdoctor.net/2010/08/the-successful-match-getting-into-emergency-medicine/. Accessed January 25, 2012.

[39]Emergency Medicine Residents' Association. Available at: http://www.emra.org/. Accessed January 25, 2012.

[40]The Health Journal. "Cynthia Romero, MD: Making Patient Care a Family Affair. Available at: http://www.thehealthjournals.com/archive.php?id=252. Accessed January 25, 2012.

[41]Virtual Family Medicine Interest Group website. Available at: http://fmignet.aafp.org/online/fmig/index.html. Accessed January 25, 2012.

[42]The Future of Primary Care. Available at: http://emc.org/body.cfm?id=41&category=6&subcategory=23&action=detail&ref=1626. Accessed January 26, 2012.

[43]ACP-ASIM Observer. Available at: http://www.acpinternist.org/archives/2000/11/namechange.html. Accessed January 25, 2012.

[44]ACP Mentoring Database. Available at: http://www.acponline.org/residents+fellows/mentors/. Accessed January 25, 2012.

[45]Ohio State University Department of Medicine. Available at: http://internalmedicine.osu.edu/education/students/summerresearch/. Accessed January 25, 2012.

[46]Uniformed University of the Health Sciences Internal Medicine Interest Group. Available at: http://www.usuhs.mil/imig/imigopportunities.html. Accessed January 25, 2012.

[47]Virginia Commonwealth School of Medicine "Exploring Career Options in Medicine." Available at: http://www.medschool.vcu.edu.studentaffairs.counseling/documents/careers.pdf. Accessed January 25, 2012.

[48]University of Iowa Medicine Alumni Society. Available at: http://www.healthcare.uiowa.edu/alumni/interviews/richerson_george.html. Accessed January 25, 2012.

[49]Student Interest Group in Neurology Reference Manual. Available at: http://www.aan.com/globals/axon/assets/7999.pdf. Accessed January 25, 2012.

[50]American Academy of Neurology. Available at: http://www.aan.com. Accessed January 23, 2012.

[51]Women In Neurosurgery "So, You Want to be a Neurosurgeon." Available at: http://www.neurosurgerywins.org/career/SYWTBANS.pdf. Accessed January 25, 2012.

[52]Fox B, Hassan A, Patel A. Fulkerson D, Suki D, Jea A, Sawaya R. Neurosurgical rotations or clerkships in US medical schools. *J Neurosurg* 2011; 114(1): 27-33.

[53]NYU Department of Neurosurgery. Available at: http://www.med.nyu.edu/neurosurgery/education/students/summer.html. Accessed January 25, 2012.

[54]Medical College of Georgia. Available at: http://www.mcghealth.org. Accessed July 12, 2011.

[55]Pauletta and Denzel Washington Family Gifted Scholars Program in Neuroscience. Available at: http://www.cedars-sinai/edu/Patients/Programs-and-Services/Neurosurgery/Washington-Family-Scholars-Program.aspx. Accessed January 25, 2012.

[56]Scott and White Healthcare. Q & A with Dr. Mark Rowe. Available at: http://www.sw.org/women-health/obgyn-waco/qa-rowe. Accessed January 26, 2012

[57]Bienstock J, Laube D. The recruitment phoenix: strategies for attracting medical students into obstetrics and gynecology. *Obstet Gynecol* 2005; 105: 1125-7.

[58]Schnatz P, Humphrey K. Reasons and principles for starting an obstetrics and gynecology scholars group. *Obstet Gynecol* 2008; 111(4): 953-8.

[59]The Successful Match: Getting into Obstetrics and Gynecology Available at: http://studentdoctor.net/2010/05/the-successful-match-getting-into-obstetrics-and-gynecology/. Accessed January 26, 2012.

[60]Research Programs Open to Jefferson Medical College Students. Available at: http://jeffline.tju.edu/Researchers/StudentResearch/jmc.html Accessed January 26, 2012.

[61]Pacific Eye. Available at: http://www.paceyemd.com/optometrist/abroms.cfm. Accessed January 26, 2012.

[62]Association of University Professors in Ophthalmology 2004 Survey on Medical Student Teaching. Available at: http://www.aupo.org.

[63]The Successful Match: Getting into Ophthalmology. Available at: http://studentdoctor.net/2009/08/the-successful-match-interview-with-dr-andrew-lee-ophthalmology/. Accessed January 26, 2012.

[64]Methodist Sports Medicine. Available at: http://www.methodistsports.com/physicians/stephen_ritter/index.html. Accessed January 26, 2012.

[65]Bernstein J, DiCaprio M, Mehta S. The relationship between required medical school instruction in musculoskeletal medicine and application rates to orthopedic surgery residency programs. *J Bone Joint Surg* 2004; 86: 2335-8.

[66]Stern P, Riley L, Johnson D, Boyer M. Educational opportunities for medical students and young orthopedic surgeons. *J Bone Joint Surg* 2003; 85: 573-5.

[67]Reilly C, Stothers K, Broudo M, Perdios A, Tredwell S. An orthopedic career fair: a novel recruitment event. *Can J Surg* 2007; 50(3): 168-70.

[68]Wake Forest University Department of Orthopedic Surgery. Available at: http://www.wakehealth.edu/School/Orthopaedic-Surgery/Tips-for-Medical -Students-Year-1-3.htm. Accessed January 26, 2012.

[69]UC Irvine Career Guidance Handbook: Orthopedic Surgery. Available at: http://www.meded.uci.edu/education/residencyselection/orthosurgery.html. Accessed January 26, 2012.

[70]Children's Hospital of Philadelphia Research Institute. Available at: http://stokes.chop.edu/programs/ortho/opportunities.php. Accessed February 9, 2012.

[71]St. Joseph's Candler. Available at: http://www.sjchs.org/drdavidoliver. Accessed January 26, 2012.

[72]Haddad J, Shah J, Takoudes R. A survey of US medical education in otolaryngology. *Arch Otolaryngol Head Neck Surg* 2003; 129: 1166-9.

[73]Drexel University College of Medicine Career Development Center. Available at: http://webcampus.drexelmed.edu/cdc/medSpecialtyOtolaryngology.asp. Accessed January 26, 2012.

[74]University of Virginia School of Medicine Student Handbook. Available at: http://www.med-ed.virginia.edu/handbook/orgs/clubService.cfm. Accessed on January 26, 2012.

[75]University of Rochester Medical Center. Available at: http://www.urmc.rochester.edu/news/story/index.cfm?id=1966. Accessed January 26, 2012.

[76]Johns Hopkins Pathology. Available at: http://apps.pathology.jhu.edu/blogs/pathology/why-i-became-a-pathologist. Accessed January 28, 2012.

[77]Holland L, Bosch B. Medical students' perceptions of pathology and the effect of the second-year pathology course. *Hum Pathol* 2006; 37(1): 1-8.

[78]Hung T, Jarvis-Selinger S, Ford J. Residency choices by graduating medical students: why not pathology? *Hum Pathol* 2011; 42(6): 802-7.

[79]University of Massachusetts Department of Pathology. Available at: http://www.umassmed.edu/pathology/first_and_second_year_teaching/index.aspx#observerships Accessed January 28, 2012.

[80]University of Chicago Pritzker School of Medicine Residency Process Guide 2011. Available at: pritzker.uchicago.edu/current/students/ResidencyProcessGuide.pdf Accessed January 28, 2012.

[81]American Society of Investigative Pathology. Available at: www.asip.org/pubs/pathways/Sept2008.pdf . Accessed July 23, 2011.

[82]Where. What. When. Community Spotlight. Available at: http://www.wherewhatwhen.com/archive/2006/08/community-spotlight/. Accessed January 29, 2012.

[83]Texas Pediatric Society General Pediatric Preceptorship Program. Available at: www.txpeds.org. Accessed January 29, 2012.

[84]White C, Waller J, Freed G, Levine D, Moore R, Sharkey A, Greenberg L. The state of undergraduate pediatric medical education in North America: The COMSEP survey. *Teach Learn Med* 2007; 19(3): 264-70.

[85]American Academy of Pediatrics. Available at: http://www2.aap.org/sections/ypn/ms/getting_involved/PIG.html. Accessed January 29, 2012.

[86]Georgetown University Medical Center. Available at: http://gumc.georgetown.edu/news/75433.html. Accessed January 29, 2012.

[87]Pediatric Interest Group Resource. Available at: http://www.aap.org/sections/ypn/ms/getting_involved/PIGResourceGuide.pdf. Accessed January 29, 2012.

[88]American College of Osteopathic Pediatricians Student Chapter Manual. Available at: http://www.acopeds.org/students/clubs.iphtml. Accessed January 29, 2012.

[89]Medical College of Georgia Department of Pediatrics. Available at: http://www.mcg.edu/pediatrics/scholars.html. Accessed January 29, 2012.

[90]Mayo Clinic. Available at: http://www.mayo.edu/msgme/profiles-knievel.html. Accessed January 29, 2012.

[91]American Academy of Physical Medicine and Rehabilitation. Available at: http://www.aapmr.org/medstu/medstudi.htm. Accessed January 29, 2012.

[92]Galicia A, Klima R, Date E. Mentorship in physical medicine and rehabilitation residencies. *Am J Phys Med Rehab* 1997; 76(4): 268-75.

[93]Association of Academic Physiatrists. Available at: http://www.physiatry.org. Accessed January 29, 2012.

[94]Reliant Medical Group. Available at: http://www.reliantmedicalgroup.org/meet-the-doctor/le-trung. Accessed January 29, 2012.

[95]Greene A, May J. Applying to plastic surgery residency: factors associated with medical student career choice. *Plast Reconstr Surg* 2008; 121(3): 1049-53.

[96]Janis J, Hatef D. Resident selection protocols in plastic surgery: a national survey of plastic surgery program directors. *Plast Reconstr Surg* 2008; 122(6): 1929-39.

[97]Association of Women Surgeons. Available at: http://www.womensurgeons.org/CDR/PlasticSurgery.asp. Accessed January 29, 2012.

[98]Becoming a Plastic Surgeon Blog. Available at: http://www.becomeplasticsurgeon.blogspot.com/. Accessed January 29, 2012.

[99]LaGrasso J, Kennedy D, Hoehn J, Ashruf S, Przybyla A. Selection criteria for the integrated model of plastic surgery residency. *Plast Reconstr Surg* 121(3): 121e-125e.

[100]Super Scholar. Available at: http://www.superscholar.org/interviews/sarah-whitman/. Accessed January 29, 2012.

[101]Indiana University Department of Psychiatry. Available at: http://medicine.iu.edu/research/student-research-opportunities/. Accessed June 22, 2011.

[102]Harper A. Residents' forum: the making of a psychiatrist. *Psychiatric News* 2004; 39(9): 62.

[103]Psychiatry Student Interest Group Network. Available at: http://www.psychsign.org/. Accessed January 29, 2012.

[104]Chicago Area Cancer Care Radiation Oncologists. Available at: http://www.chicagocancer.org/ourteam_19.htm. Accessed January 29, 2012.

[105]Hirsch A, Singh D, Ozonoff A, Slanetz P. Educating medical students about radiation oncology: initial results of the oncology education initiative. *J Am Coll Radiol* 2007; 4(10): 711-5.

[106]Washingtion University School of Medicine. Available at: http://wuphysicians.wustl.edu/page.aspx?pageID=1065. Accessed January 29, 2012.

[107]American Society for Radiation Oncology Minority Summer Fellowship Award. Available at: https://www.astro.org/Research/Funding-Opportunities/ASTRO-Supported-Grants/Minority-Summer-Fellowship/Index.aspx. Accessed January 29, 2012.

[108]Atlanta magazine July 2007 Vol. 47, No. 3 published by Emmis Communications.

[109]Branstetter B, Faix L, Humphrey A, Schumann J. Preclinical medical student training in radiology: the effect of early exposure. *AJR* 2007; 188: W9-W14.

[110]Sonners A. Value of a radiology research rotation: a medical student's perspective. *Acad Radiol* 2002; 9(7): 805-7.

[111]Amorosa J. Medical student education: how do I mentor medical students interested in radiology? *Acad Radiol* 2004; 11(1): 91-5.

[112]Fricke B, Gunderman R. Creating and enhancing radiology student interest groups. *Acad Radiol* 2010; 17 (12): 1567-9.

[113]Washington University School of Medicine. Available at: http://wuphysicians.wustl.edu/page.aspx?pageID=1168. Accessed January 29, 2012.

[114]Riboh J, Curet M, Krummel T. Innovative introduction to surgery in the preclinical years. *Am J Surg* 2007; 194(2): 227-30.

[115]Bland K. The recruitment of medical students to careers in general surgery: emphasis on the first and second years of medical education. *Surgery* 2003; 134: 409-13.

[116]The Cardiothoracic Surgery Network. Available at: http://www.ctsnet.org/sections/residents/newhorizons/article-26.html. Accessed January 29, 2012.

[117]University of Colorado School of Medicine Surgical Society. Available at: http://www.ucdenver.edu/academics/colleges/medicalschool/education/studenta ffairs/studentgroups/SurgicalSociety/Pages/FAQ.aspx. Accessed January 29, 2012.

[118]Guzman P, Schecter W. Global health opportunities in surgery: a guide for medical students and faculty. *J Surg Educ* 2008; 65(5): 384-7.

[119]Operation Giving Back. Available at: http://www.operationgivingback.facs.org/. Accessed January 29, 2012.

[120]Johns Hopkins Medicine Dome. Available at: http://www.hopkinsmedicine.org/dome/0702/feature3.cfm. Accessed January 29, 2012.

[121]American College of Surgeons. Available at: http://www.facs.org/residencysearch/specialties/urology.html. Accessed January 29, 2012.

[122]Association of Women Surgeons. Available at: http://www.womensurgeons.org/CDR/Urology.asp. Accessed February 9, 2012.

[123]Loughlin K. The current status of medical student urological education in the United States. *J Urol* 2008; 179(3): 1087-90.

[124]Bellask J. Specialty spotlight: urology. *Journal of Andrology* 2005; 26(6): 673-4.
[125]University of California Davis Department of Urology. Available at: http://www.ucdmc.ucdavis.edu/urology/education/residency_program/. Accessed January 29, 2012.

An excerpt from the best-selling book:
Success on the Wards:
250 Rules for Clerkship Success

By Dr. Samir P. Desai
and Dr. Rajani Katta

Chapter 1

Introduction

Rule # 1   **You came to medical school to be a great doctor. That process begins now.**

Why did you become a doctor? There may be a number of reasons, but the most important one is the same across the board: to take care of patients. You will read startling amounts of information during medical school, and your training will include many procedures and new techniques, but all of it is in the service of patient care. You are here to make each and every individual patient better.

That process starts now.

It is an amazing privilege to take care of patients. You can read about a disease all that you want, but to be able to speak to and examine a patient with that disease is an unsurpassed learning experience. It is an incredible responsibility as well. You will be asking patients the most intimate and intrusive types of questions. You will be asking patients to offer their arm for a needle, to disrobe for an exam, to let you literally poke and prod at their body. In return, you are responsible for protecting them from harm, and for healing them.

Starting as a medical student, and progressing to a respected physician, is a long, difficult, and intense process. It takes years of education, and years of training. The privileges granted to physicians are remarkable. In return, you have a great responsibility. Your education is in the service of patient care. You have a responsibility to make the most of that education.

What does it take to be a great doctor? There is an impressive body of research devoted to medical student education, and to the factors and interventions that ensure good doctors. Medical educators work hard to ensure that students master these different facets of the practice of medicine.

Why are clerkships so important to the process of producing great doctors?

The areas emphasized in clerkships are those that are integral to becoming a great physician.

Patient care requires the daily use of many skills. On a daily basis, a physician may need to:

- Obtain an accurate medication history.
- Detect a heart murmur.
- Create a differential diagnosis for the patient with abdominal pain.
- Interpret an elevated alkaline phosphatase.
- Formulate a management plan for the patient with a myocardial infarction.
- Communicate that plan through oral discussions and written documentation.
- Utilize the talents of an entire health care team to maximize patient care.
- Manifest their concern for the patient in every interaction.

Clerkships teach students how to accomplish these difficult, vital skills.

If you don't learn certain skills in medical school, you may never learn them.

Clinical clerkships provide the foundation of successful patient care. They represent a critical time in your education. If you want to become proficient in exam skills, you have to learn now. These aren't skills you can learn from reading a textbook. You need to evaluate patients with these findings, and you need to have a teacher that can demonstrate these findings. You need to be able to ask questions freely in order to learn all the finer points of physical exam skills. This isn't something you can easily do as a resident, and certainly not as a board-certified physician. If you don't know how to assess jugular venous distention by the end of medical school, you may never learn.

While you would assume that medical school teaches you everything you need to know to function well as a resident, that isn't true for all students, particularly those who take a passive approach to learning or those who focus their education on textbook learning. You need to maximize your learning experiences and teaching opportunities on the wards. Passive learning has real consequences.

In one eye-opening study, internal medicine residents were tested on cardiac auscultatory skills. They listened to 12 prerecorded cardiac events. American residents demonstrated poor proficiency, with mean identification rates of only 22%.[1] In another study of resident skills, ECG proficiency was measured. Surprisingly, 58% of residents wrongly diagnosed complete heart block, and only 22% were certain of their diagnosis of ventricular tachycardia.[2] In a study of radiologic proficiency, participants included mainly residents, with some students. In x-rays representing emergency situations, pneumothorax was misdiagnosed by 91% of participants overall, while a misplaced central venous catheter was missed by 74%.[3]

Skills in patient examination, interpretation of tests, synthesis of information, and medical decision-making are honed through years of practice. Clerkships are only the first step, but provide an invaluable education, with supervisors there to demonstrate, to model, and to teach skills. The best medical students regard clerkships as a unique and invaluable learning experience, difficult to replicate in residency or later through seminars and conferences.

If you don't learn it now, you may have problems as a resident.

Medical school is the time to learn and develop your clinical skills. It's also the time to develop and hone the learned attributes and attitudes that predict success as a physician. In a study of residents with problematic behavior, investigators sought to determine if there were prognostic indicators in their medical school evaluations.[4] The short answer is yes.

Students whose evaluations indicated that they were timid, had problems in organization, displayed little curiosity, and had difficulty applying knowledge clinically, among other types, were more likely to become problem residents. The authors "found a rather robust multilevel correlation between residents who have problems, major or minor, during or after residency, and negative statements, even subtle ones, in the dean's letter." The predictive statements noted in the dean's letter included:

Very nervous, timid initially/ Displayed little curiosity/ Had difficulty applying knowledge clinically/ He came across as confrontational/ Maybe somewhat overconfident for his level of training/ Lack of enthusiasm and problems in organization/
Needs to read more on her own/ Lots of effort, uneven outcome

Difficulties during clerkships may predict difficulties as a physician, including disciplinary actions by the State Medical Board.

Clerkships are the foundation of successful patient care. During clerkships, medical students also develop and hone the attributes and attitudes that are required of successful physicians. These are referred to collectively as medical professionalism. "The specific attributes that have long been understood to animate professionalism include altruism, respect, honesty, integrity, dutifulness, honour, excellence and accountability."[5] –Dr. Jordan Cohen, President Emeritus, Association of American Medical Colleges

If you don't hone these traits during medical school, you may have problems as a physician. Unprofessional behavior in medical school is a possible predictor of future disciplinary action. A particularly notable study was performed by Dr. Maxine Papadakis, associate dean for student affairs at the UCSF School of Medicine. She and her team examined the medical school records of 235 graduates of three medical schools. Each of these physicians had been disciplined by one of 40 state medical boards over a 13-year period. The disciplined physicians were three times more likely than a control group to have negative comments about their professionalism documented in their medical school record.[6]

Another study sought to identify the domains of unprofessional behavior in medical school that were associated with disciplinary action by a state medical board.[7] Three domains of unprofessional behavior were significantly associated with future disciplinary action: poor reliability and responsibility, poor initiative and motivation, and lack of self-improvement and adaptability.

Your core clerkship grades may either limit or expand your future career options.

The skills and traits reflected in core clerkship grades are considered so important to future success as a resident that residency programs use these grades as a major criteria in the selection process. Program directors are decision-makers in the residency selection process. In a survey of over 1,200 residency program directors across 21 medical specialties, grades in required clerkships were ranked as the # 1 factor used in the selection process.[8]

Studies across multiple specialties have supported the predictive nature of clerkship grades. In one study, researchers sought to determine which residency selection criteria had the strongest correlation with performance as an orthopedic surgery resident. The authors concluded that the "number of honors grades on clinical rotations was the strongest predictor of performance."[9] In a study of physical medicine and rehabilitation residents, "clinical residency performance was predicted by clerkship grade honors."[10] In one study of internal medicine residents, performance as a resident was significantly associated with the internal medicine clerkship grade.[11]

In the next 400 plus pages, we review each of the areas that students need to master in clerkships. The book contains a great deal of in-depth content across a range of areas vital to medical student success. It's also arranged to ensure ease of use. The first sections serve as straightforward how-to guides for each of the core clerkships. If you're starting your Pediatrics clerkship, and aren't sure how to write the daily patient progress note, Chapter 4 walks you through that process. If you're starting the Ob/Gyn clerkship, and don't know how to write a delivery note, Chapter 6 provides a template and sample note that details exactly what you'll need to include. The latter chapters provide more wide-ranging content. If you'll be presenting in rounds for the first time, you can turn to the chapter on oral case presentations and review the features you'll need to include. If you are committed to fully protecting your patients from the hazards of hospitalization, Chapter 8 Patients includes several tables that outline the steps that medical students can take, even at their level, to protect their patients. Chapter 22 reviews the impact of collaborative care on patient outcomes, and provides recommendations that students can implement.

The recommendations presented here are based on discussions with numerous faculty members, residents, and students, as well as our own experiences. We've also focused our efforts on evidence-based advice. This evidence-based advice is based on our review of the substantial medical literature in the area of medical student education. The book includes over 400 references from the relevant literature.

Over the next 400 plus pages, you'll learn how to maximize your education during core clerkships, as well as your performance. Your success on the wards will become the foundation of outstanding patient care.

Patients

We begin this chapter with one of the most famous quotes in the history of medicine. "First, do no harm." From ancient times onwards, medical practice has posed dangers to patients. In modern times, those dangers are shockingly common. Medical error is thought to be the third leading case of death in the US.[12] Those errors include the unbelievable: one report described an average of 27 cases in one year, per New York hospital, of invasive procedures performed on the wrong patient.[13] Some of those dangers have become so commonplace that we consider them routine. When a patient develops a hospital-related infection, we document it as a nosocomial infection and treat the infection without questioning why it occurred. However, many of those infections are preventable, and should never have occurred at all. In this chapter, we document a number of specific measures that medical students can implement to protect their patients, from the use of standardized abbreviations to ensuring that patients receive venous thromboembolism prophylaxis when indicated. We outline how medical students can identify the hazards of hospitalization, thus ensuring that you can act to mitigate those hazards. We review nosocomial infections, and how you may be a culprit through your hands, your clothing, and even your stethoscope.

We also review the type of skills that ensure that patients feel comfortable with your care. The best medical care necessitates that patients trust their physicians and have confidence in both their abilities and the fact that the physician cares about the patient, not just the illness. In this chapter, our focus is on the patient, and how medical students can improve the care provided to patients. We outline steps that students can take, even at their level, to protect their patients from physical harm. We emphasize the different ways in which medical students can enhance patient care, patient education, and patient counseling. On a daily basis, you have the opportunity and the power to enhance the care provided to your patients.

Internal Medicine Clerkship

The field of internal medicine (IM) has a broad impact on all fields of medicine. "Learning about internal medicine – the specialty providing comprehensive care to adults – in the third year of medical school is an important experience, regardless of what specialty the medical student ultimately pursues," says Dr. Patrick Alguire, the Director of Education and Career Development at the American College of Physicians.[14] Through this clerkship, you will hone your skills in history and physical examination, diagnostic test interpretation, medical decision-making, and management of core medical conditions. These skills are important ones for all physicians, even if you ultimately decide to enter radiology, pathology, emergency medicine, or another field. Overall, internal medicine does stand as the most frequently chosen specialty in the residency match. In 2010, over 3,000 allopathic and osteopathic medical students matched into an internal medicine residency program.

Your IM clerkship grade can impact your career. It's a factor in the residency selection process for all specialties, not just internal medicine. In a survey of over 1,200 residency program directors across 21 medical specialties, grades in required clerkships were ranked as the # 1 factor used in the selection process.[8] "Do well in your clerkship," writes the Department of Medicine at the University of Washington. "Yes, this is obvious – and easier said than done – but it's also important. Most residency programs look closely at the third-year clerkship grade when selecting applicants."[15]

Many medical students find this clerkship formidable. A lack of knowledge isn't the main factor. The main factor is a lack of preparation for your many responsibilities. How do I evaluate a newly admitted patient? What do I need to include in a daily progress note? What information do I need to include in a comprehensive write-up? How do I present newly admitted patients to the attending physician?

In this chapter, templates and outlines are included for each of these important responsibilities. You'll also find a number of tips and suggestions on how to maximize your learning and performance during this rotation. You'll find detailed information that will help you effectively pre-round, succeed during work rounds, deliver polished oral case presentations, create well-written daily progress notes, and generate comprehensive write-ups.

For students interested in a career in internal medicine, this chapter also details how to strengthen your application. You'll learn how to identify potential mentors and obtain strong letters of recommendation. You'll learn about recommended electives and sub-internships, as well as specifics that detail how to maximize the impact of your application.

Surgery Clerkship

The surgery clerkship provides significant exposure to common surgical problems, and allows you to evaluate the specialty as a potential career choice. Although the bulk of your education will take place on the general surgery service, most rotations provide the opportunity to explore several surgical subspecialties. A surgical clerkship education is very valuable, whether or not you choose to practice in a surgical field. Primary care physicians must be familiar with the evaluation and management of patients in the pre-operative and post-operative settings. An understanding of core surgical principles is important across many fields, including ones such as anesthesiology, dermatology, and emergency medicine. From a personal standpoint, you or a family member is likely to undergo surgery in your lifetime, and you'll find that an understanding of the pre-operative, operative, and post-operative stages will be valuable.

Regardless of your chosen career, your surgery clerkship grade will be a factor used in the residency selection process, due to an emphasis on core clerkship grades in the residency selection process. In a survey of over 1,200 residency program directors across 21 medical specialties, grades in required clerkships were ranked as the # 1 factor used in the selection process.[8] The University of Colorado Department of Surgery writes that "most surgery programs look very favorably on an 'Honors' grade in your MS3 surgery clerkship rotation and may factor in the grades you received in your Medicine and Ob/Gyn rotations."[16] It's not easy to honor the clerkship. In a survey of medical schools across the country, Takayama found that only 27% of students achieve the highest grade in the surgery clerkship.[17]

Many students approach the surgery clerkship with considerable anxiety. In one study, students were most concerned about fatigue, long hours, workload, insufficient sleep, lack of time to study, mental abuse (getting yelled at or relentless pimping), and poor performance.[18] Unfamiliarity with the operating room environment was also concerning.

In the Surgery Clerkship chapter, we provide tips for operating room success, a checklist for thorough pre-rounding, a step-by-step guide to presenting patients, and time-saving templates for the pre-op, post-op, and op notes. This information will maximize your education as well as your performance.

In 2010, approximately 2,500 allopathic and osteopathic medical students matched into general surgery or related surgical specialty, such as ophthalmology, orthopedic surgery, otolaryngology, plastic surgery, or urology. This chapter includes recommendations for those students interested in pursuing general surgery as a career. When should you do a sub-internship? Should you do an away elective? What are considered negatives in a residency application? These questions, and others, are answered.

Excerpted from the book *Success on the Wards: 250 Rules for Clerkship Success*.

Read more of the first chapter at www.MD2B.net.

An excerpt from the best-selling book:
The Successful Match:
200 Rules to Succeed in the Residency Match

By Dr. Rajani Katta
and Dr. Samir P. Desai

The Application

What does it take to match successfully? What does it take to match into the specialty and program of your choice?

In the 2007 Match, over 40% of all U.S. senior applicants failed to match at the program of their choice. In competitive fields such as dermatology and plastic surgery, over 37% of U.S. senior applicants failed to match at all.

Percentage of U.S. senior applicants who failed to match in 2007	
Specialty	% of U.S. seniors failing to match
Dermatology	38.8%
Plastic surgery	37.5%
Urology	31.3%*
Ophthalmology	30.7%*
Neurological surgery	28.3%*
Orthopedic surgery	19.7%
Otolaryngology	18.4%
Radiation oncology	18.4%
Radiology	9.2%
*All applicants (U.S. seniors + other applicants)	
From www.nrmp.org, www.sfmatch.org, www.auanet.org.	

The numbers are significantly worse for osteopathic and international medical graduates:

- 28.4% of the 1,900 osteopathic students and graduates who participated in the 2008 Match failed to match at all.
- 55% of the 10,300 international medical graduates who participated in the 2008 Match failed to match at all.

Did you know...

Applicants who fail to match may participate in the Scramble. During the Scramble, applicants try to secure a first-year residency position in a program that failed to fill during the Match. In 2008, over 12,000 applicants scrambled for one of only 1,300 positions.

What does it actually take to match successfully? The issue is a hotly debated one, and surveys of students, reviews of student discussion forums, and discussions with academic faculty all find sharp divisions on the topic. In the following 400 plus pages, we answer the question of what it takes to match successfully. We also provide specific evidence-based advice to maximize your chances of a successful match.

Our recommendations are based on data from the full spectrum of sources. We present evidence obtained from scientific study and published in the academic medical literature. The results of these studies can provide a powerful impetus for specific actions. We present anecdotal data and advice that has been published in the literature and obtained from online sources. We also provide an insider's look at the entire process of residency selection based on our experiences, the experiences of our colleagues in the world of academic medicine, and the experiences of students and residents with whom we have worked.

Who actually chooses the residents? We review the data on the decision-makers. What do these decision-makers care about? We review the data on the criteria that matter to them. How can you convince them that you would be the right resident for their program? We provide concrete, practical recommendations based on this data. At every step of the process, our recommendations are meant to maximize the impact of your application.

In Chapter 2, starting on page 21, we present specialty-specific data. Given the high failure to match rates for certain specialties, is there any literature available to applicants to guide them through the residency application process? For each specialty, we present the results of those studies. For example, in radiology, a 2006 survey of residency program directors obtained data from 77 directors on the criteria that programs use to select their residents (Otero). Which criteria did these directors rank as most important in deciding whom to interview? Which selection factors were most important in determining an applicant's place on the program's rank order list? What were the mean USMLE step 1 scores among matched and unmatched U.S. seniors? What percentage of U.S. seniors who matched were members of the Alpha Omega Alpha Honor Medical Society (AOA)? This powerful evidence-based information is data that you must have to develop an application strategy that maximizes your chances of a successful match.

We review each component of the application in comprehensive detail in the following chapters. Each single component of your application can be created, modified, or influenced in order to significantly strengthen your overall candidacy. We devote the next 400 plus pages to showing you, in detail, exactly how to do so.

LETTERS OF RECOMMENDATION

Letters of recommendation are a critical component of the residency application. Since you won't be directly writing these letters, it may seem as if you have no control over their content. In reality, you wield more influence than you realize. In our chapter on letters of recommendation, we detail the steps that you can take in order to have the best possible letters written on your behalf. These steps include choosing the correct letter writers and asking in the correct manner. We also discuss the type of information to provide, and the manner in which to provide it, in order to highlight those qualities that you hope your letter writer will emphasize.

The purpose of these letters is to emphasize that you have the professional qualifications needed to excel. The letters should also demonstrate that you have the personal qualities to succeed as a resident and, later, as a practicing physician. Since these letters are written by those who know you and the quality of your work, they offer programs a personalized view. In contrast to your transcript and USMLE scores, they supply programs with qualitative, rather than quantitative, information about your cognitive and non-cognitive characteristics.

What do the faculty members reviewing applications look for in a letter of recommendation? The first item noted is the writer of the letter. In a survey of program directors in four specialties (internal medicine, pediatrics, family medicine, and surgery), it was learned that a candidate's likelihood of being considered was enhanced if there was a connection or relationship between the writer and residency program director (Villanueva). "In cases where there was both a connection between the faculty members and in-depth knowledge of the student (i.e., personal knowledge), the likelihood was that the student's application would be noted." In a survey of 109 program directors of orthopedic surgery residency programs, 54% of directors agreed that the most important aspect of a letter was that it was written by someone that they knew (Bernstein).

In another study, the academic rank of the writer was found to be an important factor influencing the reviewer's ranking of the letter (Greenburg). 48% of the reviewers rated it as important. A survey of physical medicine and rehabilitation (PM&R) program directors asked respondents to rate the importance of letters of recommendation in selecting residents (DeLisa). The study showed that the "most important letters of recommendation were from a PM&R faculty member in the respondent's department, followed by the dean's letter, and the PM&R chairman's letter." Next in importance were letters from a PM&R faculty member in a department other than the respondents', followed by a clinical faculty member in another specialty. The University of Texas-Houston Medical School Career Counseling Catalog gives this advice: "letters of recommendation from private physicians or part-time faculty, and letters from residents are generally discounted."

For internal medical graduates (IMGs), this issue becomes even more important. A survey of 102 directors of internal medicine residency programs sought to determine the most important predictors of performance for IMGs (Gayed). When rating the importance of 22 selection criteria, the lowest rated criterion was letters of recommendation from a foreign country, with 93% of program directors feeling that such letters were useless.

What else do the faculty members reviewing applications look for in a letter of recommendation? They seek evidence of an applicant's strengths and skills. Most applicants assume that their letter writers know what to say and what information to provide in a letter to substantiate their recommendation. However, that's a dangerous assumption. In an analysis of 116 recommendation letters received by the radiology residency program at the University of Iowa Hospitals & Clinics (O'Halloran), reviewers noted that:

- 10% of letters were missing information about an applicant's cognitive knowledge
- 35% of letters had no information about an applicant's clinical judgment
- 3% of letters did not discuss an applicant's work habits
- 17% of letters did not comment on the applicant's motivation
- 32% of letters were lacking information about interpersonal communication skills

In another review of recommendation letters sent during the 1999 application season to the Department of Surgery at Southern Illinois University, writers infrequently commented on psychomotor skills such as "easily performed minor procedures at the bedside," "good eye-hand coordination in the OR," "could suture well," and so on (Fortune).

Our chapter on letters of recommendation, starting on page 159, reviews strategies to locate those letter writers who will be most helpful to your candidacy. We review how to identify these writers and how to approach them. Most importantly, we discuss the type of evidence you can provide to the writer and the professional manner in which to provide it. Your letter writers want to write the best letter possible, and you can do much more than you realize to make this a reality.

Excerpted from the book *The Successful Match: 200 Rules to Succeed in the Residency Match.*

Read more of the first chapter at www.MD2B.net.

Clinician's Guide to Laboratory Medicine: Pocket

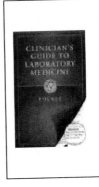

By Samir P. Desai, MD

ISBN # 9780972556187

In this book, you will find practical approaches to lab test interpretation. It includes differential diagnoses, step-by-step approaches, and algorithms, all designed to answer your lab test questions in a flash. See why so many consider it a "must-have" book.

"In our Medicine Clerkship, the Clinician's Guide to Laboratory Medicine has quickly become one of the two most popular paperback books. Our students have praised the algorithms, tables, and ease of pursuit of clinical problems through better understanding of the utilization of tests appropriate to the problem at hand."

- Greg Magarian, MD, Director, 3rd Year Internal Medicine Clerkship, Oregon Health & Science University

"It provides an excellent practical approach to abnormal labs."

- Northwestern University Feinberg School of Medicine Internal Medicine Clerkship website.

Success on the Wards: 250 Rules for Clerkship Success

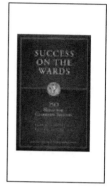

By Samir P. Desai, MD and Rajani Katta, MD

ISBN # 9780972556194

This is an absolute must-read for students entering clinical rotations.

The authors of *The Successful Match: 200 Rules to Succeed in the Residency Match* bring their same combination of practical recommendations and evidence-based advice to clerkships.

The book begins as a how-to guide with clerkship-specific templates, along with sample notes and guides, for every aspect of clerkships. The book reviews proven strategies for success in patient care, write-ups, rounds, and other vital areas.

Grades in required rotations are the most important academic criteria used to select residents, and this critical year can determine career choices. This book shows students what they can do now to position themselves for match success. An invaluable resource for medical students - no student should be without it.

"*Success on the Wards: 250 Rules for Clerkship Success* is an excellent reference for any 3rd year medical student and some is probably great reading for advanced students and even residents and interns…Given the heavy importance of being successful on the wards as a student for future residency, it's really easy to recommend this book."

- Review by Medfools.com

"*Success on the Wards* is easily the best book I have read on how to succeed in clerkship. It is comprehensive, thorough and jam-packed with valuable information. Dr. Desai and Dr. Katta provide an all encompassing look into what clerkship is really like."

- Review by Medaholic.com

The Successful Match: 200 Rules to Succeed in the Residency Match

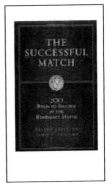

By Rajani Katta, MD and Samir P. Desai, MD

ISBN # 9780972556170

What does it take to match into the specialty and program of your choice?

The key to a successful match hinges on the development of the right strategy. This book will show you how to develop the optimal strategy for success.

Who actually chooses the residents? We review the data on the decision-makers. What do these decision-makers care about? We review the data on the criteria that matter most to them. How can you convince them that you would be the right resident for their program? We provide concrete, practical recommendations based on their criteria.

At every step of the process, our recommendations are meant to maximize the impact of your application. This book is an invaluable resource to help you gain that extra edge.

"Drs. Rajani Katta and Samir P. Desai provide the medical student reader with detailed preparation for the matching process. The rules and accompanying tips make the book user-friendly. The format is especially appealing to those pressed for time or looking for a single key element for a particular process."

- Review in the American Medical Student Association journal, *The New Physician*

The Successful Match website

Our website, TheSuccessfulMatch.com, provides residency applicants with a better understanding of the residency selection process. There, you'll find:

- Match statistics for every specialty
- Conversations with program directors about the selection process
- Important information about the future of each specialty, including current challenges
- Factors that led physicians to pursue different specialties
- Resources to help you succeed in clerkships

Consulting services

We also offer expert one-on-one consulting services to medical students. Whether you seek an overall strategy for match success, accurate assessment of your candidacy for a particular specialty or program, review of your curriculum vitae or personal statement, or thorough preparation for interviews, you can rest assured we have the knowledge, expertise, and insight to help you achieve your goals.

If you are interested in our consultation services, please visit us at www.TheSuccessfulMatch.com. The website provides further details, including pricing and specific services.

MD2B Titles

The Successful Match: 200 Rules to Succeed in the Residency Match

Success on the Wards: 250 Rules for Clerkship Success

Success in Medical School: Insider Advice for the Preclinical Years

Clinician's Guide to Laboratory Medicine: Pocket

Available at www.MD2B.net

Bulk Sales

MD2B is able to provide discounts on any of our titles when purchased in bulk. The discount rate depends on the quantity ordered. For more information, please contact us at info@md2b.net or (713) 927-6830.